The Blood Sugar Fix

How to Achieve Optimal Blood Sugar Levels and Insulin Sensitivity for a Healthier and Longer Life

Dr. James DiNicolantonio

Author of The Salt Fix

&

Siim Land

Author of Metabolic Autophagy

2023

D1528368

DISCLAIMER

You agree to accept all risks of using the information presented inside this book. You need to consult a professional medical practitioner in order to ensure you are both able and healthy enough to participate in this program.

Jacket design by James DiNicolantonio and Siim Land

Table of Contents

About the Authors

Dr. James DiNicolantonio

As a cardiovascular research scientist and Doctor of Pharmacy, Dr. James J. DiNicolantonio has spent years researching nutrition. A well-respected and internationally known scientist and expert on health and nutrition, he has contributed extensively to health policy and medical literature. Dr. 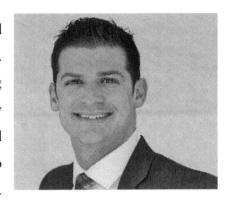 DiNicolantonio is the author of 8 best-selling health books, The Salt Fix, Superfuel, The Longevity Solution, The Immunity Fix, The Mineral Fix, WIN, The Obesity Fix and The Collagen Cure.

His website is www.drjamesdinic.com. You can follow Dr. DiNicolantonio on Twitter and Instagram at @drjamesdinic and Facebook at Dr. James DiNicolantonio.

He is the author or co-author of more than 300 medical publications, including several high-profile articles related to nutrition, including a December 2014 opinion piece about sugar addiction in *The New York Times* that was the newspaper's most emailed article during the 24 hours following its publication. Dr. DiNicolantonio has testified in front of the Canadian Senate regarding the harms of added sugars and serves as the Associate Editor of British Medical Journal's (BMJ) Open Heart, a journal published in partnership with the British Cardiovascular Society. He is also on the Editorial Advisory Board of several other medical journals, including Progress in Cardiovascular Diseases and International Journal of Clinical Pharmacology & Toxicology.

Siim Land

Siim Land is an author, speaker, content creator and renown biohacker from Estonia. Despite his young age, he is considered one of the top people in the biohacking and health optimization community with thousands of followers worldwide. Siim Land has written books like Metabolic Autophagy, Stronger by Stress, The Immunity Fix, The Mineral Fix and WIN. His website is www.siimland.com. 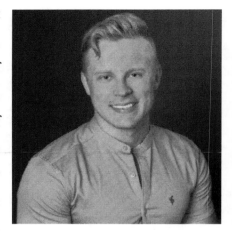 You can follow Siim on Instagram @siimland and as Siim Land on YouTube.

Siim started researching and doing self-experiments with nutrition, exercise, and other strategies to improve his performance and health after high school when he enrolled in the military for a year. He then obtained a bachelor's degree in anthropology at Tallinn University and University of Durham in the UK. By now he has written several books about diet, creates content online, and keeps himself up to date with the latest knowledge in science.

Introduction: The Diabetes Epidemic

Diabetes is one of the most widespread modern diseases. **It's estimated that up to 400 million people in the world have diabetes**[1,2]. The most dramatic rise in diabetes is seen in low- to middle-income countries[3]. Over half of U.S. adults have diabetes or pre-diabetes[4]. Type 2 diabetes makes up 90% of the adult diabetes cases worldwide[5]. Type 1 diabetes contributes to only 5-10% of all diabetic cases[6]. This reflects the rising obesity rates that have occurred in parallel with increasing rates of Type 2 diabetes[7]. Being overweight and having excess visceral fat is a major risk factor for Type 2 diabetes, as obesity promotes insulin resistance and pancreatic beta cell dysfunction[8,9,10,11,12]. Thus, the major reason for such a high number of Type 2 diabetics worldwide is poor diet and lifestyle that predisposes them to weight gain and impaired glucose tolerance[13]. **The World Health Organization predicts that by the year 2030, diabetes will be the 7th leading cause of death in the world**[14]. Based on that estimate, global expenditure on diabetes and its related healthcare will exceed $1 trillion[15].

The estimated global cases of diabetes in 2000 and projections for 2030[16]:

Country	2000	2030
India	31.7%	79.4%
China	20.8%	42.3%
U.S.	17.7%	30.3%
Indonesia	8.4%	21.3%
Japan	6.8%	8.9%

Pakistan	5.2%	13.9%
Brazil	4.6%	11.3%
Bangladesh	3.2%	11.1%

It's estimated that 3.4 million people across the globe died due to the consequences of an elevated fasting blood sugar in 2004[17]. **Diabetics have an overall risk of death twice as high as those without diabetes[18]. Diabetes increases the risk of cardiovascular disease and stroke by up to 1.8 to 6-fold**[19,20,21]. Up to 50% of diabetics die from cardiovascular disease[22]. Diabetes is also the main cause of kidney disease and kidney failure[23]. Furthermore, diabetes is linked with dementia and neurodegenerative diseases like Alzheimer's disease[24]. Diabetic retinopathy can lead to blindness and impaired vision, whereas diabetic neuropathy in the limbs can result in amputation[25,26]. Thus, diabetes is one of the worst of the modern diseases, as it increases the risk of all the other major killers. Even if a person dies from cardiovascular disease, this may have been caused by their diabetes. Hence, a major focus for every person should be to avoid lifestyle-induced Type 2 diabetes.

One of the earliest and best ways to diagnose Type 2 diabetes is using a post prandial insulin assay. Essentially, you drink 75-100 grams of an oral glucose solution in a fasted state and see if you have an elevated insulin response over the next 2-4 hours.[27,28]. Unfortunately, most doctors don't order this test and by the time someone gets diagnosed with impaired glucose tolerance they have lost up to 50% of their beta cells that produce insulin[29]. Both Type 1 diabetes and Type 2 diabetes start at a fasting blood sugar of ≥ 7.0 mmol/l (126 mg/dl) or when your 2-hour plasma glucose after an oral glucose tolerance test is ≥ 11.1 mmol/l (200 mg/dl)[30,31]. Another method of diagnosis is looking at glycated hemoglobin

(HbA1c or A1C). If your A1C is ≥48 mmol/mol (6.5% or higher) then you're diagnosed with diabetes[32]. The main physical symptoms of diabetes are dry mouth, thirst, fatigue, hair loss, blurry vision, frequent urination, and peripheral neuropathy.

	Fasting Glucose		2-Hour Glucose		A1C	
Unit	mmol/L	mg/dL	mmol/L	mg/dL	mmol/mol	%
Normal	<5.6	<100	<7.8	<140	<42	<5.7
Impaired Glucose Tolerance	5.6–7.0	100–125	≥7.8	>140	42–46	5.7-6.4
Diabetes Mellitus	≥7.0	≥126	≥11.1	≥200	≥48	≥6.5

You can pause for a moment and consider whether your own biomarkers meet the criteria presented here for diabetes or impaired glucose tolerance. Prevention, as we'll discuss shortly, is the best medicine.

Is Diabetes Preventable?

In the past, it wasn't clear whether maintaining tight glycemic control could help to prevent the development of diabetic complications. There were two landmark clinical trials published a few decades ago that revealed the truth.

From 1983 to 1993, the NIH conducted a large multicenter study called the Diabetes Control and Complications Trial (DCCT), which sought to assess whether glycemic control can prevent or decrease long-term diabetic complications[33]. They included 1441 volunteers between the ages of 13-39 from 29 U.S. centers. Participants had Type 1 diabetes for at least 1 year but not longer than 15 years. They were divided into 2 groups: (1) The Primary Prevention group or Type 1 diabetics of 1-5 years without any diabetic complications and (2) the Secondary Intervention group who had Type 1 diabetes for 1-15 years with mild diabetic neuropathy and retinopathy. Participants from both groups were randomly assigned to get either intensive (use of hypoglycemic oral agents and insulin) or conventional therapy (just diet and pharmaceuticals if needed). In the intensive therapy group, they intended to keep pre-meal blood glucose between 70-120 mg/dl and post-meal glucose below 180 mg/dl. In the conventional therapy group, the goal was to avoid diabetic symptoms. By the end of the study, **the A1C of the intensive group patients was nearly 2% lower than the ones in the conventional group.** The average blood sugar level of the intensive group patients was 155 mg/dl compared to the 231 mg/dl of the conventional group patients. Intensive therapy decreased retinopathy by 76%, the development of neuropathy by 69% and the development of early neuropathy by 34%. During the 11-year follow-up, the intensive group subjects showed a 57% decrease in the risk of non-fatal myocardial infarction, stroke or death from cardiovascular disease compared to the conventional therapy group[34].

The second trial called The United Kingdom Prospective Diabetes Study was concluded in 1998 and it was the largest study of Type 2 diabetes patients. There were 5102 participants with newly diagnosed Type 2 diabetes who were followed for an average of 11 years. They were divided into 2 groups: intensive therapy (insulin and pharmaceuticals) and conventional therapy (only diet and pharmaceuticals as needed). The average A1C in the intensive group was 7.0% compared to 7.9% in the conventional group. The intensive group saw a 12% reduction in diabetes-related endpoints (stroke, sudden death, death from hyperglycemia or hypoglycemia, fatal or non-fatal myocardial infarction, heart failure, renal failure, amputation, etc.). However, they didn't see a significant reduction in individual cardiovascular events[35]. **Maintaining tight blood pressure control (~144/82 mmHg) compared to less strict control (~154/87 mmHg) significantly decreased the risk of micro- and macrovascular complications by 37% and 34%, respectively[36].** Higher blood pressure was strongly linked to diabetic complications and the lowest risk was observed with a systolic blood pressure below 120 mmHg. Metformin, a diabetic drug, was associated with a reduced risk of diabetes-related deaths and all-cause mortality in overweight subjects[37].

It's further been shown that Type 2 diabetes is preventable. There is an inverse relationship between physical activity and the rate of developing diabetes[38]. The National Health Interview Survey found that diabetics are less likely to partake in regular exercise compared to non-diabetics[39]. In Finland, individuals on a consistent diet and exercise program have only a 10% incidence of diabetes compared to 22% for individuals who've met their physician or dietician only once a year over the course of a 4-year follow-up[40].

A 6-year randomized controlled trial found that exercise reduced the incidence of diabetes by 46% in patients with impaired glucose tolerance[41]. Engaging in vigorous exercise at least once a week reduces the risk of diabetes by 46% among middle-aged women without diabetes, cardiovascular disease, or cancer[42]. In the same study, even more leisurely activity, like walking and taking the stairs, is inversely associated with developing Type 2 diabetes, especially among those at the highest risk.

These studies among others showed that metabolic control can reduce the risk of developing diabetes-related complications. Thus, it's well documented the power of proper lifestyle that maintains tight control over one's blood sugar levels, blood pressure and other biomarkers. This book doesn't replace medical advice, but it does compile the most evidence-based and optimal ways to improve one's metabolic health and glucose control.

Chapter 1: The History of Diabetes

Diabetes is one of the oldest diseases of civilization ever described. Long before we knew about heart disease, Alzheimer's disease, osteoporosis, or cancer, we've known about diabetes. The first recorded description of diabetes dates to 1500 BC when an Ancient Egyptian medical manuscript named Ebers Papyrus described a condition of "too frequent emptying of the urine".[43] The paper was excavated in 1862 AD from an ancient grave in Thebes, Egypt, and released to the public by the Egyptologist Georg Ebers in 1874. Before the 20th century it was considered an unknown fatal disease of excessive thirst, frequent urination, and weight loss. Ancient Egyptians unfortunately tried treating this condition with wheat grains, fruit, and sweet beer[44,45]. Thus, humans have suffered from diabetes for at least three millennia and long before modern society.

Diabetes was first named in 230 BC Greece by Apollonius Memphites[46]. The Greeks considered this to be a disease of the kidneys and recommended bloodletting and dehydration as one of the treatments. Nowadays, the technical term is *diabetes mellitus*, derived from the Greek word 'diabetes', which means 'siphon' or 'to pass through'. John Rollo in the 18th century added the Latin word 'mellitus', meaning 'honeyed' or 'sweet'[47]. That's because diabetic urine has excess amounts of sugar and tastes sweet. The Swiss doctor Paracelsus (1493-1541 AD), who is called the father of toxicology, confused the white substance in the urine with salt instead of sugar[48]. However, in 1776, a British physiologist Matthew Dobson showed that the urine of diabetics indeed had excess sugar, which made it sweet[49].

A Roman physician Aulus Cornelius Celsus (30 BC–50 AD) was the first to give a full clinical description of diabetes in his *De medicina*[50]. In Ancient Rome, diabetes was quite a rare disease. The Roman physician Galen wrote he had encountered only two cases of such a condition during his entire career[51]. He called diabetes 'diarrhea of the urine' as he attributed it to the demise of the kidneys[52].

It was the Greek physician Aretaeus of Cappadocia who worked in Rome and Alexandria during the 2nd century AD who first distinguished between diabetes mellitus (diabetes characterized by chronically elevated blood sugar levels) and diabetes insipidus (a condition characterized by a large amount of diluted urine and increased thirst)[53].

Aretaeus wrote in his *On the Causes and Indications of Acute and Chronic Diseases*[54]:

> *Diabetes is a dreadful affliction, not very frequent among men, being a melting down of the flesh and limbs into urine. The patients never stop making water and the flow is incessant, like the opening of the aqueducts. Life is short, unpleasant and painful, thirst unquenchable, drinking excessive and disproportionate to the large quantity of urine, for yet more urine is passed... If for a while they abstain from drinking, their mouths become parched and their bodies dry; the viscera seem scorched up, the patients are affected by nausea, restlessness and a burning thirst, and within a short time they expire.*

Indian physicians Sushruta and Charaka around 400-500 AD conducted the first clinical test for diabetes and differentiated between two different types of diabetes. They saw that the urine of diabetics attracted flies and ants because of the sweetness, which is why they called the disease 'madhumeha' or *honey urine*[55]. Sushruta and Charaka observed that thin individuals who ended up with diabetes started developing its symptoms already at a young age as opposed to heavier individuals who developed it later in life and who lived longer after the diagnosis than the younger thin diabetics. Nowadays, we know that the former describes Type 1 diabetes and the latter Type 2 diabetes.

- **Type 1 Diabetes (T1D) is an autoimmune disease wherein the pancreas doesn't produce enough insulin because the insulin-producing beta cells in the pancreas are destroyed by the immune system**[56,57,58]. Insulin's role is to direct glucose into the cells and without treating type 1 diabetes, blood sugar levels can stay chronically elevated, which is a major health hazard. T1D is often genetic, and most Type 1 diabetics are children, which is why it's often called juvenile diabetes.

- **Type 2 Diabetes (T2D) is a medical condition wherein there is an imbalance between blood sugar levels and insulin production**[59]. It's characterized by insulin resistance and elevated blood sugar levels. In other words, the cells have become resistant or tone deaf to the effects of insulin and won't open themselves up to let the glucose in. As a result, blood sugar levels stay elevated for longer, resulting in damaged health. Although some individuals are more genetically predisposed to get T2D, it's most often caused by lifestyle, which is why it's called adult-onset diabetes.

- **Type 3 Diabetes (T3D) is a name of glucose intolerance seen in Alzheimer's disease** because it mimics insulin resistance in the brain and Type 2 diabetics have a significant two-fold higher risk of developing Alzheimer's disease[60,61,62,63].

The sugar in the urine of diabetics was proven to be glucose by Eugene Chevreul in 1815 Paris. Von Fehling created a test for measuring glucose in the urine, which enabled the acceptance of glucosuria (glucose in the urine) to become a viable diagnostic tool for diabetes[64]. Claude Bernard (1813-1878) connected the dots between the role of the pancreas in diabetes and also discovered that the liver stores glycogen. He concluded that this excess release of glycogen into the bloodstream by the liver is what contributes to diabetes[65]. Before the discovery of insulin, diabetes was treated primarily with low-calorie and low carbohydrate diets[66]. That was due to the belief that diabetics couldn't utilize food that well and limiting eating would improve the condition[67]. Interestingly, deaths from this kind of starvation-like diets were rare.

In 1921, Frederick Banting and Charles Best from the University of Toronto discovered insulin by isolating it from the pancreas of dogs[68]. This revelation showed that diabetics had a deficiency of insulin and was responsible for their pathology. At first, their extracts had issues with impurities, which caused inflammation. However, one of their collaborators, James Collip later purified the extract on January 23, 1922, and administered it to a young diabetic patient, L. Thompson, which improved their condition. After this monumental discovery, Eli Lilly started to produce insulin commercially, followed by the Danes and Brits. Today, insulin saves the lives of millions of diabetics worldwide. Banting and another professor in Toronto were awarded the Nobel Prize in Physiology or Medicine in 1923, which both shared with Best and Collip. Nicolae Paulescu, who was a professor of Biology in Bucharest, Romania, also came quite close to discovering insulin but Banting and Best beat him to the punch. Paulescu's contribution to the discovery of insulin was recognized only after his death in 1931[69].

Before the production of human insulin, diabetics mostly used bovine or porcine insulin. Although bovine insulin differs by only 3 amino acids from human insulin and porcine insulin by just 1 amino acid, it's enough to trigger an immune response in some. Frederick Sanger's structural formula of bovine insulin was published in 1955[70]. He received a Nobel Prize for this in 1958. Porcine insulin's three-dimensional structure was described by Dorothy Hodgkin in 1969 with X-ray crystallography[71]. **In 1978, Genentech, Inc. and City Hope National Medical Center in California successfully produced human insulin from *E. coli*, using recombinant DNA technology**[72]. After that, in 1982, Genentech's insulin named Humulin, became the first genetically made FDA-approved drug[73].

Here is a timeline of diabetes discoveries[74]:

- 1500 BC, Ebers Papyrus – First written record of a diabetes-like disease in Ancient Egypt.

- 230 BC, Apollonius of Memphis, Greece – Giving of the name *diabetes 'to pass through'* to the disease.

- 1st century AD, Aulus Cornelius Celsus – First clinical description of diabetes.

- 4-5th century AD, Susruta and Charaka, India – First differentiation between type-1 and type-2 diabetes.

- 1776 AD, Matthew Dobson, England – Showed that the sweetness of diabetic urine is because of sugar.

- 1788 AD, Thomas Cowley, England – Was the first to connect diabetes and the pancreas.

- 1869 AD, Paul Langerhans, Germany – Discovered small cell clusters in the pancreas, later named 'islets of Langerhans', which weren't drained by the pancreas.

- 1889 AD, Oscar Minkowski and Joseph von Mehring, Germany – They removed the pancreas in dogs, which instantly gave them diabetes.

- 1893 AD, Edouard Laguesse, France – Claimed the islets of Langerhans might be the producing an anti-diabetic substance.

- 1907 AD, Georg Zuelzer, Germany – Produced a pancreatic extract called 'acomatol', which reduced glucosuria and raised the blood pH in dogs.

- 1921-1922 AD, Frederick Banting, Charles Best, James Collip and J.R. Macleod, Canada – Pancreatic extracts from dogs decreased glucosuria and the first successful administration of the extract to a diabetic patient. Eli Lilly Company begins to work on making commercial insulin.

- 1923 AD, Banting, Best, Collip and Macleod get the Nobel Prize in Physiology or Medicine.

- 1958 AD, Frederic Sanger, Great Britain – Received the Nobel Prize in Physiology or Medicine for the structural formula of bovine insulin.

- 1966 AD, University of Minnesota, USA – First successful transplant of the pancreas.

- 1978 AD, Robert Crea and David Goeddel, USA – Production of human insulin using recombinant DNA technology.

- 1993 AD, Diabetes Control and Complications Trial, USA – Metabolic control of Type 1 diabetes related to the development of diabetic complications.

- 1998 AD, United Kingdom Prospective Diabetes Study, Great Britain – Metabolic control of Type 2 diabetes related to the development of diabetic complications.

- 2001 AD, Diabetes Prevention Program, USA – Diet and exercise related to the development of Type 2 diabetes in high-risk populations.

- 2003 AD, Human Genome Project – The human genome gets sequenced.

- 2007 AD, First Genome-Wide Association Studies for Diabetes – Novel genetic loci get identified in relation to Type 2 diabetes.

What Caused the Diabetes Epidemic?

There has been a dramatic rise in the prevalence of Type 2 diabetes over the last 100 years or so. Today, diabetes is prevalent among 8.8% of adults globally, whereas in 1980 it was only 4.7%[75]. That's almost a 2-fold increase in the global prevalence of diabetics over the past 40 years. The worldwide cases of diabetes are predicted to rise 48% from 2017 to 2045[76].

The primary reason for the rise in diabetes is rising rates of obesity, which is reflected in increased calorie consumption and sedentary lifestyle[77,78,79]. Excess bodyweight, especially visceral fat (fat in and around the liver and intestines), is linked to increased risk of diabetes and impaired glucose tolerance. In the U.S., fast food consumption has tripled between 1977 and 1995[80]. People in the United States consumed on average 200 calories more a day in 1996 compared to 1977[81]. From 1977 to 1996, total daily calorie consumption in 19–39-year-olds jumped from 1,840 to 2,198. Global food production is estimated to reach 3,000 kcal per capita by 2030, which is double compared to 1977[82]. **The biggest amount of those calories come from refined carbohydrates, sugar-sweetened beverages, added vegetable oils and ultra-processed food in general**[83]. Up to 20% of all calories in the American diet come from soybean oil[84] and soft drinks account for up to 25% of the total daily calories in U.S. adults[85,86,87,88]. The CDC estimates that less than 30% of the U.S. population doesn't meet adequate levels of physical activity, 30% are physically active but insufficiently and 40% are completely sedentary[89]. The number of children who commute to school on foot or a bike has decreased from 41% in 1969 to 13% in 2001[90].

Consumption of refined sugars is linked to weight gain, fatty liver disease, visceral fat accumulation, Type 2 diabetes, insulin resistance, hypertension, and cardiovascular disease[91,92,93,94,95,96,97,98,99,100,101]. In the U.S., over 1 out of

10 adults get 25% of their daily calories from added sugars hidden in packaged food[102]. That's anywhere from 24-47 teaspoons of sugar a day. Around 300 years ago, the average person consumed only a few pounds of sugar per year[103,104]. Today the average U.S. adult consumes between 77-152 pounds of sugar per year[105,106]. Children also consume excessive amounts of sugar per day[107]. A study on 1,000 American adolescents 14-18 years old found that their average daily sugar intake was 389 grams for boys and 276 grams in girls[108]!

Sugar Consumption Past VS Present

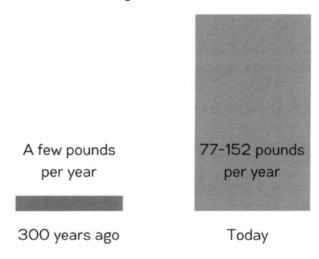

A few pounds per year

77-152 pounds per year

300 years ago

Today

Adapted From: DiNicolantonio and Lucan (2014); Storm (2012)

Even in the 1940s, sugar intake per person was only 22.5 pounds per year[109]. However, by the 1970s, that number had doubled to 44 pounds per year. Between 1970 to 2000, sugar intake has increased 3-fold – from 44 pounds to 120-152 pounds per person per year[110,111]. During that time, obesity rates in adults had also doubled[112]. From 1950s to 2000, there has been a 4-fold increase in obesity, which correlates with a 4-fold increase in the intake of sugar. Correlation does not equal causation but there are countless studies linking sugar consumption with weight gain[113,114,115,116].

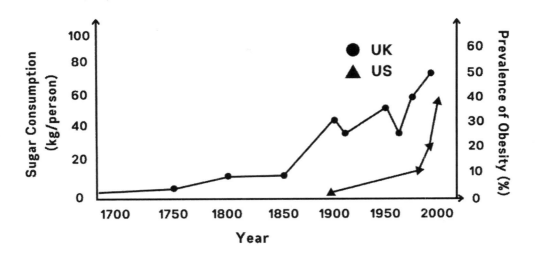

Adapted From: Johnson et al (2007)

Image Taken From: DiNicolantonio and Land (2022) 'The Obesity Fix'

Most of the added sugar in people's diets comes from soft drinks and sugar-sweetened beverages and sugar-sweetened beverages are one of the biggest drivers of obesity and Type 2 diabetes in the United States[117,118]. In the U.S. the intake of soft drinks between 1955 and 1995 has increased 5-fold, going from around 10 gallons to 47 gallons per person per year[119]. The intake of soft drinks doubled from 1970 to 1997 – from 22 gallons per person to 41 gallons per person per year[120,121]. Sugar, especially its fructose component, is even worse for causing impaired glucose tolerance in humans compared to other refined carbohydrates like starch or glucose, even when the calories are matched[122,123,124].

From 1955 to 1995, Soft Drink Intake Increased nearly 5-fold and Obesity Rates in Adults Increased ~ 4-fold[125,126]

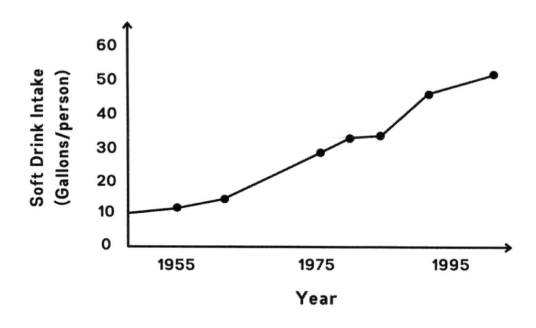

Adapted From: Bray and Popkin (2014)

Image Taken From: DiNicolantonio and Land (2022) 'The Obesity Fix'

Refined carbohydrates are also linked to weight gain and diabetes, although not as much as added sugars. Animals who have their food full of starch replaced with sugar see increased fasting insulin, worsened insulin sensitivity, and higher glucose levels[127,128,129,130,131,132,133]. **In men, replacing wheat with sugar raises fasting insulin, the insulin to glucose ratio and the insulin response to a given sucrose load[134].** This effect is linear, meaning that the more sugar you replace the wheat with, even when calories are equated, the worse outcome you get in terms of fasting insulin[135].

Prevalence of obesity in U.S. increased with increased refined carbohydrate intake[136]

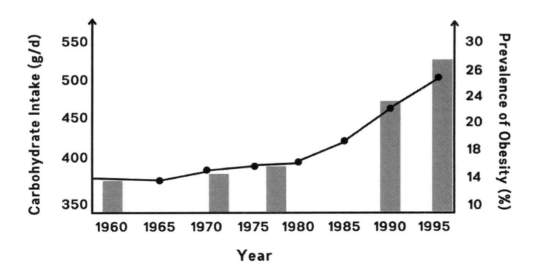

Adapted From: Gross et al (2004)

Image Taken From: DiNicolantonio and Land (2022) 'The Obesity Fix'

Besides refined carbohydrates and added sugars, people are eating significantly more refined omega-6 seed oils[137]. Humans have ancestrally consumed an omega-6-to-3 ratio of around 4-1:1[138,139]. That ratio is optimal for overall health. However, today, we consume 20-50 times more omega-6 fatty acids than we do omega-3s[140]. **The intake of soybean oil from 1909 to 1999 has increased by over 1000-fold[141]. Americans today get around 20% of their calories from soybean oil alone[142]!** Linoleic acid intake, which is the main omega-6 fat in industrial seed oils, has risen from 2% of our total calorie intake in the early 1900s to 8-10% in more recent years[143]. This tremendous rise of omega-6 fats in our diet has paralleled the rise in diabetes and obesity[144,145]. An excess omega-6/3 ratio promotes inflammation and visceral fat accumulation[146,147]. On the flip side, omega-3s alleviate insulin resistance and lower visceral fat in animals[148,149,150,151,152].

% Caloric Intake from Linoleic Acid in the United States[153]

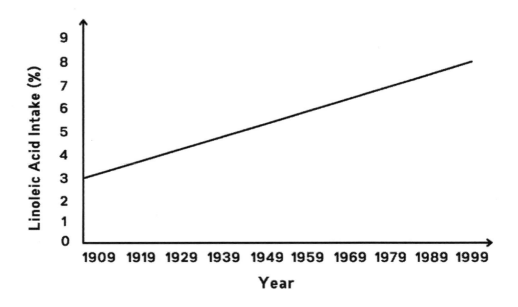

Adapted From: Blasbalg et al (2011)

Image Taken From: DiNicolantonio and Land (2022) 'The Obesity Fix'

Overall, the biggest contributors to the rise in obesity and diabetes are added sugars and refined carbohydrates, usually in the form of sugar-sweetened beverages, soft drinks, and packaged foods. This has led to a significantly greater number of calories consumed per day by the average person. Thus, the biggest problem is the consumption of ultra-processed foods that are high in added fats, sugars, and calories, which typically results in consuming on average 500-600 extra calories a day, mostly from fats and carbohydrates[154]. These foods tend to also be more hyperpalatable and easier to overconsume, which perpetuates the cycle[155]. In the case of diabetes, it's more likely the bigger culprit are sugar-sweetened beverages and refined carbohydrates because of the way they affect glucose and insulin levels.

Chapter 2: Insulin, Glucagon, and Insulin Resistance

Type 2 diabetes has many different causes. However, when it comes to Type 1 diabetes, genetics is the most important factor. However, there are also environmental factors that trigger Type 1 diabetes and genetically predisposed individuals are more susceptible to being affected by these triggers[156]. Nevertheless, **Type 1 diabetes makes up only 5-10% of all diabetes cases worldwide[157]. Type 2 diabetes comprises the remaining 90% and that's predominantly a lifestyle disease[158],** which is why it's called adult-onset diabetes. Of course, the same interplay between environment and genetics exists here as well, but nearly all Type 2 diabetes cases are preventable.

The reason for insulin's failure to bring glucose into the cell varies: in Type 1 diabetes, the pancreas doesn't produce enough insulin but in type-2 diabetes the cells have become resistant or tone deaf to insulin's actions. In both cases, the result is chronically elevated blood sugar levels that leads to all the diabetic complications, such as atherosclerosis, neuropathy, retinopathy, kidney failure, central obesity, and cardiovascular disease[159,160,161,162,163]. It is important to note, that chronically elevated insulin levels occur prior to elevated blood glucose levels in Type 2 diabetes, which drives numerous health issues in and of itself. In this chapter, we're going to address the root of the problem in those with Type 2 diabetes, which is insulin resistance and chronically elevated insulin levels, as well as Type 1 diabetes.

Insulin's Role in Insulin Resistance

Insulin is a peptide hormone produced by the pancreatic beta cells. In fact, it was the first peptide hormone discovered[164]. Insulin's primary role is to attach to the insulin receptors on the cell surface and open them up for glucose to enter the cell from the bloodstream[165]. The glucose gets stored as glycogen in the liver and in skeletal muscle for future use. Thus, insulin regulates energy metabolism and nutrient storage. Insulin is also the body's main anabolic hormone that promotes growth[166].

Beta cells in the pancreas detect blood sugar levels and release insulin when blood glucose rises above a certain threshold[167]. Insulin then promotes glucose uptake into the cells, which lowers blood glucose levels. When blood sugar levels are too low, the beta cells inhibit insulin production. Once that happens, the neighboring alpha cells in the pancreas stimulate the secretion of glucagon. Glucagon is supposed to raise blood sugar levels by stimulating glycogenolysis (breakdown of stored glycogen stores into glucose) and gluconeogenesis (creation of new sugar from amino acids and fats). Thus, glucagon and insulin work in a seesaw – when blood sugar is too low glucagon rises and when blood sugar gets too high insulin rises and vice versa. In Type 2 diabetes, there is an accumulation of amyloid in the pancreatic islets, which disrupts their function[168]. There is also some damage to the beta cells themselves.

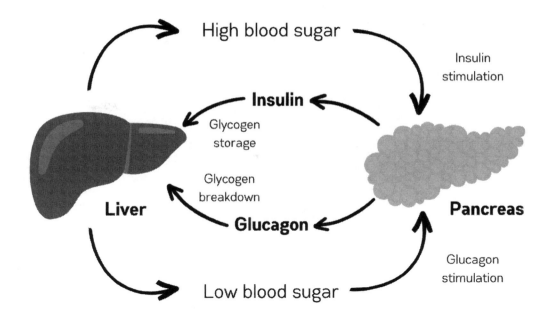

Insulin resistance (IR) describes a situation during which your cells are not responding to the message of insulin. As a result, glucose doesn't get into the cell and stays elevated in the bloodstream[169]. Fat cells can also become insulin resistant, resulting in high circulating fatty acids, which perpetuate insulin resistance further[170,171,172]. This also accelerates visceral fat storage and weight gain[173]. There are different scenarios where insulin resistance can occur and not all of them immediately lead to Type 2 diabetes. However, eventually prolonged insulin resistance will cause Type 2 diabetes and hyperglycemia[174,175]. Hyperinsulinemia is when insulin levels are elevated, which is both the driver and result of insulin resistance[176]. Hyperinsulinemia is linked to hypertension, diabetes, obesity and metabolic syndrome[177].

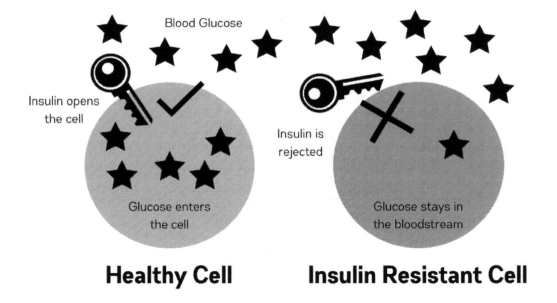

Healthy Cell   Insulin Resistant Cell

The Brain's Role in Insulin Resistance and Diabetes

The brain is also susceptible to insulin resistance. Alzheimer's disease after all is sometimes referred to as Type 3 diabetes[178,179]. Unlike skeletal muscle, the brain doesn't need insulin for glucose uptake. However, **the brain has a lot of insulin receptors and insulin regulates learning, memory and protects neurons against oxidative stress**[180,181]. Insulin gets into the brain via the blood brain barrier (BBB) and the brain also makes some of its own insulin[182,183,184]. Although your brain contains 20-25% of your body's entire cholesterol, zero dietary cholesterol crosses the blood brain barrier and the cholesterol inside the brain gets produced with insulin[185]. Cholesterol from diet has zero impact on the cholesterol content of the brain and its functions inside the brain – it's insulin and insulin sensitivity that does.

An insulin sensitive brain supports weight management, satiety, loss of abdominal fat and diet adherence because insulin in the brain affects

signaling hormones and neuropeptides that regulate the central nervous system and eating behavior[186,187,188,189,190,191,192,193,194,195]. Insulin in the brain lowers the desire to eat, snack and promotes the feeling of being satiated[196]. It's even been observed that an insulin sensitive brain responds better to healthy lifestyle interventions like exercise and various dietary protocols[197]. It's also been shown that administrating insulin to an insulin sensitive brain suppresses glucose production by the liver[198,199,200,201,202]. Thus, central insulin resistance (in the brain) has a major impact on peripheral insulin resistance (in the body).

In one study, **giving intranasal insulin to obese women after eating reduced their dessert consumption and cravings, and they rated chocolate chip cookies less desirable compared to not getting the insulin**[203]. However, the same effect wasn't seen in lean women probably due to their lower baseline desire for food and less baseline insulin resistance. There might be sex-specific differences as well as normal men receiving intranasal insulin immediately eat fewer calories, but normal weight women don't[204]. When men and women are given intranasal insulin for 8 weeks, the men lose 1.3 kg of weight and 1.4 kg of body fat, but women don't see this effect[205].

Regardless of sex, insulin is needed for reproductive health and sex hormone production in both men and women as insulin participates in the surge of Luteinizing hormone (LH) by the hypothalamic-pituitary-gonadal axis[206,207]. LH is a precursor to the other sex hormones like testosterone and estrogen[208]. In women, the surge of LH is what triggers ovulation[209].

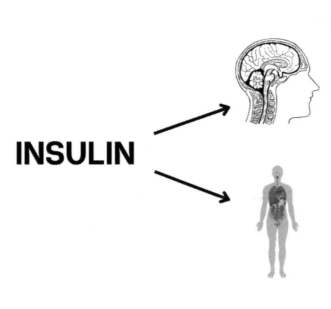

Effects on the brain
- Improves cognition
- Facilitates memory
- Improves satiety
- Lower food intake
- Cholesterol production

Effects on the body
- Lowers blood sugar
- Improves fat distribution
- Supports sex hormones
- Supports muscle growth

Adapted From: Agrawal et al (2021)

Brain insulin resistance or central insulin resistance develops when brain insulin signaling is impaired and it stops responding to insulin signaling like the rest of the body. As a result, cognitive function decreases, you experience more brain fog, inflammation, anxiety, and accelerated neurodegeneration[210,211,212]. In Alzheimer's disease, insulin resistance impairs the activation of the PI3K-Akt pathway, which is needed for survival and growth of cells, including neurons[213]. Due to lack of repair and regeneration, the brain tissue accumulates more damage and begins to degenerate even faster[214].

What Causes Insulin Resistance?

Insulin and leptin (the satiety hormone) resistance in the brain is driven by consuming a highly processed food diet that leads to intestinal permeability and endotoxemia (low-grade elevations in plasma lipopolysaccharide or LPS), creating inflammation and oxidative stress[215,216]. This is what contributes to out-of-control hunger, obesity, and peripheral insulin resistance[217,218].

Additionally, too frequent releases of insulin will eventually desensitize the cells to insulin's effects, causing insulin resistance. In 1985, a study took 12 non-obese men and injected them with insulin at increasing doses over the span of 40 hours[219]. As a result, the men saw a 15% drop in glucose tolerance. In other words, they became 15% more insulin resistance. Another study on 15 healthy non-diabetic men found that giving them normal doses of insulin over the course of 96 hours reduced their insulin sensitivity by 20-40%[220]. Thus, hyperinsulinemia or frequently high levels of insulin eventually causes insulin resistance. Granted, there are different thresholds and circumstances it can occur but at the center of human physiology, hyperinsulinemia does lead to insulin resistance.

Here are the main drivers of insulin resistance and glucose intolerance:

- Excess consumption of refined carbohydrates, added sugars, ultra-processed foods, refined omega-6 seed oils and trans fat.
- Lack of exercise, especially resistance training
- Sedentary lifestyle
- Sleep deprivation
- Circadian rhythm mismatches (exposure to light at night)[221]
- High inflammation and cortisol levels
- Smoking[222,223]
- Excess alcohol intake[224,225,226]

- Lack of vitamin D[227]
- Low salt or potassium intake[228]
- Lack of magnesium[229,230]
- Lack of vitamin C[231]
- Lack of chromium[232]
- Lack of thiamine[233,234,235,236,237,238]

The biggest risk factors for insulin resistance include sedentary lifestyle, overconsumption of high fat-high carb foods, vitamin D deficiency and circadian rhythm mismatches[239,240,241,242,243,244]. Certain nutrient deficiencies, such as magnesium, potassium, chromium, and thiamine, predispose the body to reduced glucose tolerance and insulin resistance[245,246,247,248,249]. Low magnesium status is both the cause and result of elevated insulin[250,251,252]. Higher magnesium intake is linked to a reduced risk of diabetes[253]. There are even medications, such as corticosteroids, antipsychotics and protease inhibitors that promote insulin resistance[254,255].

Physical activity and muscle mass are the biggest determinants of your insulin sensitivity[256]. Muscle contraction causes glucose transporters, primarily GLUT4, to translocate to the cell membrane, improving uptake of glucose into the cell[257]. The more muscle you have, the bigger your storage capacity for glucose is as muscle glycogen. **Staying physically active for over 90 minutes a day (walking, exercise, chores, etc.) can reduce the risk of diabetes by 28%**[258]! Thus, any movement matters in terms of managing your blood sugar levels. However, resistance training is by far the most powerful thing for increasing insulin sensitivity and activating GLUT4 receptors.

In Type 2 diabetics, resistance training (such as lifting weights on machines or free weights) improves glycemic control during early stages of glucose intolerance[259]. Even a single bout of exercise helps to translocate GLUT4 to the cell surface without insulin signaling[260,261]! Thus, even with already existing insulin resistance or impaired glucose tolerance, you can still improve your condition with regular exercise[262,263]. Chronic stress impairs GLUT4 activation, which worsens glucose disposal and can lead to insulin resistance[264,265]. At the same time, stress-reducing activities like mindfulness meditation and yoga improve insulin resistance likely by reducing stress[266].

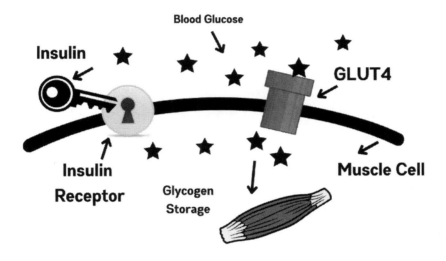

Redrawn From: Ishiguro et al (2016)

Insulin Resistance and the Randle Cycle

Insulin resistance and Type 2 diabetes can also occur when the body is struggling to burn different fuel sources[267,268]. In 1963, Randle et al discovered that glucose and fatty acids compete in what's called 'glucose fatty acid cycle' or The Randle Cycle[269,270,271]. Your body is always burning a mix of glucose, fatty acids, ketones, amino acids, lactate etc. but the most readily available one gets preferential treatment. To not waste anything, the body inhibits and upregulates the use of the other fuel sources, depending on the situation. For example, **insulin and glucose rapidly inhibit fat burning**[272]. Eating something that raises insulin slows down fat oxidation because the body is more in a storing mode. With a drop in insulin and a rise in glucagon the body switches more towards fat burning. **High triglycerides (derivatives of glycerol and free fatty acyds) in the blood are implicated in insulin resistance**[273,274]. The reason has to do with reduced glucose disposal when your body is burning fat instead of glucose and the hyperglycemia that ensues[275]. There's also evidence that free fatty acids in high amounts may cause pancreatic beta-cell dysfunction[276,277]. Accumulation of lipids in the tissue disrupt insulin signaling and decrease GLUT4 translocation[278]. Too high glucagon levels are also linked to Type 2 diabetes because of the high glucose levels – glucagon keeps breaking down glycogen into glucose uncontrollably, resulting in chronically elevated blood sugar levels[279]. Essentially, when you eat a lot of carbs and fat at the same time the body has a hard time utilizing both fuels at once.

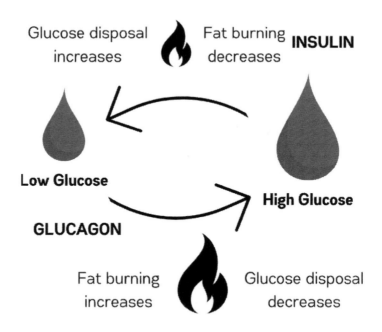

Adapted From: Hue and Taegtmeyer (2009)

36

Fast food is high in both sugar and fat, raising your blood glucose, insulin and triglycerides, and promotes insulin resistance[280]. This kind of 'energy toxicity' disrupts The Randle Cycle and leads to impaired utilization of all fuel substrates. Ultra-processed food tends to also be high in trans fats and added sugars, which promote insulin resistance as well[281]. The fructose in sugar-sweetened beverages is the primary diet-related reason for the high prevalence of Type 2 diabetes and obesity in the United States[282]. Fructose consumption (from processed foods, not fruit) raises cortisol and damages the liver, which raises triglycerides much more than eating fat and causes insulin resistance[283,284].

Metabolic Flexibility = Metabolic Freedom

The key to preventing The Randle Cycle from disrupting your glucose homeostasis and insulin sensitivity is metabolic flexibility. It refers to being able to swap between different fuel sources when transitioning from a fasted state into a fed one without experiencing poor glucose metabolism or insulin resistance[285]. **Lack of metabolic flexibility is implicated in insulin resistance, obesity, Type 2 diabetes, and metabolic syndrome**[286]. With poor metabolic flexibility, your body can't inhibit the oxidation of fat once insulin rises and suppress glucagon stimulating glucose secretion. As a result, you get elevated free fatty acids (as insulin can't store fat as readily), hyperglycemia, insulin resistance and hyperlipidemia. Because the mitochondria are in a particular type of 'gridlock', they start building up reactive oxygen species, causing oxidative stress and inflammation[287,288,289]. This is what leads to metabolic syndrome.

In obese and diabetic individuals, metabolic inflexibility manifests itself as[290]:

- Failure to secrete insulin in response to eating.

- Failure of muscles to switch between using fats in the fasted state and carbs in the fed state.

- Impaired transition from burning fatty acids to storage after eating a meal.

The biggest cause of metabolic inflexibility is overeating (driven by an ultraprocessed food diet) and the ensuing weight gain[291]. To achieve metabolic flexibility, you need to maintain insulin sensitivity and efficient mitochondrial function with a physically active lifestyle, weight loss and calorie moderation[292,293]. Things like intermittent fasting and cold exposure have been also shown to improve markers of metabolic flexibility and insulin sensitivity[294,295,296]. Intriguingly, exercise is the most powerful thing for increasing metabolic flexibility and it also boosts glutathione levels and improves the body's overall antioxidant defense[297,298].

Exercise can also override The Randle Cycle by preventing fatty acid-inhibition of glucose oxidation and making the body use up all the fuel sources it can find[299]. This is mediated by an energy sensor called AMPK (AMP-activated protein kinase) that gets activated during physiological stressors, such as fasting, exercise, sauna, cold exposure or calorie restriction[300,301,302]. During exercise, the demand for energy generally exceeds the supply and with activated AMPK your body will use both glucose and fat for fuel. Thus, metabolic inflexibility and the insulin resistance that it causes are predominantly caused by a state of energy overabundance or energy toxicity. Using up that excessive energy is what protects against the glucose intolerance and hyperlipidemia and

Marzullo, Kaitlyn H

16984

Thursday, June 22, 2023

31183213719799   The blood sugar fix : how

can be accomplished with increasing physical activity or reducing energy input. Simply put, you need to limit your intake of foods that disrupt the Randle Cycle while at the same time staying physically active. It also means that with a physically active lifestyle and good body composition that facilitates good insulin sensitivity, you can get away with eating more of these ultra-processed foods because your body just 'gobbles up' everything you feed it. However, if you start gaining weight or go into an energy surplus, this ability becomes increasingly diminished.

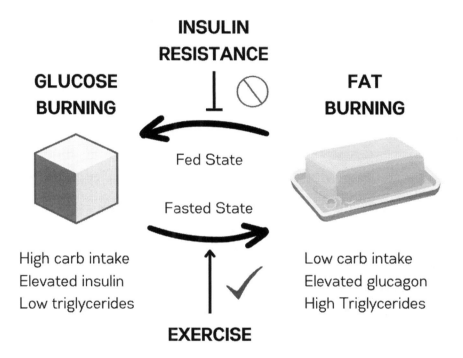

Athletes may have a higher deposition of intramyocellular triacylglycerol (IMTG) content and still maintain insulin sensitivity, which usually correlates with insulin resistance, hence the term Athlete's Paradox[303]. Endurance athletes can have much more muscle lipid content than Type 2 diabetics[304]. This might be explained by the fact that low intensity exercise, especially cardio, burns predominantly fat for fuel and endurance athletes would burn it up preferably over glucose. Type 2 diabetics appear to store intramuscular lipids in type-2 muscle fibers, whereas endurance athletes do so in type-1 muscle fibers, which is what are activated during endurance activities[305]. Because of their insulin sensitivity and GLUT4 activation from exercise, these individuals can maintain good metabolic flexibility and avoid insulin resistance. While the intramuscular lipids in athletes are in constant flux and being used for energy, in obese and Type 2 diabetics, they are stagnant.

Insulin resistance also occurs as a protective response under different metabolic conditions, such as pregnancy, fasting, ketosis or starvation[306]. In these cases, the muscles become insulin resistant as to preserve glucose for the brain. Indeed, it's been observed that ketogenic diets in humans and mice cause a state of quasi-insulin resistance[307,308,309]. There is no pathological sign of insulin resistance reflected in bloodwork – insulin and fasting glucose levels are normal – but after an oral glucose tolerance test the blood sugar stays elevated for a longer period of time. Categorically, this would mean insulin resistance but given everything else is normal, it's not pathological. Insulin sensitivity and glucose clearance resume back to normal after returning to a regular way of eating. This is more described as 'decreased glucose demand' or 'glucose sparing' because the muscles only have blocked the request for glucose[310]. Nevertheless, this is not optimal for metabolic flexibility in the long term and you should always maintain some intake of carbohydrate cycling to keep your body adept to using glucose. In the short term, ketosis is great and can actually improve metabolic flexibility, especially in terms of enhanced fat oxidation, but in the long term it's recommended to do it cyclically. You should also be careful with eating a large amount of carbohydrates immediately after fasting or when having been on a ketogenic diet for weeks.

Here are the things that promote metabolic inflexibility:

- Overnutrition and excess calorie intake

- Obesity and weight gain

- Sedentary lifestyle

- Chronically high refined carbohydrate intake

- Chronically low carbohydrate intake

- Diabetes and insulin resistance

Here are the things that promote metabolic flexibility:

- Regular exercise and physical activity

- Resistance training

- Periodic carbohydrate restriction

- Cyclical ketosis

- Intermittent fasting/time-restricted eating

Chapter 3: How Sugar and Fructose Make You Fat on the Inside and Drive Insulin Resistance

Sugar has been cultivated for at least a few thousand years, since Ancient India[311,312]. The oldest historical reference to sugar cane dates to an 8th century BC Chinese paper that pinpoints the origins of using sugarcane to India[313]. In the past, people got exposed to sugar only through chewing raw sugar cane or eating honey. Sugar refinement became possible around the 5th century BC in the Indian Gupta Empire[314]. The Indians started making crystallized sugar, which they called *khanda* (where the word *candy* is derived from) and spread it to China and the Middle East[315]. Buddhist monks were the ones who took sugar crystallization technologies to China[316]. China built its first sugar cane plantations in the 7th century AD[317]. At first, sugar wasn't used for cooking purposes that much and was thought to help with colds, stomach problems and lung issues[318].

In the 4th century BC, Alexander the Great was the first European to come in contact with sugar during his military campaigns to India[319]. Sugar was brought back to Europe after the crusades in the Middle East, which they called 'sweet salt'. Back then, the only sweetener available was honey[320]. The chronicler William of Tyre wrote in the 12th century that sugar was *"very necessary for the use and health of mankind"[321]*.

Widespread cultivation of sugar began in the middle of the 15th century when Europeans, primarily Spaniards and Portuguese, colonized the Canary Islands, Madeira, and São Tomé[322]. Cristopher Columbus brought sugar cane to the Caribbean Sea in the early 1500s where it began to be cultivated much more extensively[323,324]. Before the 19th century, sugar was considered a luxury good in Europe because of its lack of accessibility. All of that changed in the mid-1800s when Prussia began to extract sugar from beets[325,326]. The first beet sugar facility was built in Prussia in 1801 after which sugar became much more commonly found in European households[327]. Beets became the main source of sugar by 1880, replacing the need for sugar cane grown in the Americas. Global sugar consumption since 1850 has increased by over 100-fold[328].

Today, the sugar we know has been refined to such an extent that it can be added into virtually every packaged or processed food, increasing the sugar content of those foods to unnatural levels[329]. Since sugar is refined in a crystalline form, it can have drug-like qualities[330,331]. Indeed, the sugar we consume today is more like a drug than food because it leaves the body more depleted than before while providing no real nutritional value besides empty calories. It also consumes essential vitamins and minerals for it to be metabolized in the body[332,333]. Added sugars that come in the form of high-fructose corn syrup (HFCS), pure crystalline sugar and others cause a massive glycemic load on the body, overwhelming its ability to deal with it, resulting in hyperglycemia, hyperinsulinemia, and oxidative stress[334].

In this chapter, we're going to look at all the ways added sugars and refined carbohydrates contribute to insulin resistance. It's not that all carbohydrates are harmful. Instead, carbohydrates that have been refined and stripped from their fiber and micronutrients overburden the body, leading to metabolic dysfunction and glucose intolerance. Reducing the intake of refined carbohydrates is effective in improving glycemic control, especially in insulin resistant individuals[335,336,337]. However, as we've discussed in the previous chapter, long term ketosis isn't optimal for the best metabolic flexibility. That's why we aren't going to demonize all carbohydrates but rather show you how certain refined carbohydrates harm your health.

All the Different Types of Sugars

The term *sugar* refers to many different types of carbohydrates. They are divided into monosaccharides or simple sugars, such as glucose and fructose; disaccharides, such as sucrose, maltose, and lactose; and oligosaccharides[338]. Most commonly, sugars end with *-ose* like glucose or fructose.

- **Glucose** is the most abundant monosaccharide and the primary product of photosynthesis in plants. It's also the exact molecule in your bloodstream. Naturally, you get glucose from vegetables, tubers, and some fruits. When you digest starch, it gets broken down into glucose. Glucose syrup is a processed liquid used in a lot of processed foods and it has a much bigger impact on your blood sugar levels than glucose from natural sources. Dextrose is another naturally occurring form of glucose, which technically should be called D-glucose[339]. You can get it from corn syrup, grape sugar, and honey.

- **Fructose** is the predominant fruit sugar that you get from fruit, such as apples, pears, bananas, pineapple, etc., as well as berries, such as blueberries, cranberries, strawberries, etc., although in much smaller amounts. Honey also contains fructose. Fructose is found in refined sugars like table sugar and high-fructose corn syrup (HFCS)[340]. Compared to regular corn syrup, HFCS contains more fructose than glucose.

- **Sucrose** is the correct name for table sugar. It's made of 50% glucose and 50% fructose. You do get sucrose from some natural foods and fruits, but most of your exposure comes from processed foods. Sucrose tastes sweeter than glucose alone but less sweet than fructose. Fructose has the sweetness of about 1.5x of table sugar.

Glucose is absorbed directly through the small intestine into the bloodstream[341]. Because of that, it raises your blood sugar levels faster than other sugars, stimulating the release of insulin. Once absorbed, glucose is either burned for immediate energy or stored as glycogen, whether in the muscle or liver[342,343]. When your blood sugar gets too low, glucagon begins breaking down glycogen to raise glucose levels.

Fructose, like glucose, gets directly absorbed through the small intestine into the bloodstream[344]. **In contrast to glucose, however, fructose doesn't raise blood sugar and insulin as much[345].** However, large amounts of fructose can still have a negative effect on your metabolic health and increase the risk of metabolic syndrome and fatty liver disease[346]. The body can only handle a small amount of fructose at once and overconsumption can lead to visceral fat accumulation. Your muscles can store up to 400-500 grams of glycogen from glucose and the liver can store around 100-150 grams of glycogen. If you're already eating a diet with a lot of glucose coming in, then it's very easy to exceed your body's capacity to store glucose. Excess consumption of fructose will be converted into triglycerides that then increase the risk of fatty liver as well as insulin resistance and hyperlipidemia[347,348].

Sucrose begins to be broken down already in your mouth into glucose and fructose. However, the absorption still occurs in the small intestine[349]. The lining of the small intestine produces an enzyme called sucrase, which breaks sucrose into glucose and fructose[350]. Glucose and fructose are then assimilated in the bloodstream as previously discussed. **Having glucose present increases the amount of fructose that gets absorbed and releases more insulin, which may imply that consuming fructose and glucose together at the same time is more harmful than eating them alone[351].** This is why table sugar and high-fructose corn syrup are one of the worst types of sugars for your health.

How Sugar Causes Metabolic Syndrome and Hyperlipidemia

The intake of large amounts of added sugars is linked to the development of metabolic syndrome, which is characterized by elevated triglycerides, low HDL cholesterol, high blood pressure, high blood sugar levels and weight gain around the midsection[352,353,354,355,356]. Added sugar overconsumption also promotes premature death, cardiovascular disease, fatty liver disease and heart disease[357,358,359,360,361,362,363]. The primary reason the overconsumption of added sugars causes these issues has to do with insulin resistance and interfering with the Randle cycle[364,365]. When your body is under hyperglycemia and hyperinsulinemia from metabolizing the sugar you consumed, you suppress fat oxidation, which results in high plasma triglyceride levels. Over time those excess triglycerides begin to interfere with insulin production and cause insulin resistance[366].

Here are the things that raise your triglyceride levels:

- High fructose intake
- High sucrose intake
- High carbohydrate intake
- High fat intake
- Alcohol consumption[367,368]
- Lack of physical activity
- Lack of aerobic exercise[369,370,371]
- Obesity
- Diabetes
- Low fiber intake[372,373]
- Low vitamin D levels[374]
- Eating too frequently (6x vs 3x a day)[375]

A 2020 review concluded that people who regularly consumed sugar-sweetened beverages were over 50% more likely to have high triglycerides, compared to non-regular drinkers[376]. High triglyceride levels are indicative of poor glycemic control in Type 2 diabetics[377]. The overconsumption of sugar, and in particular fructose, increases de novo lipogenesis in the liver, which increases the production of very-low density lipoproteins (VLDL) elevating triglyceride levels[378]. Additionally, the hyperglycemia and hyperinsulinemia induces insulin resistance. **That's why carbohydrate restriction, even in the presence of a higher fat intake, can lower triglyceride levels – the triglycerides are being burned for energy because insulin is low**[379,380]. A low carb diet has been shown to result in a greater reduction in triglycerides than a low-fat diet because the body is burning more fat instead of glucose[381]. However, someone on a low-fat high carb diet can still have normal triglycerides if they're not eating a lot of fat. Their body just isn't getting that much fat from food and/or they're burning it for fuel during physical activity. A 2007 study discovered that individuals on a vegan diet had about half the triglycerides compared to omnivores (81.67 vs 155.68)[382]. **Switching from an omnivorous diet to a plant-based one generally results in a drop in cholesterol and triglycerides**[383], **most likely because the total fat intake in the diet also decreases as well as their higher fiber intake**[384]. Simultaneously, a low carb diet lowering triglycerides is also because the carbohydrate intake has been reduced. **Thus, mixing high carb and high fat foods is not optimal for insulin resistance and metabolic syndrome because it disrupts The Randle Cycle.** That's why ultra-processed food consumption (which contains both large amounts of carbs and fat) is generally linked to diabetes and insulin resistance. This is supported by studies on vegan individuals that eat more processed foods – their triglycerides are still high because their food is high in both carbs and fats[385]. The only exception that can give some room for freedom is exercising a lot or being in a calorie deficit, as AMPK activation enables the body to burn all the fuels simultaneously.

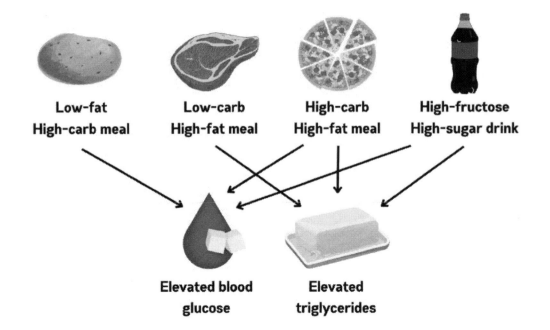

Low-fat High-carb meal **Low-carb High-fat meal** **High-carb High-fat meal** **High-fructose High-sugar drink**

Elevated blood glucose **Elevated triglycerides**

The type of fats consumed can also affect triglyceride levels. **It's been shown that replacing trans fats with omega-3 fats found in fish can dramatically lower triglyceride levels**[386]. Eating salmon twice a week decreases triglycerides[387]. Olive oil decreases triglycerides as well but not as much as other plant oils[388]. A study on the Indigenous people of Alaska found that saturated fat intake was associated with higher levels of blood triglycerides and polyunsaturated fat intake was linked to lower levels[389]. However, this is caused by the western dietary habits that these people have adopted. They're eating large amounts of processed foods together with saturated fat, which is the worst combination for maintaining optimal triglyceride levels and insulin sensitivity. To achieve the best outcome for your triglyceride levels, replace all trans fats and saturated fats from processed foods with saturated fats from whole foods, olive oil and marine fats[390]. If you're eating saturated fat from whole foods like beef or pork, then limit the carbohydrate content of that meal as to not disrupt the Randle Cycle.

How Sugar Causes Insulin Resistance

High sugar intake alone, even without an excessive intake of fat, is still harmful to your energy production and overall health. In fact, **sugar metabolism can deplete your ATP levels because it strips phosphates from the ATP molecule** (ATP being adenosine triphosphate)[391,392,393,394,395]. Experiments on animals show that adding refined sugar to a low nutrient diet leads to their malnourishment and death[396]. Replacing starch with sugar has also been shown to shorten lifespan of animals, which suggests that it's not natural carbohydrates but refined sugars that are the bigger issue[397,398,399]. Fructose metabolism also depletes ATP in the liver by damaging the mitochondria and causing oxidative stress[400,401,402]. As a result, you may get increased appetite and hunger due to lower ATP levels[403]. In reality, you have obtained calories from the sugar but because it's a net negative on energy reserves and nutrient status, you feel deprived and get the signal to continue seeking food for more energy. It's estimated that the average person consumes around 400-800 calories of sugar every day, which equates to 20-40% of calories out of a 2000 calorie diet[404,405]. That's about 1/3rd of daily calories being empty calories with no nutritional value. The World Health Organization suggests that reducing sugar consumption to 5-10% of total calories would have great benefits to public health (and we agree)[406].

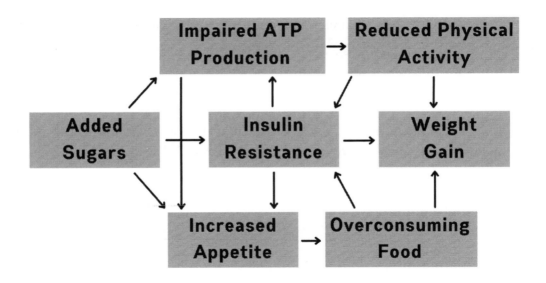

Taken From: DiNicolantonio and Land (2022) 'The Obesity Fix'

Overconsuming refined sugars also increases your insulin production, which in excess is one of the primary drivers of insulin resistance and diabetes[407]. Refined **sugars and refined carbohydrates have a very high glycemic index, meaning they raise blood sugar and subsequently insulin a lot more than lower glycemic foods[408].** The Glycemic Index (GI) is a measurement tool to assess how much a particular food raises blood sugar 2 hours after consumption[409]. It scales from 0 to 100 with pure glucose being 100. 'High GI' foods (70 or more) are generally refined carbohydrates and sugars with little to no fiber, whereas 'low GI' foods (55 or less) are fibrous vegetables with fewer carbs and fats. Proteins are generally on the lower end of 'medium GI' foods (56-69)[410]. The glycemic index isn't going to predict every person's blood sugar response to a particular food because there are many other variables at play, such as their individual insulin sensitivity, metabolic condition, and the entire meal composition[411]. Also, you rarely eat one type of food alone, with the exception of maybe fruits as a snack. Thus, your blood sugar and insulin response will always be determined by all the foods eaten together. That's why it has been proposed that the Glycemic Load (GL) is more relevant. The Glycemic Load is calculated by multiplying the GI of the food eaten by the amount of carbohydrates in the serving. A single unit on the GL scale is the equivalent of consuming 1 gram of glucose[412]. There's also the Insulin Index (II) that reflects how much insulin gets released within 2 hours after eating[413].

Here is the glycemic index chart of common foods[414,415,416]:

Food	Glycemic Index	Insulin Index
Glucose	100	100
Mashed Potatoes	87	121
Rice Crackers	87	79
Rice Milk	86	-
Cornflakes	81	75
Instant Oat Porridge	79	40
Mars Bar	79	122
Rice Porridge	78	79
Potato Boiled	78	121
Mango	76	-
White Bread	75	100
Grapes	74	82
Cookies	74	92
White Rice, Boiled	73	79

Whole Wheat Bread	72	96
Watermelon	72	-
Unleavened Wheat Bread	70	56
Wheat Flake Biscuits	69	96
Brown Rice, Boiled	68	62
Millet Porridge	67	40
Couscous	65	-
Pop Corn	65	54
Table Sugar	65	-
Pumpkin, Boiled	64	-
French Fries	63	74
Sweet Potato, Boiled	63	-
Doughnuts	63	74
Wheat Roti	62	-
Lentils in Tomato Sauce	62	58
Honey	61	-
Pineapple	59	-
Soft Drink/Soda	59	-
Muesli	57	46

Apricot	57	
Potato Chips	56	61
Porridge, Rolled Oats	55	40
Plantain/Green Banana	55	-
Cheese	55	45
Specialty Grain Bread	53	56
Taro, Boiled	53	-
Rice Noodles	53	79
Chapatti	52	-
Sweet Corn	52	-
Banana, Yellow	51	81
Mango	51	-
Ice Cream	51	89
Orange Juice	50	-
Spaghetti, White	49	40
Strawberry Jam/Jelly	49	-
Vegetable Soup	48	-
Corn Tortilla	46	-
Orange	43	60
Peaches	43	-

Dates	42	-
Eggs	42	31
Apple Juice	41	-
Yogurt	41	-
Chocolate	40	-
Carrots, Boiled	39	-
Milk, Full Fat	39	-
Skim Milk	37	-
Apple	36	59
Soy Milk	34	-
Lentils	32	-
Barley	28	-
Fish	28	59
Chickpeas	28	-
Kidney Beans	24	-
Cherries	22	-
Beef	21	51
Soya Beans	16	-
Fructose	15	-
Peanuts	12	20
Cabbage	10	-

High GI: ≥ 70; Medium GI: 56-59; Low GI: ≤ 55

Persistent stimulation of insulin leads to the insulin receptors on the cell surface to become desensitized to insulin's actions, resulting in insulin resistance[417]. Thus, if you're spiking your insulin multiple times a day with sugar-sweetened beverages or other foods that have a high glycemic index, you're eventually going to experience insulin desensitization or insulin resistance[418,419]. It's been found that in humans, continuous 40-hour hyperinsulinemia significantly decreases glucose utilization[420]. In contrast, **pulsatile insulin instead of hyperinsulinemia prevents insulin resistance in both diabetic humans and animals**[421,422,423,424]. The less frequent insulin release also increases the efficiency of glucose clearance and blood sugar decrease, meaning the more frequent insulin release the smaller effect it has on reducing blood sugar levels, whereas less frequent insulin release decreases blood sugar levels more. In vitro studies show that insulin receptor expression is significantly greater in liver cells exposed to insulin in a pulsatile manner as opposed to a continuous exposure[425]. Thus, the frequency at which you stimulate insulin appears to be more important for maintaining insulin sensitivity.

Refined carbohydrates and flours also create larger spikes and blood sugar and insulin than whole grains[426]. Before the late 1800s, grains were stone ground instead of ground with the steel roller mill. The steel roller mill enables the complete refinement of the grain and removal of the fiber. As a result, the highly refined flour causes a much larger spike in blood sugar and insulin. Most of the breads and flour people eat nowadays is highly refined white flour with no fiber. This can lead to elevations in insulin several times a day and decreased glucose tolerance. The intake of refined carbohydrates from flour and cereal foods in the U.S. has increased from 135.1 pounds per person per year in the 1970s to 200 pounds by the year 2000[427]. At the same time, the rates of diabetes in the U.S. have increased from 1-2% of the total population to 8% in 2015[428]. In 2018, over 10% of the U.S. population were diagnosed with diabetes[429].

Milled smooth grain leads to higher spikes in insulin vs. coarse grain:

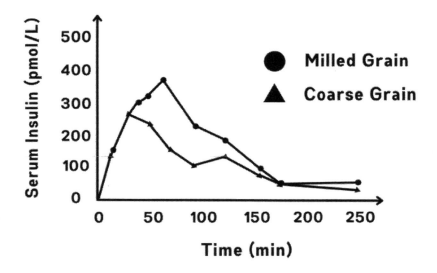

Redrawn From: Edwards et al (2015)

Milled smooth grain leads to higher spikes in glucose and higher risk for low blood sugar:

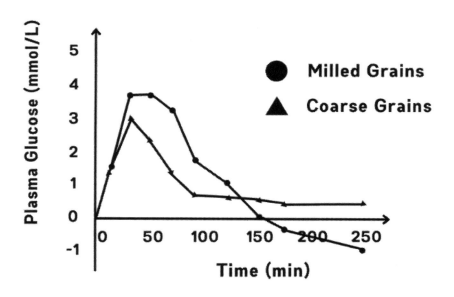

Redrawn From: Edwards et al (2015)

Excess refined carbohydrate intake can still cause insulin resistance but it's still not as harmful as sugar. Animals replacing starch with sugar see worse insulin sensitivity, higher fasting insulin, and higher glucose levels[430,431,432,433,434,435,436]. Compared to other refined carbohydrates, added fructose in humans also promotes more glucose intolerance even when the calories are matched[437,438,439]. Men who replace wheat with sugar show significantly higher fasting insulin, insulin to glucose ratio and raise insulin a lot more when given sucrose[440]. The more sugar they replace the wheat with, the worse fasting insulin and glucose responses they see even with matched calories[441]. That's because of the higher glycemic index of sugar and its 50-50 glucose/fructose composition.

How Fructose Makes You Fat on the Inside

Out of all sugars, added fructose, especially high-fructose corn syrup, might be the worst for your health by overburdening the liver and causing insulin resistance[442,443,444,445,446]. **Although fructose has a lower glycemic index than glucose, fructose is more harmful in terms of diabetes, obesity, and atherosclerosis**[447,448]. Consuming fructose-sweetened beverages is linked to weight gain[449,450,451,452,453]. A 10-week study saw that people who drank fructose-sweetened beverages experienced an 8.6% increase in belly fat compared to the 4.8% of those who drank glucose-sweetened beverages[454]. This kind of weight around the midsection is associated with a greater risk of heart disease, diabetes, and overall mortality than weight around the hips[455].

If someone looks skinny on the outside but with a popping belly, then they have a lot of visceral fat in and around the organs of the abdominal cavity (stomach, liver, and intestines). This phenomenon is called 'thin on the outside, fat on the inside' or TOFI or just 'skinny fat'[456,457]. About 12-14% of the population has this kind of 'normal weight but metabolically obese' phenotype[458,459,460,461]. Visceral adipose tissue (VAT) is the internal fat in and around the organs as opposed to subcutaneous adipose tissue (SCAT) that's just underneath the skin. VAT is associated with diabetes and insulin resistance much more so than subcutaneous adipose tissue[462,463,464,465,466,467,468,469,470,471,472]. Neck fat accumulation is also linked to higher mortality[473]. In small amounts, visceral fat has a purpose to protect the internal organs but in excess it begins to spread pro-inflammatory cytokines and oxidative stress[474]. Visceral fat also produces more free fatty acids and triglycerides that begin to interfere with glucose uptake and insulin sensitivity[475].

The biggest promoters of visceral fat accumulation are high cortisol and insulin levels[476,477]. Individuals with higher urinary cortisol levels have higher waist to hip ratios[478]. According to the World Health Organization, an optimal waist to hip ratio for women is <0.80 and for men <0.95. A waist circumference above 40 inches in men and above 35 inches in women is a risk factor for heart disease, diabetes, and premature death[479]. Insulin resistance and poor glucose control promote visceral fat gain[480] and visceral fat itself contributes to developing insulin resistance[481,482,483]. Fructose affects both insulin resistance and visceral fat gain by promoting liver fattening and hyperinsulinemia much more so than glucose[484,485,486,487].

Here are the mechanisms by which added fructose makes you fat on the inside:

- Excess fructose consumption releases glucocorticoids and cytokines that promote the production of triglycerides and visceral adiposity[488,489].

- Fructose reduces insulin sensitivity, which eventually leads to insulin resistance[490,491].

- Fructose increases 11B-hydroxysteroid dehydrogenase-1 (11β-HSD), which elevates intracellular cortisol inside subcutaneous fat cells[492,493,494,495]. As a result, they turn insulin resistant and fewer fatty acids can enter the subcutaneous fat cells and instead they get stored as visceral fat around the organs[496,497].

Fructose can also store fat in the liver and muscles instead of the adipose tissue[498,499]. Intracellular lipids in the liver and muscle promote insulin resistance[500].

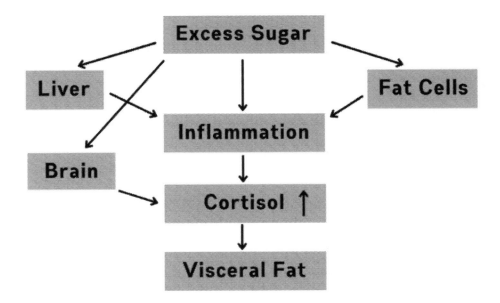

Redrawn From: DiNicolantonio et al (2018)

Added fructose became more predominant in processed foods around the 1950s[501]. In 2004, the average American consumed 50 grams of fructose a day[502]. Today, it's closer to 83.1 grams a day with 20% of the population even exceeding 100 grams of fructose per day[503]. Most of that fructose comes from soft drinks and sugar-sweetened beverages that can be comprised of up to 65% fructose[504,505,506]. We want to make a clear differentiation between added fructose and the fructose you get from natural sources, such as berries, fruit and vegetables. These foods are not linked to obesity or insulin resistance because they contain a lot less fructose and come with fiber and water. In fact, fruit and vegetable consumption is one of the most common themes in longevity, health, and a reduced risk of obesity[507,508].

High-fructose corn syrup (HFCS) is the most worrisome because it can contain more fructose than glucose, exacerbating hyperlipidemia and oxidative stress on the liver[509]. Soft drinks typically contain HFCS 55 (55% fructose and 45% glucose), whereas other processed foods like breakfast cereal or baked foods are HFCS42 (42% fructose)[510]. Despite having 10% more fructose, HFCS55 has a comparable sweetness to sucrose[511,512]. HFCS is commonly used over regular sugar because it's cheaper and easier to handle[513]. Indeed, HFCS has almost fully replaced table sugar as a sweetener in most ultra-processed foods[514]. HFCS is the main ingredient in most syrups because it's cheaper than maple syrup and often used to adulterate honey[515].

HFCS began to be used in the United States in the 1970s as a replacement to table sugar[516]. From 1980 to 1999, domestic production of HFCS in the U.S. increased from 2.2 million tons to 9.5 million tons a year. Since the year 2000, HFCS production has declined about 19% with 2019 production being at 7.9 tons a year[517]. Although in the U.S., HFCS is used equally as much as sucrose, the rest of the world uses sucrose for 90% of their sweeteners. Coca-Cola and Pepsi use sucrose as the sweetener in their drinks in other nations but in the U.S., they've been using HFCS since 1984[518]. Overall, total corn sweetener consumption (HFCS, glucose syrup and dextrose) has dropped from 85.7 lb. per person in 1999 to 55.3 lb. in 2021. At the same time, refined sugar intake exceeded corn sugars in 2011, reaching 69.7 lb. per person in 2021[519]. In the end, sugar is sugar as both have the same deleterious effect on your insulin sensitivity, visceral fat composition and metabolic health.

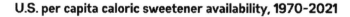

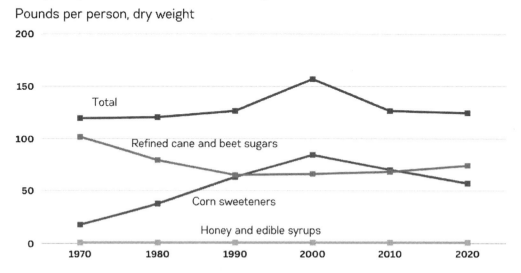

Redrawn From: USDA (2022)

Whether or not fructose and HFCS impact cardiometabolic health when replaced for sucrose has been controversial for some time now[520]. A 2021 review on 25 studies involving 1744 subjects concluded that substituting sucrose for fructose or HFCS had no effect on cholesterol, apolipoproteins or fasting triglyceride levels when calories were matched[521]. Meaning, fructose isn't particularly worse than table sugar in terms of altering your lipids but it doesn't mean it's better either. However, other **studies show that fructose is worse than glucose (even when matched for calories) regarding insulin resistance, visceral fat gain and**

hyperlipidemia[522]. There's a long history of other studies linking fructose and sugar consumption to diabetes, insulin resistance and obesity. Granted, that's primarily because these individuals are consuming an excess amount of calories, which gives them insulin resistance. However, it would be absurd to claim that because fructose isn't worse than regular sugar that it's somehow safe and healthy. In reality it's quite evident that consuming added sugar makes it more likely that someone goes into an energy surplus. It's true that being in a calorie deficit can avoid the excess body fat accumulation from overconsuming sugar, however, **eating a normal amount of calories but with higher levels of added sugars leads to worsening insulin resistance**[523,524]. Thus, **you don't necessarily have to overconsume calories to get insulin resistance, this can occur if the diet is high enough in added sugars (usually around 15% of total calories or more).**

The Personal Fat Threshold

It's been observed that individuals have a different threshold for developing insulin resistance and metabolic syndrome. **Some people can become severely obese before developing metabolic syndrome, particularly people of Caucasian and African descent, whereas others, especially people of Indian and Asian descent, can get diabetes and metabolic syndrome even at lower bodyweights**[525]. In the U.S., more than 1 out of 5 people have diabetes but among Asian Americans that number is 1 out of 3[526]. Over half of Asian Americans and nearly half of Hispanic Americans with diabetes go undiagnosed probably because they tend to not be as overweight as the average American[527]. Why is that? It's hypothesized that this is because Asians tend to be shorter and thus the regular BMI measurements in their case are misleading[528]. However, there might be some cultural and genetic variables as well, which make it more likely that

Asian Americans store more of their fat as visceral fat around the organs as opposed to as subcutaneous fat like the Caucasians do[529]. It's estimated that by 2030, most people with diabetes in the world will live in Asia and Africa[530].

Why some people get diabetes faster than others is refered to as the Personal Fat Threshold Theory (PFTT). In 2015, Roy Taylor and Rury Holman published a paper called *'Normal weight individuals who develop type 2 diabetes: the personal fat threshold'*[531], which showed that **everyone gets sick from excess bodyweight only after they've exceeded their limit for storing subcutaneous fat underneath the skin and they start to store fat as visceral fat**[532]. This threshold is partly genetic and depends on ethnicity as shown by the higher prevalence of diabetes in Asian Americans. The underlying pathology is the same for everyone – insulin resistance and visceral fat accumulation – but *when* those things develop differs.

To know your personal fat threshold, you have to look at your biomarkers and assess your overall metabolic health. Metabolic syndrome is a condition in which you meet at least 3 or more of the 5 requirements: (1) high blood pressure, (2) visceral obesity, (3) high fasting triglycerides, (4) high blood glucose and (5) low serum HDL cholesterol[533]. In the U.S., about 25% of the population has metabolic syndrome[534]. Metabolic syndrome promotes cardiovascular disease and Type 2 diabetes[535]. It also doubles the risk of cardiovascular disease and increases all-cause mortality by 1.5-fold[536].

Here's how to assess whether or not you have metabolic syndrome:

- **Fasting Blood Glucose:** Normal ranges: <100 mg/dl (5.3 mmol/L), prediabetes: 100-125 mg/dl (5.6-6.9 mmol/L), diabetes: >126 mg/dl (7 mmol/L).

- **Blood pressure:** Normal blood pressure is <120/80 mmHg. 130-139/80-89 mmHg is considered stage 1 hypertension. Stage 2 hypertension is ≥140/90 mmHg.

- **Triglycerides**: Normal range: <150 mg/dl (1.7 mmol/L); borderline-high levels: 150-200 mg/dl (1.8 to 2.2 mmol/L); high levels: 200-500 mg/dl (2.3 to 5.6 mmol); very high levels: >500 mg/dl (5.7 mmol/L or above).

- **HDL Cholesterol:** Normal fasting HDL is between 40-60 mg/dl. Optimally, it should be between 50-80 mg/dl. HDL <40 mg/dl can be problematic and a sign of either dyslipidemia or metabolic syndrome.

- **Waist to Hip Ratio (for assessing visceral fat)**: Optimal ratio for women is <0.80 and for men <0.95. Moderate risk for women is 0.81–0.85 and for men 0.96–1.0. High risk for women is >0.86 and for men >1.0. A waist circumference over 40 inches (men) or 35 inches (women) is problematic and increases risk of heart disease, diabetes, and premature death[537].

Health Risk	Women	Men
Low	0.80 or lower	0.95 or lower
Moderate	0.81–0.85	0.96–1.0
High	0.86 or higher	1.0 or higher

If you have 3 or more of the 5, then you're categorized as having metabolic syndrome. You would also likely have a degree of insulin resistance and Type 2 diabetes under this definition. At this point, you have to start fixing your diet, exercise and improve your overall lifestyle. The biggest culprits for metabolic syndrome are excess calorie intake, being sedentary, consuming too many added sugars, fats, alcohol, and soft drinks[538,539,540,541,542].

How to Reduce Visceral Fat

Being in a calorie deficit is the main requirement for losing weight but it makes you lose predominantly subcutaneous fat over visceral fat[543]. That's still very important – you need to lose excess body fat across the board to not get metabolic syndrome and diabetes. However, there are more specific means to target visceral fat specifically. And those means will also make you lose subcutaneous fat as well.

Here are the things that will make you lose visceral fat:

- **Limit added sugars and added fructose.** These are the biggest culprits of visceral adiposity and insulin resistance. Individuals who consume more added sugars have more visceral fat[544,545,546]. Fructose in the form of HFCS is easily converted into visceral fat[547,548]. Replacing added fructose with starch has been found to reduce liver fat by 3.4% and visceral fat by 10.6% in just 10 days[549]. A 2018 review concluded that reducing sugar-sweetened drink and fructose consumption can decrease liver fat accumulation[550].

- **Avoid alcohol.** Drinking alcohol promotes visceral fat storage[551,552]. The reason has to do with the alcohol overburdening the liver when you consume it beyond the liver's ability to detoxify it. Even modest alcohol consumption is linked to having more visceral fat[553,554]. A 2003 study found that those who drank <1 drink per drinking day had the lowest average abdominal circumference compared to weekly drinkers (4 or more drinks per drinking day) who had the largest[555]. Thus, consuming a lot of alcohol at once is worse for visceral fat accumulation because you're exposed to a larger amount of alcohol in one sitting. After a certain threshold, the liver can't handle the alcohol anymore, and you begin to store it as visceral fat. If you do prefer to have a few drinks every now and then, keep the amounts to a minimum. Based on this, frequent but lower doses of alcohol might be better for central adiposity than infrequent or biweekly episodes of overconsuming alcohol.

- **Avoid trans fats.** Besides causing many other health problems, trans fats can also promote visceral adiposity[556,557]. A 6-year study on monkeys found that the monkeys on a trans-fat diet gained 33% more visceral fat compared to those consuming monounsaturated fat, despite consuming the same number of calories[558]. In 2015, the FDA determined Partially Hydrogenated Oils (PHOs), including margarine and other trans fats, to not be Generally Recommended as Safe (GRAS)[559]. As of June 18, 2018, PHOs and trans fats are forbidden from being added to food products. However, trans fats can be formed during high heat cooking of vegetable oils, such as canola oil and sunflower oil as well. Thus, limit your intake of fast food and restaurant foods, which are almost always cooked in these oils.

- **Exercise** has a greater effect on visceral fat reduction than calorie restriction[560]. To see a decrease in visceral adiposity, you need at least 10 hours of aerobic exercise a week, which includes brisk walking, jogging or cycling[561]. Combining modest calorie restriction with either aerobic exercise or resistance training results in significant decreases in both subcutaneous fat and visceral fat with a preference towards losing visceral fat[562]. Both resistance training and calorie restriction can help to reduce visceral fat[563]. However, resistance training combined with calorie restriction isn't more effective in reducing visceral fat than resistance training alone. Strength training also improves insulin sensitivity[564].

- o **High intensity exercise is one of the most powerful ways to reduce abdominal visceral fat**[565,566]. However, **aerobic exercise** should also be implemented because it **preferentially targets visceral fat even without calorie restriction**[567,568,569].

- **Getting enough sleep.** Insufficient sleep promotes visceral fat gain[570,571,572,573]. Sleep apnea is also associated with higher visceral fat[574,575,576]. On the flip side, **sleeping longer can help to cut down on visceral fat**. A 6-year study on 293 people discovered that sleeping 7-8 hours instead of 6 hours reduced visceral fat by about 26%[577].

  - o **Sleep deprivation also promotes insulin resistance and glucose intolerance**. Sleeping just 4.5 hours per night for 4 nights is enough to decrease insulin sensitivity by 16% and make fat cells 30% more insulin sensitive and more likely to store fat[578].

  - o It's recommended for adults to get 7-9 hours of sleep per night and children 10-12 hours. Unfortunately, up to 40% of people report that they get less than 7 hours of sleep[579].

- **Intermittent fasting** helps to target visceral fat and promotes insulin sensitivity[580,581]. Intermittent fasting can reduce visceral fat by 4-7% in just 6-24 weeks[582].

- **Carbohydrate restriction** and low carb diets have been shown to be more effective in decreasing visceral fat than low fat diets[583,584,585]. An 8-week study among 69 overweight men showed that those who followed a low carb diet lost 10% more visceral fat than those on a low fat diet[586].

  - For weight loss, low carb diets haven't been found to be superior to high carb diets when calories are matched[587,588,589,590]. Claims that ketogenic diets are more effective and that you can lose weight even without being in a calorie deficit have been proven to be wrong[591,592]. These claims are based on inaccurate self-reporting[593,594,595], which can be underestimated by up to 14%[596]. People who lose weight on a low carb diet do so primarily because of replacing their carbs with protein and fiber that makes them undereat calories due to higher satiety[597]. For helping with hyperglycemia and glucose control, some aspects of low carb diets might be effective but in the long term it isn't optimal for insulin sensitivity.

- **Fiber intake** decreases the risk of gaining visceral fat by up to 3.7%[598]. In epidemiological studies, dietary fiber intake is associated with lower bodyweight because it's very filling and is low in calories[599,600,601,602,603,604]. Fiber also reduces fat absorption, helping to create a bigger calorie deficit[605,606].

  - Some probiotic strains from the *Lactobacillus* family can help to decrease visceral fat[607,608]. A 2013 study on 210 healthy Japanese women saw that taking *Lactobacillus gasseri* for 12 weeks resulted in a 8.5% reduction in visceral fat[609]. After they stopped taking the supplement they regained all the initially lost visceral fat.

- **Higher protein intake** is linked with lower waist circumferences[610,611]. That's primarily because protein has a high thermic effect and you burn a lot of calories digesting it, helping to create a calorie deficit[612,613].

Overconsuming added sugars is one of the main culprits causing diabetes and insulin resistance. They also promote visceral fat storage and impaired glucose tolerance. Theoretically, someone who's very physically active and has a good amount of skeletal muscle can consume a fair amount of sugar and stay healthy. However, the frequency of raising insulin and the occasional situations of going into an energy surplus would over the course of many years lead to a slow accumulation of visceral fat and wear and tear on the pancreas.

Chapter 4: Omega-6 Seed Oils, Free Fatty Acids, and Insulin Resistance

Insulin resistance can also develop for other reasons besides wearing out the pancreas' ability to produce insulin as occurs with the overconsumption of high glycemic carbohydrates and sugars. The second reason this may occur is an **excess supply of free fatty acids that cause worsening glucose control and decrease in beta-cell mass**[614,615,616,617,618,619,620]. **This is exemplified by human studies that show elevated levels of free fatty acids predict declining glucose tolerance**[621,622]. Isolated beta-cells exposed to fatty acids for longer than 24 hours exhibit a blunted insulin response to glucose[623,624,625,626,627,628].

Acute exposure to fatty acids increases beta-cell mass to compensate for the insulin insensitivity but during chronic exposure the beta-cell mass decreases, reducing insulin secretion and causing lipotoxicity[629]. In high amounts, fatty acids, especially palmitate, are toxic to beta-cells[630,631]. The biggest reason for this is due to disruptions in the Randle Cycle[632]. If the body isn't burning fat due to hyperglycemia, then the triglycerides begin to stay elevated, leading to worsening glucose control. However, defects in insulin production can occur even when beta-cells lack a working Randle Cycle[633]. Thus, fatty acids can also cause beta-cell dysfunction through altering gene expression and signal transduction[634,635,636,637].

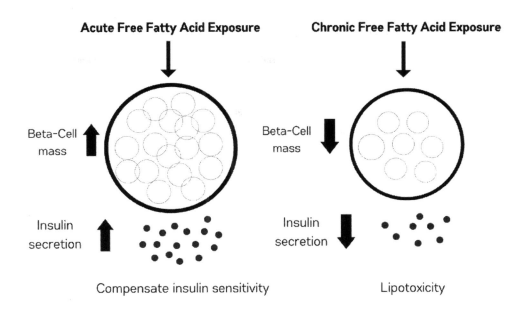

Acute Free Fatty Acid Exposure

Chronic Free Fatty Acid Exposure

Beta-Cell mass

Insulin secretion

Compensate insulin sensitivity

Lipotoxicity

Adapted From: Oh et al 2018

The effect of fatty acids on insulin secretion depends on the length of the carbon chain. **Saturated fats with a long length of over 16 carbon atoms [palmitate (C16:0) or stearate (C18:0)] appear to be more toxic to beta-cell function than shorter lengths [myristate (C14:0) or laurate (C12:0)][638].** Prolonged exposure to palmitate inhibits beta-cell capacity to secrete insulin and impairs insulin gene expression[639]. Certain unsaturated fats like arachidonic acid, docosahexaenoic acid (DHA, C22:6) and eicosapentaenoic acid (EPA, C20:5) can enhance insulin secretion,[640,641,642] which can enhance glucose clearance. However, hyperinsulinemia can still lead to the pathology of insulin resistance over time. Thus, the goal should be to maintain an optimal balance between glucose levels and insulin secretion. What's more, **certain unsaturated fats like polyunsaturated omega-6 seed oils are implicated in insulin resistance and diabetes**[643]. In this chapter, we're going to look at the effects of all fats on the risk of diabetes and insulin resistance.

Fanning the Flame with Oxidized Fats

Omega-3 and omega-6 fats are notorious in the context of cardiovascular disease (CVD) and atherosclerosis. It's commonly thought that omega-3 fatty acids from fish and seafood are protective to heart health and can improve blood lipids[644]. Indeed, there's a long epidemiological history between fish consumption and a reduction in risk of cardiovascular disease[645]. People who eat fish once or twice a week have been observed to have 50% fewer strokes, 50% lower CVD risk and 34% lower CVD mortality risk compared to those eating no fish[646,647]. Omega-3 supplements may also decrease mortality from cardiovascular disease[648]. Fish oil reduces risk factors for cardiovascular disease and has been shown to improve mortality in those who have recently experienced a heart attack or have heart failure[649,650,651,652]. Omega-3 fatty acids have been shown to have anti-inflammatory effects and they can improve insulin resistance[653]. In rats, insulin resistance can be alleviated with fish oil thanks to the anti-inflammatory effects of omega-3s[654]. Fish oil-fed rats also have less visceral fat and insulin resistance compared to those fed lard or corn oil[655].

Omega-6 fats like those found in nuts, seed oils and grain-finished meat, on the other hand, are thought to contribute to heart disease and numerous other health ailments. While some **systematic reviews and meta-analyses of randomized controlled trials, including Mendelian randomization studies have not found that omega-6 polyunsaturated fats significantly affect CVD mortality and morbidity risk**[656,657]. Other systematic reviews of randomized controlled trials that have appropriately eliminated trials that had a combined increase in omega-3 and omega-6 and only looked at studies that increased omega-6 intake have found trends for an increase in mortality and cardiovascular mortality with omega-6 polyunsaturated fats[658,659]. Furthermore, the Sydney Diet Heart study found a higher rate of death as well as significantly higher cardiovascular disease and coronary heart disease with omega-6 polyunsaturated fat[660]. Some studies find that higher circulating and tissue levels of linoleic acid (the parent omega-6 fat) are linked to a lower risk of cardiovascular events[661]. However, this is likely because omega-6 in the blood can readily oxidize and higher omega-6 levels may simply reflect lower inflammation and oxidative stress. This also would likely be why there has been no link between linoleic acid levels in humans and Type 2 diabetes[662] and even an inverse association to hyperinsulinemia[663]. However, when we look at other studies testing more reliable indicators of omega-6 intake (that would not be so readily affected by inflammation), such as linoleic acid levels in adipose tissue or platelets, we find positive associations with linoleic acid and coronary artery disease[664]. Additionally, linoleic acid in serum cholesteryl esters and phospholipid fatty acids are higher in patients with cornary artery disease compared to those without coronary artery disease[665]. Regardless, several clinical studies suggest that overconsuming omega-6 seed oils can increase death and coronary heart disease[666]. In regards to insulin levels, fasting insulin and the incremental two-hour post-prandial insulin over the fasting insulin has been shown to be lowest on a diet high in saturated fat (8 uU/ml and 10 uU/ml), moderate on an omega-3 diet (12 uU/ml and 14 uU/ml) and highest on the omega-6 polyunsaturated fat diet (14 uU/ml and 25 uU/ml)[667]. Thus, a diet high in omega-6 may promote elevated levels of insulin and potentially insulin resistance. More studies are certainly warranted but what does appear to be important is whether the omega-6 seed oils have been heated or not, the former being much worse than the latter. Thus, consuming non-heated, cold-pressed omega-6 seed oils, would be much less harmful versus consuming heated omega-6 seed oils.

As noted previously, the state in which a fat is consumed matters – whether it's oxidized or not. **Lipid peroxidation or the oxidation of fatty acids is implicated in insulin resistance, cardiovascular disease, cancer, and neurodegeneration**[668,669,670]. Polyunsaturated fatty acids (PUFAs) found in fish, seed oils and nuts, for example, get oxidized very easily when exposed to heat, light, oxygen and pressure. This causes lipid peroxidation, which promotes inflammation and insulin resistance. People with diabetes have elevated levels of lipid peroxidation that begins to oxidize the lipids and cholesterol in their bloodstream[671].

Virtually all omega-6 fats used in food processing and as cooking oils are oxidized because they get exposed to high heat and pressure during the manufacturing and extraction processes. This damages their PUFA chains, causing lipid peroxidation. Thus, it's not recommended to be eating high amounts of canola oil, sunflower oil, grapeseed oil and soybean oil as they get the most industrial processing. Another important point to note, is even if omega-6 seed oils are not oxidized when ingested, the acidity of the stomach will start to oxidize them and this effect is enhanced further in the presence of iron (red meat)[672,673]. Roasted nuts and seeds still in their natural form experience less lipid peroxidation because they're not directly heated for long periods of time. However, they will still go through some lipid peroxidation when sitting on store shelves etc. Even fish and other healthy fats like olive oil can start to oxidize when exposed to too much heat, oxygen, or sunlight. However, the difference is that we don't cook with fish oil and only small amounts are consumed (1-3 grams) versus omega-6 seed oils (20-50 grams).

How to Protect Against Lipid Peroxidation

Fortunately, the human body is quite adaptable and has defense mechanisms against lipid peroxidation. In small amounts, your body can protect itself even against an occasional exposure to oxidized fats. However, chronic consumption can overwhelm the body's defense mechanisms and cause chronic health issues.

Here are the things to do to keep your body resilient against lipid peroxidation:

- **Avoid Oxidized Fats** – Do not cook with corn oil, peanut oil, canola oil (rapeseed), cottonseed oil, safflower oil, sunflower oil, soybean oil, and don't use margarine as this will contribute to lipid peroxidation and promote oxidative stress[674]. All polyunsaturated fats (seed oils, nuts, fish, seeds) are more prone to oxidation than saturated fats (butter, lard, tallow, coconut oil) and monounsaturated fat (olive oil, avocado, certain nuts like almonds, cashews, hazelnuts and macadamia).

  - Although extra virgin olive oil doesn't have the highest smoking point, it's generally protected against lipid peroxidation due to its high polyphenol content[675]. Unfortunately, many commercial olive oils either don't have a high polyphenol content or are mixed with canola oil. The peppery taste of olive oil is a good indication of the polyphenol content (oleocanthal). Only buy olive oil that comes in a dark bottle and store it in a cool, dark place and consume it within a few weeks after opening.

  - Certain commercial fish oils can be oxidized, especially if they are not formulated with antioxidants or vitamiin E[676]. According to consumerlabs.com rancid fish oil supplements are quite common but not all of them are oxidized[677]. You have to find a reputable brand and better yet ones that come in a dark glass bottle and hasn't been sitting on the store shelf for months. If your fish oil or cod liver oil smells bad and tastes rancid, then it's likely oxidized. A lot of companies also use flavorings and odors like strawberry or lemon to mask the rancid taste.

- **Take Vitamin C and E** – Suppressing lipid peroxidation-induced inflammation with vitamin C alleviates insulin resistance in type 2 diabetics[678]. Vitamin E can alleviate lipid peroxidation as well[679,680]. Supplemental vitamin C and vitamin E can both protect against lipid peroxidation to a similar extent but combining them together doesn't appear to have any extra benefits beyond either supplement alone[681].

- **Exercise Regularly** – Intense exercise causes oxidative stress and lipid peroxidation but this drops during recovery[682]. Peak lipid peroxidation peaks above 60% of VO2 max but also rises below 50%[683,684]. Thus, any exercise at reasonable intensities causes lipid peroxidation to a certain degree. It's our body's recovery from this stress that makes exercise healthy for us. Creatine, resveratrol, vitamin C as well as ginger supplementation has been shown to attenuate the rise in oxidative stress and lipid peroxidation that occurs from intense exercise[685,686,687,688]. Regular exercise is linked to lower inflammation levels overall[689]. Physical activity is the biggest protective factor to cardiovascular disease and diabetes because of improved insulin sensitivity and reduced metabolic syndrome[690]. So, you should definitely keep exercising regularly as it will bolster your body's antioxidant defense systems.

- **Don't Over-Cook Your Food** – High-heat cooking, grilling, deep-frying and sauteing can lead to a certain degree of oxidation. This applies especially to vegetable oils that are repeatedly heated[691]. The most vulnerable to oxidation are fish and seed oils, whereas the least vulnerable are butter, lard, coconut oil and olive oil. Canned seafood like tuna, sardines, anchovies should be limited because they get exposed to high heat during the canning process.

- **Excess Iron Intake** – Iron in the presence of polyunsaturated fats can cause lipid peroxidation through production of reactive oxygen species[692]. Having high iron levels increases the susceptibility for lipids to become oxidized because of this interaction. Excess iron promotes oxidative stress and is linked to arthritis, cancer, diabetes, heart failure and liver damage[693,694,695]. One of the biggest reasons for iron overload is not consuming enough copper (found in liver, oysters and shellfish). Additionally, most cereals and grains are fortified with iron.

- **Carotenoids** from colorful vegetables like carrots, turnips, yams and beetroot as well as pastured animal fats can inhibit lipid peroxidation[696,697]. In PUFA-enriched membranes, however, certain carotenoids (lycopene and beta-carotene) given separately may increase lipid hydroperoxides[698]. Astaxanthin has the opposite effect and reduces lipid peroxidation because it can counteract PUFA oxidation but certain isolated carotenoids may make things worse (think isolated beta-carotene supplements increasing lung cancer in cigarette smokers). You find astaxanthin from algae, wild salmon and pink/red seafood.

- **Spirulina** – Spirulina decreases serum malondialdehyde (MDA), which is a marker of lipid peroxidation[699]. When rats are given oxidized vegetable oils their health deteriorates but spirulina can alleviate those harmful effects thanks to its antioxidant properties and inhibition of lipid peroxidation[700]. Consuming 2-3 grams of spirulina or chlorella with your meals may protect against the harm of oxidized fats.

- **Crushed Garlic** – Garlic's main bioactive compound is called allicin that gets activated once you crush the garlic. In one study, swallowing whole garlic had no effects on lipid levels but crushed garlic did lower cholesterol, triglycerides, blood pressure and serum malondialdehyde (MDA), which is a marker of oxidized polyunsaturated fat[701].

- **Turmeric** – Curcumin in turmeric can reduce lipid peroxidation by promoting antioxidant enzymes such as superoxide dismutase (SOD) and catalase[702]. These antioxidant enzymes reduce reactive oxygen species and repair DNA damage that occurs due to lipid peroxidation[703]. Turmeric also chelates iron, making it a good supplement or spice to absorb less iron if needed.

- **Coffee, Cacao, Olive Oil, Red Wine, Tea, Spices & Avocado** reduce lipid peroxidation in cooked animal foods[704,705,706,707,708,709,710,711]. Polyphenols in general have a protective effect on lipid peroxidation. In type 2 diabetics, pomegranate polyphenols lower lipid peroxidation but not in healthy adults[712]. Drinking either 4 cups of green tea a day or taking a green tea extract for 8 weeks has been shown to significantly lower blood lipids and lipid peroxidation in subjects with metabolic syndrome[713]. Both caffeine and coffee inhibit lipid peroxidation and decrease the absorption of lipoxidation products[714,715]. However, note that green tea, black tea, and coffee can inhibit thiamine absorption.

- **Glycine (and possibly glutamine)** – Glycine can protect against the damage from oxidized seed oils and reduces lipid peroxidation caused by alcohol[716,717]. Supplementing glycine propionyl-L-carnitine with aerobic exercise lowers lipid peroxidation in subjects with normal lipid levels[718]. Glycine can be useful for inflammatory conditions as it can boost glutathione and antioxidant defenses[719,720,721].

They say a best defense is a good offence, but in the context of lipid peroxidation the best defense is avoidance. Nevertheless, you can't avoid lipid peroxidation completely. Either due to exercising too hard or just going out to dinner at a restaurant. You shouldn't be stressed out about this if it's only an occasional occurrence. The best defense against lipid peroxidation is having your body's own antioxidant defense systems working properly.

How to Balance Omega-3 and Omega-6 Fats

To keep your inflammation levels in check, you should be consuming a balanced omega-6 to omega-3 ratio. A high omega-6 intake in relation to omega-3s promotes chronic low-grade inflammation and creates excessive inflammatory responses[722]. Throughout human history, humans have been consuming an omega-6 and omega-3 fatty acid ratio of around 1:1 to 4:1[723]. After the industrial revolution in the 1800s, omega-6 consumption started to increase slowly[724]. Today, the average Westerner consumes an omega-6/3 ratio of 20:1 and even up to 50:1, favoring omega-6s[725,726,727]. That's a 30-fold increase in omega-6 intake compared to the early 1900s[728]. Up to 20% of all calories in the American diet come from soybean oil alone – with up to 9% of all the daily calories coming from linoleic acid[729].

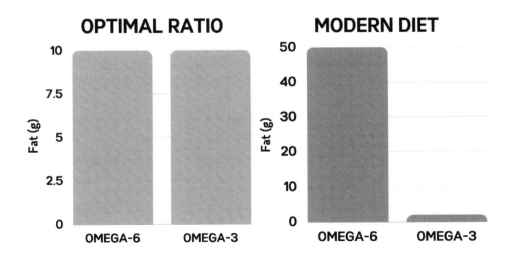

Meta-analyses up until 2020 did not find that increasing omega-3 fat intake prevents or treats Type 2 diabetes[730,731]. However, a 2020 meta-analysis of 26 randomized controlled trials concluded that omega-3 PUFAs might improve insulin sensitivity and lipid metabolism in people with already existing Type 2 diabetes[732]. The the anti-inflammatory properties of omega-3 fatty acids, especially DHA and EPA, might have a positive effect on some aspects of glucose intolerance and insulin resistance[733,734,735,736,737]. In Type 2 diabetics, supplemental curcumin and omega-3s both improve insulin sensitivity and lower triglycerides but combining them together didn't show any complimentary benefits[738]. Giving omega-3s, vitamin E and alpha-lipoic acid (ALA) to Type 2 diabetics significantly reduces their A1c[739]. In mice, omega-3s can also inhibit inflammation and insulin resistance of the adipose tissue[740]. In middle-aged overweight men, a higher omega-3 index is associated with greater insulin sensitivity and better metabolic health[741]. Supplemental omega-3s might help to alleviate gestational insulin resistance during pregnancy[742].

Whatever the case may be, getting more omega-3s as your fat intake still are one of the most researched ways to improve cardiovascular disease outcomes[743,744]. Cardiovascular disease is one of the major endpoints and causes of mortality of diabetes. **Thus, the goal to improve your fatty acid balance is also to avoid poor glucose control and diabetic pathologies leading to cardiovascular disease.**

After the American Heart Association's recommendation to increase omega-6 vegetable oil intake, heart disease started climbing[745] and our fat stores are now saturated in linoleic acid.[746] We are also sicker as a population due to higher calorie consumption, less physical activity, and more sugar intake. **It is true that linoleic acid levels in the blood are associated with lower all-cause mortality and heart disease[747,748,749]. However, inflammation oxidizes linoleic acid, producing oxidized linoleic acid metabolites, which lowers the amount of** linoleic acid in the blood[750,751]. **Studies that adjust for this factor discover that low linoleic acid levels are not linked to increased risk of death[752].** In short, inflammation lowers linoleic acid in the blood, and it is the inflammation that promotes the increased mortality risk, not the low linoleic acid. Instead of increasing linoleic acid, it's better to reduce it and keep your omega-6 in balance with omega-3.

The optimal omega-6/3 ratio is around 1:1 to 4:1[753]. It's estimated that hunter-gatherers consumed half as much linoleic acid as humans today[754]. They also got linoleic acid from whole foods, where the fats haven't been oxidized, whereas virtually all the omega-6 fats people eat today have been oxidized. Simultaneously, **the average person today gets 10 times less ALA (1.5 grams today vs. 15 grams in Paleolithic times) and 143 times less EPA/DHA (100-200 mg today vs 660-14,250 mg in Paleolithic humans)[755].** During the Paleolithic era, humans obtained 10 times more ALA than we do today (15 grams versus 1.4 grams), which provides ~ 750 mg of EPA for men and 3.15 grams of EPA for women of child-bearing age[756,757,758]. That ALA they consumed from plants and nuts was generally 3 times higher in omega-3s than omega-6s[759]. Grain-finished cattle have a 2-fold higher omega-6/3 ratio compared to 100% grass-fed cattle[760]. Grain finished animals have over twice as much fat marbling as 100% grass-fed animals. Wild-game has 2-4 times more omega-3s than grain-finished animals, and 2-3 times more than 100% grass-fed animals[761].

Here is a table that compares the current AHA recommendations for fatty acids to evidence-based recommendations that we have outlined in this chapter:

Current AHA Recommendations	Evidence-based Recommendations
Consume at least 5–10% of total daily calories as omega-6.	You need only 0.5-2% of total calories as linoleic acid to support essential bodily functions. The upper limit for linoleic acid is 3% to prevent enzymatic competition with ALA and to avoid inflammation. In any case, linoleic acid should come from only whole food sources.[762]
Industrial vegetable oils and seed oils are considered heart healthy	Avoid industrial seed oils. Omega-6 should come from whole foods like nuts, seeds, fish, eggs, poultry, etc.
No advice given about the optimal omega-6/3 ratio	The ideal omega-6/3 ratio is 1:1 but 4:1 is also acceptable
500 mg EPA/DHA a day to prevent heart disease. Those who already have heart disease should consume 1000 mg EPA/DHA	Get about 2-4 grams of EPA/DHA a day for both primary and secondary prevention of heart disease. However, EPA/DHA consumption should be titrated to maintain an omega-3 index (EPA+DHA in red blood cells) of at least 8% or more[763]

Here's a list of the different oils and their fatty acid content:

FOOD	OMEGA-6 (g)	OMEGA-3 (g)	RATIO 6:3
FISH			
Salmon (4 oz/113 g)	0.2	2.3	1:12
Mackerel (4 oz/113 g)	0.2	2.2	1:11
Swordfish (4 oz/113 g)	0.3.	1.7	1:6
Sardines (4 oz/113 g)	4.0	1.8	2.2:1
Canned Tuna (4 oz/113 g)	3.0	0.2	15:1
Lobster (4 oz/113 g)	0.006	0.12	1:20
Cod (4 oz/113 g)	0.1	0.6	1:6
VEGETABLES			
Spinach (1 cup/110 g)	30.6	166	1:5.4
Kale (1 cup/110 g)	0.1.	0.1	1:1
Collards (1 cup/110 g)	133	177	1:1.3
Chard (1 cup/110 g)	43.7	5.3	8.2:1
Sauerkraut (1 cup/110 g)	37	36	1:1
Brussels Sprouts (1 cup/110 g)	123	270	1:1.3
NUTS AND SEEDS			

Walnuts (1 oz/28 g)	10.8	2.6	4.2:1
Flaxseeds (1 oz/28 g)	1.6	6.3	1:4
Pecans (1 oz/28 g)	5.7	0.3	21:1
Poppy Seeds (1 oz/28 g)	7.9	0.1	104:1
Pumpkin Seeds (1 oz/28 g)	2.5	0.1	114:1
Sesame Seeds (1 oz/28 g)	6	0.1	57:1
Almonds (1 oz/28 g)	3.3	0.002	1987:1
Cashews (1 oz/28 g)	2.1	0.017	125:1
Chia Seeds (1 oz/28 g)	1.6	4.9	1:3
Pistachios (1 oz/28 g)	3.7	0.071	52:1
Sunflower Seeds (1 oz/28 g)	6.5	0.021	312:1
Lentils (1 oz/28 g)	0.0384	0.0104	3.7:1
OILS AND FATS			
Butter (1 Tbsp)	0.18	0.83	1:1.5
Lard (1 Tbsp)	1.0	0.1	10:1
Cod Liver Oil (1 Tbsp)	2.8	1.3	2.2:1
Grain-Fed Tallow (1 Tbsp)	3.35	0.2	16.8:1

Grass-Fed Tallow (1 Tbsp)	1.2	0.8	1.5:1
Peanut Oil (1 Tbsp)	4.95	Trace	1:0.0
Soybean Oil (1 Tbsp)	7.0	0.9	7.8:1
Canola Oil (1 Tbsp)	2.8	1.3	2.2:1
Walnut Oil (1 Tbsp)	7.2	1.4	5.1:1
Sunflower Oil (1 Tbsp)	6	0.0	6:1
Margarine (1 Tbsp)	2.4	0.04	6:1
Peanut Butter (1 Tbsp)	1.4	0.008	17:1
Almond Butter (1 Tbsp)	1.2	0.04	2.8:1
Flaxseed Oil (1 Tbsp)	2.0	6.9	1:3.5
Olive Oil (1 Tbsp)	1.1	0.1	11:1
MEAT			
Ground Pork (6 oz/170 g)	2.83	0.119	23.8:1
Chicken	2.2	0.16	13.8:1
Grain-Fed Beef	0.73	0.08	9:1
Grass-Fed Beef	0.72	0.15	4.9:1
Domestic Lamb	1.9	0.6	3.3:1
Grass-Fed Lamb	1.7	2.2	0.7:1
Farmed Salmon	1.7	4.5	0.39:1

Wild Salmon	0.3	3.6	0.08:1

The Verdict on Fat and Insulin Resistance

Although fat doesn't raise insulin or blood sugar, in excess it can still contribute to the development of insulin resistance and diabetes. If the beta-cells get damaged due to lipotoxicity and hyperlipidemia, then a decrease in their function will follow[764]. Chronic exposure to free fatty acids also causes endoplasmic reticulum (ER) stress, mitochondrial dysfunction and dysfunctional autophagy[765]. The result and cause of this is a dysfunctional Randle Cycle that promotes hyperglycemia, hyperinsulinemia and hypertriglyceridemia. To prevent this, you need to avoid a state of 'energy toxicity' for lack of a better word. Basically, to increase the body's energy demands, whether through physical activity or reducing calorie intake, that would burn through all these fuels.

Excess saturated fat lipotoxicity could be as harmful as excess omega-6 fat lipotoxicity on the pancreatic beta-cells. Palmitate appears to be the most toxic to the beta-cells[766]. You get palmitate or palmitic acid from both animal and plant fats – meat, cheese, nuts, peanut butter, fish, milk, palm oil, etc. In reality, this only matters in the context of an energy surplus by which the lipotoxicity and hypertriglyceremia can develop in the first place. Importantly, it's the carbohydrate intake that primarily determines the saturated fat (palmitic and palmitoleic acid levels) in the blood[767]. When we consume more carbs the saturated fat levels in the body increase. During energy balance and calorie maintenance, lipotoxicity cannot develop as the body is not in a state of excess fuel.

Excess calorie intake in the form of fat consumption, even during a low carb intake, could also contribute to some aspects of insulin resistance because of this.

The chronic exposure to free fatty acids over time will wear out the pancreatic beta cells and as a result insulin production decreases. We do know that insulin sensitivity and glucose tolerance return to normal after re-introducing carbs after a period of ketosis. So, it's possible to reboot insulin production by changing one's diet. Thus, for optimal insulin sensitivity and glucose tolerance, it's not recommended to stay on a very low carb ketogenic diet indefinitely. Granted, if you're not going to eat carbohydrates then it wouldn't really matter for your glucose levels if you stayed in ketosis even if you were to be physiologically insulin resistant. It's just that if you're planning to eat carbohydrates, at least occasionally, like the vast majority of people would do, then it's better to do ketosis cyclically.

What about someone who already has diabetes, insulin resistance and hyperglycemia? Should they also be eating carbohydrates? Low carb and ketogenic diets can be effective in treating patients with Type 1 diabetes, Type 2 diabetes and obesity[768,769]. **Adhering to a low carb diet for 6 months has even been shown to lead to disease remission in Type 2 diabetics without adverse side effects**[770,771]. So, we believe that going low carb for some time will definitely be useful for a lot of people. However, a plant-based, low fat, high carb diet has also been found to improve diabetes and ameliorate insulin resistance[772]. In fact, vegetarian diets are inversely associated with the risk of developing diabetes[773]. Unfortunately, the long term consequences of not eating meat outweigh any short term benefits found with vegetarian diets. Typically, if one goes on a vegetarian diet for long enough, body composition worsens (increased fat and decreased skeletal muscle), mood worsens and numerous nutrient deficiencies are likely to occur (lack of carnitine, carnosine, creatine, B12 and protein).

The key to preventing insulin resistance is not interfering with the Randle Cycle – if you're eating low carb you're primarly burning triglycerides but when you're eating low fat, high carb you're primarly burning glucose. Because there's no excess supply of both fats and glucose, insulin resistance doesn't develop. The average person's diet, however, is high in both fats and carbs, which is why over time they develop insulin resistance – i.e., disrupted Randel Cycle causing hyperlipidemia and insulin resistance. If you do choose to improve your glucose tolerance with a low carb diet, then it's highly recommended to reintroduce some carbohydrates back in. At least during certain parts of the day, such as after exercise. The frequency of when and how to do this we will be discussing in the following chapters.

Chapter 5: How Nutrient Deficiencies Promote Glucose Intolerance and Insulin Resistance

Insulin resistance and diabetes are partly caused by an oversupply of energy that desensitizes the body to insulin. Hyperglycemia is a state of excess glucose in the bloodstream. When you look at the trend of calorie consumption by the average person, you can see that it's been gradually increasing over the past century and it's estimated to keep doing so[774,775]. Unfortunately, those calories are generally not very nutritious. In the modern industrialized society, it's hard to find someone who is malnourished of calories and macronutrients – protein, carbs, and fats. However, most of the population is deficient in micronutrients, especially minerals[776]. For example, at least 30-50% of the adult population is getting suboptimal intakes of copper and magnesium[777,778].

Your body needs micronutrients for a wide range of essential functions, such as energy production, neurotransmitter synthesis and insulin production[779,780,781,782,783,784,785,786,787,788,789,790]. Deficiencies in certain minerals, such as magnesium or potassium, can promote the development of cardiovascular disease and diabetes[791,792,793,794,795,796]. Ultra-processed foods lack micronutrients, but they also require vitamins and minerals to liberate calories from them[797] and they also make your body lose micronutrients via stool and urine[798,799]. The elevated insulin levels caused by overeating these foods also makes you lose calcium and magnesium out the urine and decreases the entry of magnesium and potassium into the cell[800].

In this chapter, we're going to be talking about the role of micronutrients for optimal glucose control and insulin sensitivity. We'll also cover the role of food processing on nutrient deficiencies and cravings.

Magnesium and Insulin's Actions

Insulin gets a bad reputation when it comes to weight loss and diabetes. However, as we've already shown, diabetes is partly caused by inadequate insulin production. Type 1 diabetics suffer primarily from not being able to produce insulin. **Insulin is a peptide hormone that is essential for optimal glucose metabolism and blood sugar balance**. You need it to clear excess glucose from the bloodstream, no matter where that glucose is coming from, whether from dietary carbohydrates or the glycogen you break down in skeletal muscle. Impaired insulin production, and especially impaired insulin signaling, is implicated in Type 2 diabetes and Alzheimer's disease pathology[801,802,803].

Magnesium is one of the most important minerals for insulin's action and glucose utilization[804,805]. However, you also need insulin for magnesium uptake into the cells. Magnesium controls GLUT4 translocation to the cell surface[806], which are the receptors that take up glucose upon insulin signaling. Low magnesium levels are associated with hypertension, Type 2 diabetes, insulin resistance and cardiovascular disease[807,808,809,810,811,812]. Higher magnesium intake is associated with a reduced risk of diabetes[813]. **Type 2 diabetics have lower intracellular magnesium** and there is an inverse relationship between plasma magnesium and insulin resistance in these individuals[814]. Being deficient in magnesium also raises triglycerides and lipids, contributing to lipotoxicity-induced insulin resistance[815,816].

Magnesium is needed for insulin's actions & glucose utilization

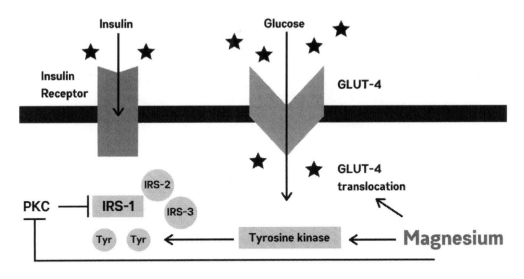

Adapted From: Takaya et al (2004) 'Intracellular magnesium and insulin resistance', Magnesium Research. 2004;17(2):126-135.

The recommended daily allowance (RDA) for magnesium in adults is around 350-420 mg per day, which up to 50% of the population does not meet[817]. The risk of Type 2 diabetes is 23% lower when getting 360-770 mg/day of magnesium compared to 150-260 mg/day[818]. A meta-analysis among 286,668 subjects and 10,912 cases of diabetes with a 6-17-year follow-up saw that **a 100 mg/day increase in magnesium intake was linked to a 15% lower risk of diabetes**[819]. Adding an extra 100 mg of dietary magnesium a day has been associated with an 8% reduced risk of ischemic stroke among 241,378 subjects[820]. Magnesium intake is inversely associated with coronary artery calcification with the risk being lowest at 450 mg/day of magnesium[821]. There are studies indicating that 180-320 mg/d of magnesium is enough to maintain a positive magnesium balance, but 107 mg/day is apparently not enough[822,823,824,825].

For someone who already has diabetes or insulin resistance, the 350-420 mg/d of magnesium may not be enough as their high insulin levels and cellular insulin resistance promote magnesium excretion[826,827,828,829]. In type-2 diabetes patients, 75% and 30.8% show magnesium depletion as reflected by serum and intracellular magnesium status, respectively[830]. It may be that individuals with magnesium deficiency, especially when combined with insulin resistance and hypertension, may need anywhere from 450 to 1,800 mg per day or more[831].

Here are the top 10 highest magnesium foods[832](keep in mind that plant sources of magnesium have a bioavailability of around 25-35%, whereas animal foods have a bioavailability of around 25-75%)[833,834,835]

Food	Mg of Magnesium per Serving	% of RDA
Pumpkin Seeds, 1 oz	156 mg	37%
Chia Seeds, 1 oz	111 mg	26%
Almonds, 1 oz	80 mg	19%
Spinach, ½ cup	78 mg	19%
Cashews, 1 oz	74 mg	18%
Lentils, 1 cup	71 mg	18%
Peanuts, ¼ cup	63 mg	15%
Soymilk, 1 cup	61 mg	15%
Black Beans, ½ cup	60 mg	14%
Edamame, ½ cup	50 mg	12%
Peanut Butter, 2 tbsp	49 mg	12%

Potato, 3.5 oz	43 mg	10%
Brown Rice, ½ cup	42 mg	10%
Yogurt, low fat, 8 oz	42 mg	10%
Fortified Cereal, 1 serving	42 mg	10%
Oatmeal, instant, 1 packet	36 mg	9%
Kidney Beans, canned, ½ cup	35 mg	8%
Banana, 1 medium	32 mg	8%
Mussels, 3 oz	31 mg	8%
Sardines, 3 oz	29 mg	7%

To know whether you need more magnesium than the RDA, you must look at several measures of magnesium status, including more optimal levels of blood magnesium, mononuclear blood cell magnesium, urinary magnesium levels as well as assess your symptoms of magnesium deficiency. **Normal blood magnesium is considered 0.7-1.0 mmol/L, but optimal levels are >0.80 mmol/L[836]. Chronic subclinical magnesium deficiency is a serum magnesium between 0.75 and 0.849 mmol/L[837].** If your serum magnesium is below 0.82 mmol/L (2.0 mg/dL) and your 24-hour urinary magnesium excretion is 40–80mg/d, that is indicative of magnesium deficiency[838]. Healthy magnesium-sufficient subjects retain only about 2-8% of intravenous magnesium[839,840]. If you retain over 10%, that's a sign of a magnesium insufficiency, and if you retain greater than 20-28% that suggests some degree of magnesium deficiency[841].

Elderly people on average retain 28% of an IV magnesium load, which suggests that older individuals tend to suffer from marginal magnesium deficiency[842].

Here are the signs and symptoms of possible magnesium deficiency[843]

- Hypokalemia and hypocalcemia[844]
- Tremors and fascilations[845]
- Arrhythmias[846]
- Migraine headaches[847].
- Spontaneous spasms and muscle cramps[848]
- Seizures[849]
- Twitching of the facial muscles upon touch
- Aggression and irritability[850]
- Pain or hyperalgesia[851]
- Photosensitivity[852]
- Tinnitus (ringing in the ears)[853]
- Hearing loss[854]
- Parathyroid resistance and impaired function[855]
- Cataracts[856]
- Coronary artery disease
- Cardiovascular disease
- Hypertension
- Weakened immune response[857,858]
- Depression[859]

There are many different forms of magnesium supplements with slightly different effects[860]. For example, magnesium threonate is the most effective at increasing brain magnesium levels[861], whereas magnesium malate improves energy and fatigue[862,863]. For insulin resistance and Type 2 diabetes, magnesium chloride has good evidence[864]. However, magnesium taurate, magnesium citrate, magnesium gluconate, magnesium orotate and magnesium arginate have all been found to improve cardiovascular function or arterial health.[865,866,867,868,869]. Thus, all types of magnesium would be of benefit to someone with magnesium deficiency just by virtue of raising their magnesium status. When supplementing magnesium, it's better to take smaller doses more frequently instead of large doses all at once because of improved absorption and less risk of diarrhea[870].

Chromium – The Secret Insulin Amplifier

In 1959, scientists discovered a protein in Brewer's yeast that they named 'glucose tolerance factor' (GTF)[871]. It was later recognized to be trivalent chromium (chromium 3+) that contains glycine, glutamic acid, cysteine, and nicotinic acid[872]. Trivalent chromium has been found to alleviate glucose intolerance caused by high sucrose consumption in rats[873]. In human diabetics, chromium-enriched yeast has been shown to reduce fasting blood glucose and insulin levels[874,875,876]. Chromium deficiency in animals leads to diabetic glucose levels and stunted growth[877,878]. Chronic maternal chromium restriction in animals promotes visceral adiposity and hyperlipidemia[879].

Chromium is an essential mineral needed for insulin production, glucose, and lipid metabolism[880]. You need chromium for insulin to bind to the cell surface and exert its effects[881]. However, to lower blood sugar through the glucose tolerance factor, chromium must work synergistically with nicotinic acid[882]. In the 1970s, chromium deficiency was associated with impaired glucose tolerance, elevated triglycerides, and neuropathy in patients with normal insulin levels on long-term total intravenous nutrition[883,884]. Getting intravenous (IV) nutrition without chromium can cause chromium deficiency and glucose regulation issues[885]. Giving IV nutrition patients just 150-250 mcg of chromium improves their glucose intolerance, neuropathy, and hyperglycemia[886,887]. That's why high dose chromium is often given to patients on total IV nutrition[888].

GLUCOSE TOLERANCE FACTOR (GTF)

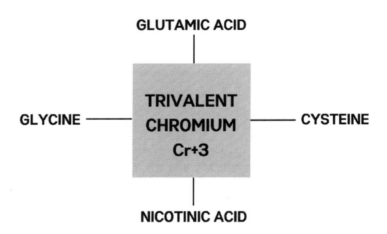

The exact way chromium improves glucose regulation is complex. Currently, it's thought that **chromium binds to a peptide to form chromodulin, which activates the insulin receptor to help with insulin's actions**[889]. Chromodulin or low-molecular-weight chromium-binding substance (LMWCr) transports chromium around the body and stimulates insulin-dependent tyrosine kinase activity, which activates the insulin receptor[890,891,892]. Thus, chromodulin amplifies insulin signaling. In vitro, chromium has been shown to increase glycolytic flux, a decrease in which contributes to glucose intolerance, metabolic inflexibility and accumulation of lactic acid[893]. A deficiency in chromium will thus decrease insulin's response on the cell and promote insulin resistance[894].

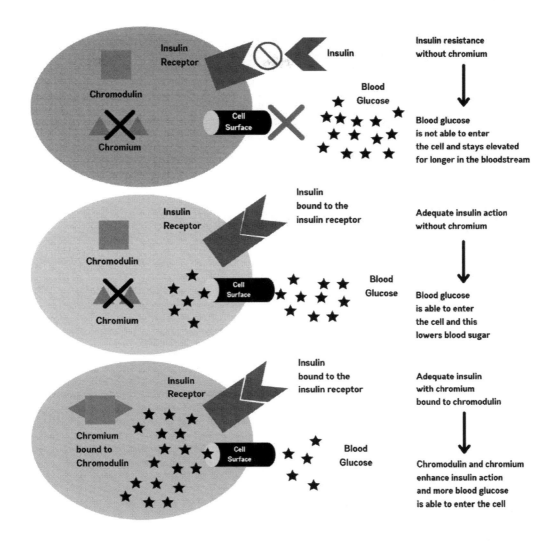

Adapted From: Phung et al (2010)[895]

The chromium found in foods and supplements is trivalent chromium (Cr 3+) but you can also find it as hexavalent chromium (Cr 6+) in the toxic by-products of steel manufacturing[896]. Inhaling hexavalent chromium is carcinogenic and mutagenic[897]. Ingestion of hexavalent chromium has also been associated with stomach tumors and allergenic dermatitis[898]. The movie Erin Brockovich is based on hexavalent chromium contamination in the water supply of a town called Hinkley in Southern California.

Chromium is deemed an essential nutrient in the U.S., India, and several other countries due to its insulin-sensitizing/modulating effects[899]. However, the European Food Safety Authority has not categorized chromium as essential[900]. **The adequate intake (AI) of chromium in the United States is set at 25-35 mcg/d for adults**[901]. In 1969, it was thought humans needed only 1 mcg/day of chromium but consuming 1 mcg/d of chromium from dietary sources would result in significantly less chromium reaching the body because **the absorption of dietary chromium is only 0.4-2.5%**[902] **and absorption of supplemental chromium chloride is 1-3%**[903]. **To meet the 1 mcg/day guidance you would have to ingest 33-100 mcg of chromium and to meet the 25-35 mcg/day AI you would need to consume up to 1000 mcg/day.** In 1980, chromium's Estimated Safe and Adequate Daily Dietary Intake (ESADDI) was lifted to 50-200 mcg/d for adults[904]. The World Health Organization claims about 33 mcg/d of chromium is enough to satisfy normal requirements[905]. In the U.S., chromium's daily value has been labeled to be 35 mcg[906].

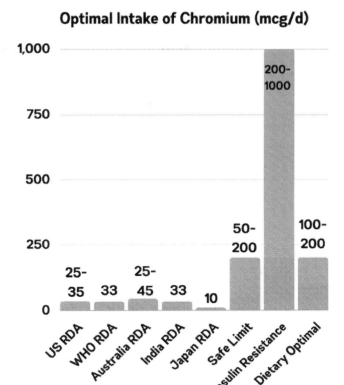

Optimal Intake of Chromium (mcg/d)

Picture Taken From: DiNicolantonio and Land (2021) 'The Mineral Fix'

The FDA has suggested that chromium picolinate supplementation may lower the risk of insulin resistance and Type 2 diabetes[907]. However, these claims are not definitive. The FDA does reject the idea that chromium could alleviate cardiovascular disease, retinopathy or kidney disease caused by high blood sugar levels[908]. The American Diabetes Association doesn't recommend supplementing chromium because of the uncertainties[909,910]. In 2010, the European Food Safety Authority (EFSA) accepted claims that chromium could help with normal blood sugar levels[911].

A 2021 study found that **chromium picolinate supplementation at a dose of 400 mcg/day for 3 months improved glycemic control, insulin resistance, triglycerides, inflammation, and insulin levels** in patients with non-alcoholic fatty liver disease[912]. Taking 600 mcg/day of chromium for 4 months improves glycemic regulation of Type 2 diabetics without affecting lipids[913]. A larger dose of 1,000 mcg/d compared to 100 mcg/d in Type 2 diabetics lowers fasting blood glucose significantly more (128 mg/dl vs 159 mg/dl, respectively)[914]. Those getting the 1,000 mcg/d dose also had a lower response to an oral glucose challenge and a lower A1c. However, **chromium supplements don't appear to improve insulin sensitivity in healthy non-obese individuals**[915,916,917]. That makes sense because these people already have well-functioning insulin production and sensitivity. Nevertheless, there's evidence to show that chromium supplementation can be beneficial in cases of poor glucose tolerance and insulin resistance.

One 2007 review paper by Balk et al claimed brewer's yeast could be the best supplemental sources of chromium:

> *Among participants with type 2 diabetes, the effects of brewer's yeast, chromium chloride, and chromium picolinate on fasting glucose were each significantly different from each other (P < 0.02), such that **studies of brewer's yeast had the greatest net effect** (−1.1 mmol/l), followed by chromium picolinate (−0.8 mmol/l) and chromium chloride (−0.3 mmol/l). Similarly, among studies of participants with normal glucose tolerance, **brewer's yeast was significantly more likely to reduce fasting glucose than chromium chloride** (−0.2 vs. +0.1 mmol/l, P = 0.01) **and to raise HDL cholesterol than chromium picolinate** (+0.21 vs. −0.02, P = 0.002).* [918]

Thanks to its effects on insulin and glucose regulation, chromium might help with polycystic ovary syndrome (PCOS), which is typically characterized by insulin resistance and dyslipidemia[919,920,921]. Giving PCOS patients chromium improves their HOMA-IR scores, which is a marker of insulin resistance[922].

Supplementing 200-1,000 mcg/d of chromium for 8-24 weeks lowers fasting glucose and bodyweight in PCOS patients but it has no significant effect on fasting glucose[923]. In a study on 84 Canadian postmenopausal women, 60% don't meet the adequate intake of chromium[924].

Chromium might assist in weight loss and muscle growth[925,926,927], but the evidence isn't clear[928]. In a 2019 meta-analysis, doses of 200-1,000 mcg/d of chromium for 9-24 weeks in 1,316 obese subjects reduced their weight by 0.75 kg compared to placebo[929]. Dietary supplements don't usually cause a weight loss any greater than 2 kgs and they only work in combination with a calorie restricted diet[930]. However, chromium can reduce appetite and hunger[931], which are the most important determinants of a sustainable diet. A study on 154 healthy and physically active individuals saw that 72 days of supplementing 200 or 400 mcg of chromium improved their body composition compared to placebo[932]. There are other studies that don't find a similar effect, which might mean that the people who do see an effect are depleted of chromium[933,934]. Indeed, you can lose a lot of chromium through urine and sweat, which athletes are especially susceptible to.

You can get chromium from many foods, starting with vegetables and ending with meat. Most foods have on average 1-13 mcg of chromium per serving[935]. However, not all of them have glucose tolerance factor (GTF), which is the more bioactive form of chromium. Foods with the most GTF are brewer's yeast, black pepper, liver, cheese, bread, and beef, whereas the lowest ones are skim milk, chicken breast, flour, and haddock[936]. Supplemental brewer's yeast of 9 grams/d (providing just 10.8 mcg of chromium) for 8 weeks improves impaired glucose tolerance, reduces serum cholesterol, and lowers the insulin response to a glucose load[937]. Different polyphenolic herbs and spices like cinnamon and rosemary improve insulin sensitivity with chromium[938].

Here are the top 20 foods that contain chromium[939,940,941,942]

Food	Mcg of Chromium per Serving	% of AI
Mussels, 3 oz	120 mcg	390%
Oysters, 3 oz	52 mcg	120%
Lobster, 3 oz	29 mcg	71%
Shrimp, 3 oz	24 mcg	67%
Broccoli, 1 cup	22 mcg	65%
Barley, ½ cup	12 mcg	36%
Turkey Ham, 3 oz	10.4 mcg	30%
Oats, ½ cup	10 mcg	30%
Grape Juice, 1 cup	7.5 mcg	21%
Waffles, 1 (75 g)	6.7 mcg	18%
Ham, 3 oz	3.6 mcg	10%
Muffin, whole wheat	3.6 mcg	10%
Chocolate Chip Cookies (4)	3.4 mcg	9%
Brewer's Yeast, 1 tbsp	3.3 mcg	9%
Potatoes, 1 cup	3.0 mcg	9%
Orange Juice, 1 cup	2.2 mcg	6%

Beef, 3 oz	2.0 mcg	6%
Lettuce, 5 oz	1.8 mcg	5%
Turkey Breast, 3 oz	1.7 mcg	5%
Barbeque Sauce, 1 tbsp	1.7 mcg	5%

Thiamine Deficiency and Insulin Resistance

The Emergence of Beri-Beri with the invention of the steel roller mill:

"With the advent of mechanical rice milling in the late 19th century, which removed the main dietary source of thiamin in rice husk, beriberi became a major public health problem in Asia, responsible for considerable mortality."[943]

Thiamine deficiency was widespread in Japan in the early 1900s and caused beriberi heart disease, which had a peak mortality reaching 26,797 in 1923[944]. This was due to the limited diet which mainly consisted of polished rice lacking in thiamine. A similar story played out in the United States and the UK. The roller mill was invented by Helfenberger around 1830 and the first roller mills were constructed in America in Connecticut around 1874[945]. Compared to stone ground wheat, modern milling caused an 11-fold reduction in the vitamin B1 content, going from 4.95 mcg/gram to 0.45 mcg/gram. Wheat flour provided around 25% or more of the total calories consumed by Americans in the early 1900s. Thus, there was a tremendous reduction in vitamin B1 intake with the increased intake of milled wheat. The preference for milled wheat over stone ground wheat was similar to what occurred in Asia with polished rice.

In the United States, from 1821 to 1931, the intake of refined sugar went from 9.9 grams/day to 134.2 g/day. Thus, wheat and sugar, which contained little to no thiamine, made up approximately 50% of the total caloric intake of Americans in the early 1930s. Jolliffe noted that 55% of the fraction of calories in the American diet of 1840 came from whole wheat, which provided a minimum of 1.8 mg of thiamine, but this was replaced with milled wheat in the late 1800s and early 1900s, which provided < $1/10^{th}$ of that amount, or just 0.150 mg[946].

In one review paper by George Cowgill, he concluded:

> *"There are grounds for believing that American dietaries as a whole are unsatisfactory with respect to the content of vitamin B1. The examination of available food statistics as well as of recently collected American dietaries, the observations of clinicians concerning the high therapeutic value of vitamin B...and the observations of the value of added vitamin B1 to the dietaries of many children all support this belief. It is believed that prosecution of a program fostering addition of vitamin B1 to staple American foods according to the principles discussed in the present report would be definitely in the interests of the public."*[947]

The writings of Dr. HM Sinclair in the Proceedings of the Royal Society of Medicine noted that an increased consumption of empty calories, particularly from alcohol and refined carbohydrates, dramatically increased the need for thiamine[948].

He wrote,

"... an unbalanced diet that is high in calories and low in vitamin B1 will produce symptoms of deficiency. Cases of "alcoholic" polyneuritis afford excellent examples, because they take a diet high in calories (most of the energy being supplied by alcohol) and low in vitamin B1 (since no form of spirits contains the vitamin). This disease, which afflicts spirit-drinkers in America but not beer-drinkers in England, has been proved to be due to deficiency of the vitamin..." [949]

The paper goes on to state:

"A number of factors increase the requirement of the vitamin. Since it is necessary both for the oxidation of carbohydrate and for its conversion to fat, the requirement will be proportional to the quantity of carbohydrate ingested. Three cases have been recorded of beri-beri following the ingestion of abnormally large amounts of carbohydrate." [950]

Two long-term (88-147 days) thiamine deficiency studies

One group of authors, Ray D. Williams, MD and colleagues from the Mayo Foundation and Rochester State Hospital performed two studies, one from April 4, 1939, until August 30 (147 days)[951] and a second thiamine restriction study that began on Dec 12, 1939 and continued until March 9, 1940 (88 days).[952]

In the first study, four young healthy women (21-29 years old) were placed on a thiamine deficient diet (< 0.1 mg per day).[953] The diet consisted of polished rice, sugar, tapioca, white bread, cornstarch, white raisins, egg whites, cottage cheese, American creamed cheese, butter, black tea, and cocoa. The total content of protein in the diet was limited but much greater than the minimal requirement. The content of carbohydrates was at no time less than 188 grams. The curves of blood sugar provided evidence of **slight but progressive impairment of tolerance for carbohydrate by all four patients**."[954] "*The deficient intake of thiamin was interrupted by the subcutaneous injection of thiamin chloride. One milligram of thiamine chloride was given on August 31, 1939, and subsequently every third day until four doses had been given. One patient (case 1) after the sixth day was given 30 mg thiamin chloride daily in order to determine the effect of large doses on electrocardiographic recovery. Nearly the maximal recovery had already occurred in response to the 2 mg of thiamin chloride.*"[955] The authors went on to note, "***The time curves of blood sugar lost all semblance of diabetic reaction and all other abnormalities incident to the period of deficiency disappeared within the twelve days in which each patient received 4 mg of thiamin chloride parenterally***."[956] The authors also noted, "*Many workers in the vitamin field have stressed the probability that a fairly large portion of the population is continually on the verge of a state of vitamin B1 deficiency and it has often been suggested that perhaps many obscure complaints arise from a chronic, mild deficiency.*"[957]

A few important key take-aways from the study include, 1.) symptoms of thiamine deficiency are vague (lack of appetite and fatigue), 2.) electrocardiogram changes can occur with thiamine deficiency, particularly diminished or inverted T waves in the apex leads, 3.) **thiamine deficiency leads to impaired carbohydrate tolerance**, 4.) **thiamine supplementation improves glucose tolerance in those who are deficient**. A key take-away from this study is that simply being deficient in vitamin B1 can lead to carbohydrate intolerance and blood glucose curves resembling a diabetic reaction. In other words, **thiamine deficiency can cause prediabetes and Type 2 diabetes.** What's mind blowing is that we've known about this since 1939, and yet most clinicians and certainly the general public have no idea.

The following is an account of the second study by Williams and colleagues performed on six healthy white women aged 21 to 46. The woman were *"...chosen on the basis of their absence of physical defects, absence of any history of abnormal nutrition and quiescence of associated mental illness. These women were active physically and were engaged in hospital housework. The group included asthenic and sthenic, hyperkinetic and sedentary, thin and well-nourished women."*[958] During thiamine deprivation the urinary thiamine excretion *"fell rapidly to remarkably low values."*[959] On a low thiamine intake (0.15 mg/day or less) **3 of the 4 subjects who received the diet low in thiamine for prolonged periods, blood sugar time curves became diabetic in type**...and lactic acid in the blood were elevated irregularly before, but particularly after, exercise...In all cases **gastric acidity**, as determined by a test meal of 100 cc. of 7 percent solution of alcohol, **was decreased, and gastrointestinal motility** as evidenced by roentgen examination after a barium meal **was impaired**.."[960]

Importantly, the authors noted that thiamine administration improved these symptoms in the following:

> *"The period of restricted intake of thiamine was terminated after eight-eight days (March 9, 1940) by giving a subcutaneous injection of 1 mg of thiamine hydrochloride. The diet low in vitamin B1 was continued until March 26. During the interval from March 9 to March 15 daily injections of small doses of thiamine hydrochloride were made, and the amount of thiamine contained in the urine was determined daily. During the eighteen days (March 9 to 26 inclusive) in which administration of thiamine hydrochloride represented the only change made, all signs and symptoms incident to the period of restriction of thiamine disappeared. The electrocardiograms became normal;* **the previously diabetic type of sugar tolerance curve was replaced by a normal curve**... "[961]

Thus, an important take away from the study was that **a thiamine deficient diet, in some instances in as little as 15 days, but especially after 2-3 months, induces prediabetes/diabetes on a dextrose tolerance test**. Numerous studies show that thiamine or thiamine related compounds (benfotiamine or thiamine tetrahydrofurfuryl disulfide) improve diabetic glucose control and diabetic symptoms[962,963,964,965,966,967,968,969,970,971].

In Type 2 diabetics:

- Thiamine at 150 mg/day significantly reduced blood glucose and leptin levels within one month in 24 drug naïve Type 2 diabetic patients.[972]
- Thiamine at 300 mg daily significantly improved microalbuminuria, A1C and decreased protein kinase C (PKC) levels (a marker of inflammation) in Type 2 diabetic patients.[973]
- Thiamine administered as a one-time 100 mg IV dose improved endothelium-dependent vasodilation in 10 Type 2 diabetics during an acute glucose tolerance test.[974]

The active form of thiamine is called thiamine diphosphate (also known as thiamine pyrophosphate), **which requires magnesium in order to form in the body**. Thiamine pyrophosphate acts as a coenzyme for three essential enzymes, transketolase, pyruvate dehydrogenase and alpha ketoglutarate dehydrogenase.[975] These three enzymes catalyze the initial steps in glucose oxidation. Therefore, thiamine (as well as magnesium) is so important for glucose control as it is required for metabolizing glucose.

Type 1 and Type 2 diabetes can lead to thiamine deficiency via a downregulation of thiamine absorption transporters in the proximal tubule of the kidney due to elevated glucose levels.[976] Essentially, an increase in thiamine loss can occur out the urine with elevated glucose levels. Numerous medications that are used to treat diabetes also increase thiamine need.

Medications that increase thiamine need[977,978,979,980,981,982]

- **Proton pump inhibitors** (decrease thiamine absorption and inhibits two thiamine dependent enzymes)
- Oral birth control (drop in erythrocyte transketolase activity)
- **Angiotensin Receptor Blockers**
  - Quinapril
- **Metformin**
- Metronidazole (formation of a thiamine antagonist interfering with thiamine metabolism)
- Trimethoprim (inhibits thiamine transporters, THTR-1 and THTR-2, which actively bring thiamine into the brain, liver, kidneys, placenta, muscle and small intestine)
- Phenytoin (increased metabolism)
- Digoxin (increased elimination out the urine)
- **Diuretics** (increased elimination out the urine)
- Chemotherapy (leads to the overutilization and destruction of thiamine)

Nutrient deficiencies can be a major determinant of mild insulin resistance in seemingly healthy non-diabetic individuals. If the person isn't overweight and their diet consists of mostly whole foods, then a very common cause for their **impaired glucose intolerance could be due to a lack of certain key nutrients, particularly thiamine, magnesium and/or chromium.** This is something that goes even deeper than insulin production or glucose regulation as there are minerals and nutrients involved with other parameters of metabolic health, namely the thyroid, which we'll cover next.

Chapter 6: Thyroid Function, Insulin Resistance and Weight Gain

Diabetes and obesity have one common cause out of many and that's an excess supply of energy. Whether it comes in the form of fats, sugars or carbs, an overabundance will eventually lead to impaired metabolic function and weight gain. A simple example of this are sumo wrestlers who have about a 20-year shorter life expectancy than the average Japanese person (60-65 vs 85)[983,984]. **Sumo wrestlers have a significantly higher mortality rate due to their high bodyweight**[985]. Although, sumo wrestlers are very strong and fit in many ways, their diet consisting of up to 10,000 calories a day still makes them metabolically unhealthy and shortens their lifespan[986]. However, the sumo wrestlers aren't eating an ultra-processed food diet with hamburgers and fries – they're eating a relatively clean diet of traditional whole foods with lots of fish, rice, vegetables, and soups. Thus, even on a whole food diet, a very large excess surplus of energy will still over time cause impaired metabolic function, insulin resistance and weight gain.

However, you don't have to be eating like a sumo wrestler to start packing on the pounds. In fact, most people are doing it at a much lower effort and calorie intake. The reason for that has to do with a lower energy expenditure and lower metabolic rate that once exceeded makes you gain weight. In this chapter, we're going to talk about everything related to metabolic rate and the link between thyroid health and weight gain, diabetes, and insulin resistance.

Thyroid Function and Insulin Resistance

One factor for developing insulin resistance and gaining weight that doesn't get talked about that much is low thyroid function or hypothyroidism. Your body regulates its energy balance by the thyroid gland located in your throat[987]. Thyroid hormones, thyroxine (T4) and triiodothyronine (T3), affect your body temperature, heart rate, and metabolic rate[988,989]. **Thyroid hormones promote glucose absorption in the gastrointestinal tract and can activate an enzyme called phosphoenolpyruvate carboxykinase (PEPCK), which enhance gluconeogenesis (the process of forming glucose in the body)**[990]. T3 is the more bioactive thyroid hormone that also regulates insulin sensitivity by mediating the actions of GLUT4 and increasing basal insulin-mediated glucose transportation[991,992]. Type 2 diabetics have significantly lower free T3 and a correlating higher A1c[993]. Thyroid hormones can also increase glucagon secretion by the alpha cells in the pancreas[994]. **Both Type 1 and Type 2 diabetes induce a state of low T3 characterized by low total and free T3, increased reverse T3 but almost normal T4 and TSH levels**[995]. This hypothyroidism reduces glucose-induced insulin secretion by the beta cells[996]. However, in hyperthyroidism, beta cells are more responsive to glucose or catecholamines which can lead to hyperinsulinemia as well as hyperglycemia[997,998]. In hyperthyroidism, the body is burning through and producing energy at a higher rate, which increases insulin demand and eventually leads to decreased insulin sensitivity[999,1000]. Hyperthyroid patients are also more susceptible to ketoacidosis from breaking down an excessive amount of fat[1001].

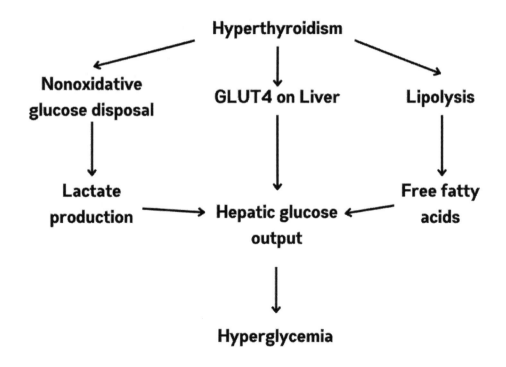

Adapted From: Wang (2013) 'The Relationship between Type 2 Diabetes
Mellitus and Related Thyroid Diseases', Journal of Diabetes Research.
Article ID 390534.

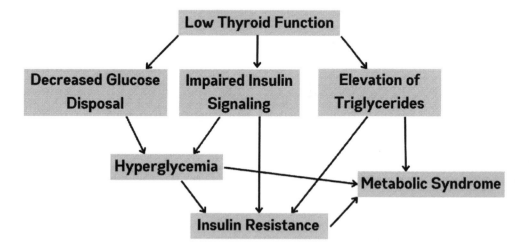

Low thyroid function or hypothyroidism increases the risk of gaining weight and obesity[1002,1003]. Thyroid hormones are needed for mobilizing adipose tissue lipids, which are used for fuel and heat production[1004]. **Thyroid disorders, both hypo- and hyperthyroidism, have been associated with insulin resistance as well[1005,1006,1007].** At the same time, insulin resistance can lead to both hypo- and hyperthyroidism[1008,1009,1010]. Because of insulin resistance, subclinical hypothyroidism impairs lipids and increases the risk of metabolic syndrome[1011,1012,1013]. Insulin resistance and hyperinsulinemia lead to the growth of thyroid tissue, which increases the risk of nodular thyroid disease and goiter[1014]. Women with pre-existing diabetes have been found to have up to a 1.38-fold increased risk of thyroid cancer[1015,1016]. Diabetes patients have a 20% increased risk of thyroid cancer[1017]. Hypothyroidism significantly raises cholesterol and triglycerides as well[1018,1019], which can contribute to lipotoxicity-induced insulin resistance. Most of thyroid disorders in diabetes patients is subclinical hypothyroidism[1020,1021]. Subclinical hypothyroidism increases the risk of diabetic neuropathy, retinopathy, peripheral arterial disease and peripheral neuropathy[1022,1023,1024].

Type 2 diabetes patients often have thyroid dysfunction[1025,1026,1027,1028]. In fact, aound 10-13% of diabetic patients have thyroid dysfunction[1029], the prevalence being 31.4% in type 2 diabetic women and 6.9% in type 2 diabetic men[1030]. **Type 1 diabetics also often have some form of autoimmune thyroid condition, such as Graves disease or Hashimoto's thyroiditis[1031].** Up to 50% of patients with Graves' disease have some degree of glucose intolerance[1032]. Graves' disease patients with Type 2 diabetes have more frequent and more severe Graves' orbitopathy also known as thyroid eye disease[1033]. A study on 50 women in a diabetic center found that 26% of them had subclinical hypothyroidism[1034]. Out of those 26%, 46% had insulin resistance. Women are 5-8x more likely to develop hypothyroidism and 8-10x more likely to develop hyperthyroidism than men[1035]. Women with gestational diabetes have a significantly higher prevalence of low T4 levels[1036], which promotes weight gain, poor lipids and worse insulin sensitivity[1037]. Children born to mothers with hypothyroidism or gestational diabetes can experience delayed neurodevelopment[1038,1039]. Hypothyroidism during pregnancy also increases the risk of diabetes later in life[1040,1041].

Hypothyroidism is diagnosed when T3 or T4 levels are low or when thyroid stimulating hormone (TSH) levels are elevated. Lower T4 levels, even with normal thyroid function, are associated with increased visceral fat and insulin resistance in humans[1042,1043,1044,1045,1046]. T3 improves glucose metabolism similar to insulin[1047,1048]. The role of TSH is to start producing thyroid hormones. If TSH and thyroid hormones are in a normal range, the thyroid is working normally. Even small increases in TSH have been linked to hypothyroidism and insulin resistance[1049,1050,1051]. Serum TSH is positively associated with weight gain and a higher BMI[1052,1053,1054,1055,1056,1057]. Rising BMI, however, is associated with lower serum free T4 levels[1058,1059,1060]. High TSH levels are implicated in raising triglycerides and cholesterol, as well as a higher risk of cardiovascular disease[1061,1062]. On the other hand, T3 increases the breakdown of fat and cholesterol[1063]. **Subclinical hypothyroidism is linked to an increased risk of coronary heart disease events and mortality, especially in those individuals with a TSH level of >10 mIU/L (normal range 0.5-5 mIU/L)**[1064]. Hashimoto's thyroiditis is diagnosed with a TSH between 5-10 mIU/L[1065]. The normal range for TSH is 0.45-4.5 mU/L and 95% of the disease-free population in the U.S. has a TSH of 0.45-4.12 mU/L[1066,1067].

Here are the normal ranges of TSH levels[1068]

Age Range	Low	Normal	High
0–4 days	<1 mU/L	1.6–24.3 mU/L	>30 mU/L
2–20 weeks	<0.5 mU/L	0.58–5.57 mU/L	>6.0 mU/L
20 weeks – 18 years	<0.5 mU/L	0.55–5.31 mU/L	>6.0 mU/L
18-30	<0.5 mU/L	0.5–4.1 mU/L	>4.1 mU/L
31–50 years	<0.5 mU/L	0.5–4.1 mU/L	>4.1 mU/L
51–70 years	<0.5 mU/L	0.5–4.5 mU/L	>4.5 mU/L
71–90 years	<0.4 mU/L	0.4–5.2 mU/L	>5.2 mU/L

Measuring your body temperature can also quickly describe your thyroid status. If you're cold all the time and you have a below normal body temperature, then it might suggest hypothyroidism because the body is trying to preserve energy for vital organ functions instead of heat production. The other symptoms of hypothyroidism include chronic fatigue, weight gain, brain fog, cold intolerance, low body temperature, joint pain, constipation, hair thinning, dry skin, puffy face, water retention, high LDL cholesterol, low resting heart rate and depression[1069,1070,1071,1072]. People without a thyroid are more susceptible to these symptoms.

Here are the risk factors for developing hypothyroidism[1073]:

- Pregnancy or lactation[1074]

- Iodine deficiency

- Excess iodine intake

- Rapidly transitioning from iodine deficiency to sufficiency[1075]

- Autoimmune conditions[1076]

- Genetic risk factors[1077,1078]

- Smoking

- Selenium deficiency[1079]

- Certain drugs and pharmaceuticals

- Infections[1080]

- Insulin resistance

Minerals for Thyroid Function

Thyroid hormones require certain minerals, especially iodine, selenium, sodium, zinc and magnesium[1081,1082,1083,1084,1085,1086]. Iodine being the most important one. Low iodine status is one of the biggest risk factors for hypothyroidism[1087]. Up to 50% of all the iodine in your body is located in the thyroid gland or thyroid hormones, whereas the remaining amount is concentrated in non-thyroid tissues[1088,1089]. Iodine makes up 65% of the molecular weight of T4 and 59% of T3.

Iodine's RDA for schoolchildren is 120 mcg and 150 mcg for adults[1090]**.** During pregnancy, the RDA rises to 220-250 mcg[1091]. According to the World Health Organization, 2 billion people worldwide aren't getting enough iodine[1092]. **There's a U-shaped connection between iodine intake and thyroid dysfunction[1093,1094]. Both high, as well as low iodine intake, can cause**

hypothyroidism or hyperthyroidism[1095,1096]. Excess iodine is a risk factor for thyroid autoimmune disease[1097,1098]. The safe upper limit of iodine is set at 1,100 mcg/day[1099]. However, intakes of ≥ 500 mcg/day for several weeks have been observed to increase the TSH response to thyrotropin-releasing hormone (TRH), which is a hormone that stimulates the release of TSH from the pituitary gland[1100]. Hypothyroid people react worse to doses ≥750 mcg/day of iodine[1101]. The maximal upper limit of 1,000 mcg of iodine a day has been deemed appropriate for everyone except those with thyroid issues or iodine sensitivity[1102]. Japanese people, however, consume 25x more than that without any apparent issues, which is likely due to their genetics[1103].

Seafood, especially seaweed, has the highest amount of iodine out of all foods. The average Japanese person consumes 1-3 mg of iodine a day from seaweed, fish and shellfish[1104,1105]. Food on a typical Western diet provides on average 3-80 mcg of iodine per 3-5 oz serving[1106,1107]. Dairy, eggs, yogurt, milk, and fish can be reliable sources of iodine on the Western diet[1108,1109]. Vegan options for iodine include iodized bread, iodized pasta, seaweeds, and potatoes[1110].

Here are the foods highest in iodine[1111,1112,1113]:

Food	Mcg of Iodine per Serving	% of RDA (150 mcg)
Seaweed, Nori, 1 oz	664 mcg	440%
Haddock, fish, 3 oz	200 mcg	134%
Whole-Wheat Bread, iodate dough, 1 slice	198 mcg	132%
Lobster, 3.5 oz	185 mcg	123%
White Bread, iodate dough, 1 slice	185 mcg	123%

Cod, cooked, 3 oz	156 mcg	106%
Iodized Table Salt, 1/2 tsp	142-152 mcg	102%
Crab, cooked, 3 oz	32.5-150 mcg	100%
Iodized Sea Salt, 1/2 tsp	148 mcg	98%
Greek Yogurt, 1 cup	116 mcg	77%
Oysters, 3 oz	93 mcg	62%
Milk, nonfat, 1 cup	85 mcg	57%
Fish Sticks, cooked, 3 oz	58 mcg	39%
Mollusks, clam, 3 oz	50 mcg	31%
Pollock, fish, 3 oz	38 mcg	26%
Milk Chocolate, 3 oz	36 mcg	25%
Salmon, fish, 3 oz	30 mcg	21%
Egg, boiled, 1 large	26 mcg	17%
Protein Powder, 1 oz	25 mcg	16%
Chorizo, pork, 3 oz	22 mcg	12%

Raw vegetables, especially cruciferous vegetables and collard greens like broccoli, kale, cauliflower, and cabbage, contain goitrogenic compounds called glucosinolates that can inhibit iodine absorption and thus lead to low thyroid function[1114]. Soy, cassava, peanuts, corn, beans, millet and strawberries also contain a certain amount of goitrogens[1115]. Thus, you should avoid eating large amounts of these foods raw. Fortunately, cooking lowers the amount of goitrogens and prevents any adverse effects on the thyroid[1116]. A study looked at the effects of cooked Brussels sprouts on the thyroid and found that after 4 weeks of eating 150 grams (5 oz) a day there was no effect on thyroid function[1117]. Thus, you shouldn't be afraid of eating cooked vegetables. Cruciferous vegetable consumption is also linked to a reduced risk of cancer and cardiovascular disease[1118]. The breakdown products of glucosinolates activate anti-cancer pathways as well[1119,1120].

The main transporter of thyroid hormones that facilitates their cellular uptake is the sodium-iodide symporter (NIS)[1121]. Its main job is to deliver iodine into the thyroid gland where it can begin producing thyroid hormones and this is the first step in thyroid hormone synthesis[1122]. This process requires magnesium, ATP, and sodium[1123,1124,1125,1126,1127,1128]. Low blood sodium levels have been found to be slightly associated with elevated TSH and hypothyroidism[1129]. Selenium controls deiodinase activity, which is the scavenging pathway of iodine, helping to recycle it and support thyroid hormone synthesis[1130]. Thus, selenium is needed for activating thyroid hormones as well as recycling them. There's been an established association between selenium deficiency and hypothyroidism since the early 1990s[1131].

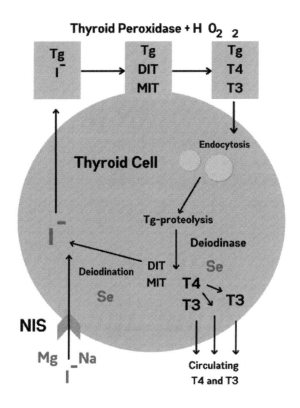

Adapted from: Zimmermann, M. B., Jooste, P. L., & Pandav, C. S. (2008). *'Iodine-deficiency disorders.'* The Lancet, 372(9645), 1251–1262.

Not getting enough sodium can also cause rapid insulin resistance even in healthy subjects[1132]**. There are at minimum 14 human studies indicating that low salt intakes worsen insulin resistance or elevate insulin levels after an oral glucose tolerance test**[1133,1134,1135,1136,1137,1138,1139,1140,1141,1142,1143,1144,1145,1146]. Restricting sodium also raises aldosterone, which may lead to chronic hypertension[1147.] Thus, not getting enough sodium impairs thyroid function by (1) inhibiting the delivery of iodine into the thyroid gland and (2) causing insulin resistance, which perpetuates thyroid dysfunction. Dietary salt raising blood pressure is an issue of salt sensitivity, which is primarily driven by insulin resistance and sympathetic nervous system dominance[1148].

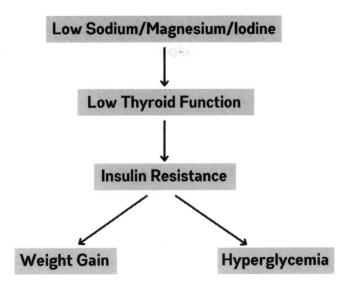

Low Sodium/Magnesium/Iodine

↓

Low Thyroid Function

↓

Insulin Resistance

Weight Gain   Hyperglycemia

Strategies for Improving Hypothyroidism

The most common thing that reduces thyroid function and suppresses the conversion of T4 into T3 is physiological stress[1149,1150]. It can come from overtraining, sleep deprivation, low calorie intake or prolonged fasting, all of which lower thyroid hormones to a certain extent[1151]. The hypothalamus-pituitary-thyroid (HPT) axis responds to nutritional challenges by regulating thyroid hormones to preserve energy during perceived starvation[1152]. Fasting for 72 hours reduces serum T3 levels by 30% and TSH by 70% in healthy men[1153]. However, T3 returns to prefasting levels after resuming eating[1154]. Thus, low thyroid is often an adaptive response to energy scarcity as to minimize the body's energy demands during times of energy shortage[1155].

Leptin is called the satiety hormone, but it also regulates your metabolic rate and energy expenditure[1156,1157]. **Low leptin levels encourage overeating and weight gain**[1158]. Raising leptin therapeutically has been used to reverse obesity and improve health biomarkers[1159,1160,1161]. When you're obese, you become leptin resistant and your brain doesn't get the signal that you're full[1162,1163,1164]. Ultra-processed foods can also cause this effect and impair satiety[1165]. With leptin resistance, leptin levels stay elevated, which is one of the biggest risk factors for weight gain[1166].

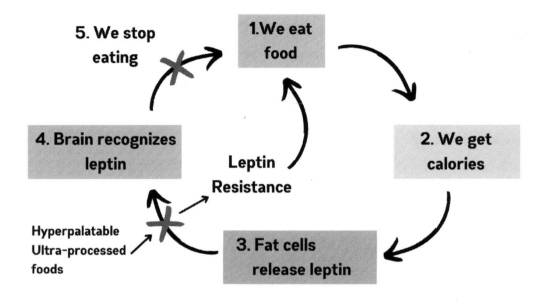

Leptin gets stimulated by TSH in the adipose tissue[1167,1168,1169]. There's a positive association between serum leptin and serum TSH in obese individuals[1170]. Leptin increases thyroid deiodinase activity, which converts T4 into T3[1171,1172]. **Thus, leptin sensitivity is vital for optimal thyroid function and metabolic rate.** Obese patients have been reported to have a small increase in total and free T3, which could be the body trying to increase its energy expenditure to mitigate fat gain[1173,1174]. Gaining fat is linked to a parallel rise in TSH and T3 independent of insulin sensitivity[1175]. Basically, the body starts burning more calories to protect against weight gain. Unfortunately, in that state, the desire to keep eating may be higher than what the body can keep up with in terms of energy expenditure. Both thyroid hormones and leptin contribute to heat production and metabolic rate[1176,1177]. **Obese people have lower TSH receptor expression on fat cells,**

which further raises TSH and T3 levels, mimicking peripheral thyroid hormone resistance[1178]. After weight loss, this normalizes[1179]. In sum, gaining weight reduces TSH receptor expression, which increases TSH, free T3 and leptin levels, whereas losing weight decreases TSH, free T3 and leptin[1180]. Weight gain can cause peripheral thyroid hormone resistance, which perpetuates weight gain.

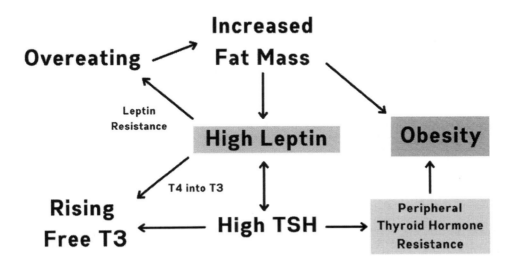

Eating less calories will downregulate your metabolic rate eventually, making you burn fewer calories[1181,1182,1183,1184]. That's why chronic low calorie intake can cause irreversible harm to the thyroid as has been shown by the participants of weight loss TV shows. A 2016 study on the competitors of The Biggest Loser found that 6 years after the show had ended, the subjects had regained up to 70% of their weight and were expending 700 fewer calories a day compared to when they started the competition[1185]. If you're familiar with the show, you know that the contestants are competing for losing the most weight, which is why they willpower through excessively long and strenuous workouts combined with minimal calorie intake. This sets them up to fail from the start as the body's counter-mechanisms for weight maintenance will eventually kick in, making them go off the rails and binge-eat at some point due to higher hunger hormone ghrelin and lower satiety hormone leptin[1186]. As a result, they rebound and can regain some or all of their weight back (and in some cases they end at an even higher weight than when they started the show). The bigger harm is that their thyroid function has also dropped slightly due to the chronic calorie restriction and it hasn't fully recovered after regaining the weight. This makes losing weight harder and weight regain easier. This kind of yo-yo dieting over time wreaks havoc to your metabolism and thyroid function and is the reason why so many people struggle with losing the weight the longer they try.

Studies have found that *intermittent* energy restriction instead of continuous energy restriction provides greater weight loss and results in less weight regain[1187]. Instead of eating at a severe calorie deficit (40-50% deficit) until you reach your goal weight, you stay at about a 25-33% calorie deficit for a 1-2 weeks and then return to maintenance calories for 1-2 weeks and repeat this cycle as long as necessary[1188]. This mitigates the drop in thyroid hormones and metabolism by keeping your satiety and leptin levels elevated. You can also mitigate metabolic adaptation as it's called by keeping a moderate calorie deficit (10-20%) instead of a severe one (20+%) and taking diet breaks[1189,1190]. Raising leptin (the satiety hormone) gives your body the signal that things are not scarce and there's no reason to go into starvation mode (i.e. low thyroid and slow metabolism). Carbohydrates have the largest effect on raising leptin and thyroid function[1191,1192].

A carbohydrate-rich diet has been shown to reverse changes in serum T3 and reverse T3 caused by prolonged fasting even when eating at a calorie deficit[1193]. Glucose is the main fuel for the thyroid gland and the brain, which is why they raise your metabolic rate more than fat as long as there's no insulin or leptin resistance[1194]. In fact, you need insulin to convert T4 into T3. Eating healthy whole food carbohydrates and spiking insulin, which raises leptin, improves insulin sensitivity and weight loss[1195]. Restoring leptin levels to normal have been shown to normalize blood sugar and insulin resistance[1196]. Ketogenic diets, however, can reduce T3 and raise reverse T3[1197], which is not optimal for thyroid function and insulin sensitivity[1198]. Thus, cyclical ketosis is better for improving metabolic health over the long term[1199]. Carbohydrate metabolism also produces more CO_2 than fat metabolism[1200,1201], which raises your metabolic rate and helps to cope with stress[1202]. Hypothyroidism lowers CO_2 production[1203]. In other words, carbohydrates can help you deal with stress by increasing CO_2 production and thyroid function.

Fructose reduces thyroid hormones similar to fasting in rats[1204,1205,1206]. In humans, fructose reduces liver T4 uptake[1207]. This is considered to be due to fructose increasing lactic acid and uric acid, which consumes ATP[1208,1209]. Without the ATP, there's no iodine uptake into the thyroid cells and hypothyroidism ensues.

Anti-diabetic drugs like metformin can alter thyroid function and anti-thyroid drugs like methimazole can alter glycemic control[1210]. Metformin improves insulin sensitivity and TSH levels[1211]. Thiazolidinediones (think Actos and Avandia) inhibit the activity of thyroid hormone receptors, which increases the risk of hypothyroidism and goiter[1212]. Methimazole and carbimazole are linked to the development of insulin autoimmune syndrome[1213]. Levothyroxine, which helps increase thyroid hormones in the body, reduces fasting and postprandial glucose levels and decreases A1C[1214].

Chapter 7: Sodium and Potassium: Insulin Resistance and Hypertension

High blood pressure or hypertension is the world's leading cause of cardiovascular disease, which contributes to stroke, coronary heart disease, myocardial infarction (heart attack), heart failure, atrial fibrillation, and kidney disease[1215,1216]. Hypertension is the main cause of mortality and morbidity worldwide[1217]. About 1.13 billion people across the globe have hypertension and 2/3rds of them are in low- to middle-income countries[1218]. NHANES data from 2005-2008 has discovered that 33.5% of U.S. adults over 20 years old have hypertension, which is essentially 1 out 3 people! There are even more people with 'pre-hypertension' or at a higher risk of becoming hypertensive. At the age of 70 or older, hypertension is found in 50% of Americans[1219]. The prevalence of hypertension in African American adults is 44%, which is the highest in the world[1220].

Most people don't know they have hypertension because there are no visible symptoms, which is why hypertension is termed 'the silent killer'. However, there are some signs that may indicate elevated blood pressure, such as headaches, pounding of the heart, blurry vision, buzzing in the ears, fatigue, nausea, chest pain, anxiety, and tremors. Measuring your blood pressure regularly is the only reliable method for assessing your blood pressure status and prevent it from rising. Blood pressure is measured by looking at two indicators: (1) systolic blood pressure, which reflects the pressure in the blood vessels while the heart beats or contracts, and (2) diastolic blood pressure, which is the pressure in the blood vessels during rest between heart beats. Hypertension is diagnosed with a systolic blood pressure $\geq$ 140 mmHg (millimeters of mercury) and a diastolic blood pressure of $\geq$ 90 mmHg on two different days.

There are many causes for hypertension, such as obesity, aging, being sedentary, excess alcohol intake, smoking and electrolyte imbalances[1221,1222,1223,1224]. However, **insulin resistance and metabolic syndrome are associated with hypertension as well**[1225,1226,1227] According to clinical studies, 80% of Type 2 diabetics have hypertension and 50% of hypertensive patients have hyperinsulinemia or glucose intolerance[1228,1229]. Furthermore, **in individuals with normal blood pressure, the higher the insulin the higher the blood pressure**[1230,1231,1232]. In this chapter, we're focusing on hypertension in the context of diabetes and insulin resistance. Specifically, how sodium and potassium affect the development of both conditions.

How Potassium Deficiency Causes Insulin Resistance and Hypertension

It's well established that insufficient potassium raises blood pressure and promotes cardiovascular disease[1233,1234,1235]. However, **not getting enough potassium also impairs insulin production and causes carbohydrate intolerance**[1236,1237]. The production of insulin by the pancreatic beta-cells is dependent on potassium[1238]. Serum potassium levels are inversely linked to fasting insulin levels[1239]. In healthy men, insulin infusions increase potassium absorption into the gastrointestinal organs and muscles, which reduces plasma potassium in a dose-dependent manner[1240,1241]. This potassium influx into the cell is caused by the sodium-potassium pump. Potassium is also needed to activate pyruvate kinase – the enzyme involved in the last step of glycolysis that's used to produce energy from glucose[1242]. A high dietary potassium intake is associated with a decreased risk in diabetes and metabolic syndrome[1243,1244,1245].

Besides its effects on glucose metabolism, insulin also causes vasorelaxation of the blood vessels by stimulating the production of nitric oxide (NO) in the endothelium[1246]. However, insulin can also have vasoconstrictive effects on the vasculature through the mitogen-activated protein kinase (MAPK) pathway[1247]. **During normal conditions, insulin stimulates NO release, which improves endothelial function, but in a state of insulin resistance, insulin-stimulated NO production is impaired, and the accompanying hyperinsulinemia activates the MAPK pathway, resulting in vasoconstriction, increased water and sodium retention, inflammation, and hypertension**[1248,1249]. Insulin controls sodium balance, which affects blood pressure, by promoting sodium reabsorption in the kidneys[1250,1251]. It has been discovered that insulin resistance can develop not only in insulin-responsive tissues like the muscles or liver but also in cardiovascular tissues and vascular tissue, which leads to hypertension and cardiovascular disease[1252,1253]. Thus, maintaining insulin sensitivity and normal insulin levels is crucial for not only preventing diabetes but also hypertension.

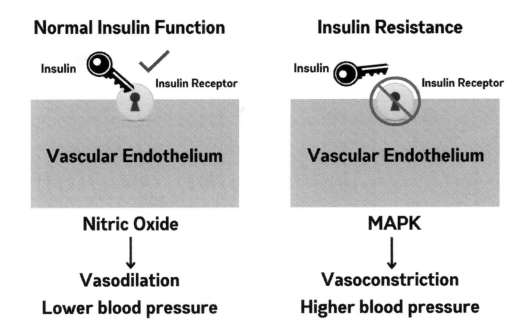

Intriguingly, **subclinical hypothyroidism is also associated with elevated blood pressure**[1254,1255,1256,1257]. About 30% of patients of hypothyroidism have elevated blood pressure[1258]. Compared to age-matched controls with normal thyroid levels, those with hypothyroidism have a 3-fold higher prevalence of hypertension[1259]. Among people with normal thyroid function, free T3 and free T4 are positively related to elevated blood pressure but among that population age and BMI are major confounding variables[1260]. Higher TSH levels (suggesting hypothyroidism) are positively associated with current hypertension in adults and children[1261,1262]. A 2018 systematic review and meta-analysis of 29 studies discovered that levothyroxine, which is a thyroid medication, reduced blood pressure in subclinical hypothyroidism patients[1263]. There's a well-known association between hypothyroidism and impaired vasodilation[1264,1265]. People with hypothyroidism have higher central arterial stiffness, which can increase atherosclerosis development[1266], and this phenomenon is reversed after T4 levels are normalized[1267,1268].

The Salt-Potassium Balance in Hypertension

We also know that sodium is needed for optimal thyroid function and **low salt intake can quickly induce insulin resistance**. Yet, excess sodium intake is well linked to an increased risk of hypertension (but a lot of this is because salt intake tracks with processed food intake)[1269,1270]. It's true, if **you consume large amounts of salt and you have insulin resistance or hyperinsulinemia, then you will retain more of the salt and water, resulting in an inevitable rise in blood pressure. The root cause of the issue isn't salt however – as salt is a vital mineral for optimal insulin sensitivity and thyroid function – but the insulin resistance that causes a state of salt retention.** Low salt intake elevates stress hormones and adrenaline, which contribute to stiffening of the arteries and systemic insulin resistance[1271,1272,1273]. Without enough salt, blood flow to muscles decreases via increased peripheral resistance[1274], reducing glucose delivery to muscles, worsening insulin resistance, and eventually causing hypertension and increasing risk of myocardial infarction (heart attack), cardiovascular disease and all-cause mortality[1275,1276,1277,1278].

In a study on moderate salt restriction (1,725 mg of sodium a day) vs a normal salt intake (5,405 mg of sodium a day) for one week, the low salt intake didn't result in reduction of blood pressure because of the aggravated systemic insulin resistance that developed due to the low salt intake[1279]. What's more, the individuals on the salt restricted diets saw their fasting plasma insulin levels more than double from 4.4 mIU/L to 9.9 mIU/L. Another study on 31 middle-aged people with essential hypertension found that one week of being on a low salt intake (782 mg of sodium a day) compared to a high-salt diet (7,866 mg/d) resulted in a significantly higher area under the curve (AUC) for glucose and insulin after an oral glucose tolerance test[1280]. There are at least 23 clinical studies in humans showing that salt restriction worsens insulin resistance, fasting insulin and/or glucose/insulin levels after an oral glucose tolerance test[1281].

Mechanisms for how low salt diets induce insulin resistance:

- Increased catecholamines which decrease insulin sensitivity and increase liver glucose production.
- Activation of the renin angiotensin aldosterone system.
- Elevation of non-esterified fatty acids.
- Increased glucose absorption from the diet.
- Reduced blood flow and insulin/glucose delivery to skeletal muscle.

It's been shown that insulin resistance enhances the blood pressure raising effects of sodium[1282]. Clinical studies suggest that both insulin resistance and hypertension are associated with salt sensitivity[1283]. Hypertensive patients with salt sensitivity show worse insulin resistance[1284,1285]. **Elevated insulin often precedes hypertension**[1286]. Insulin resistant individuals have impaired sodium excretion through the urine[1287], making them retain more water and sodium. Hyperinsulinemia activates the renin angiotensin system[1288,1289,1290], which promotes further sodium retention. Thus, hyperinsulinemia drives fluid and sodium retention[1291,1292], contributing to hypertension. Importantly, when you fix the insulin resistance you fix the "salt-sensitive" hypertension[1293,1294,1295,1296]. Thus, whatever causes elevated insulin levels and sodium retention is the culprit causing hypertension. In other words, not salt, but sugar, causes hypertension[1297,1298,1299].

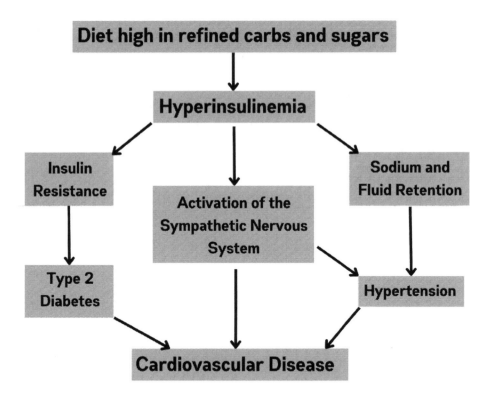

Adopted From: DiNicolantonio and O'Keefe (2022) 'Added Sugars Drive Insulin Resistance, Hyperinsulinemia, Hypertension, Type 2 Diabetes and Coronary Heart Disease', Missouri medicine, 119(6), 519–523.

High salt intake harms insulin sensitivity in salt sensitive hypertensive patients but not in those with salt resistance[1300]. This means that salt-sensitivity of blood pressure has more to do with insulin resistance (driven by an overconsumption of refined carbs and sugar) than salt per se. Thus, salt restriction may not be needed if the intake of refined carbs/sugars are reduced. In fact, salt restriction could be especially detrimental in those who are not salt sensitive and don't have insulin resistance[1301]. Salt sensitivity of blood pressure is an independent risk factor for developing cardiovascular disease morbidity and mortality. African Americans have been found to have a higher prevalence of salt sensitivity than white Americans[1302]. The reason for that could be evolutionary as humans living in hotter climates adapted to retain more salt due to sweating more, whereas humans in cooler regions adapted to higher sodium conditions[1303,1304]. Indeed, you can lose more than 1 teaspoon of salt (2,300 mg of sodium) after 1 hour of exercise in the heat.

Part of the problem is also not getting enough potassium that would keep the electrolytes and salt in balance. Industrialized societies with a lot of salty processed food usually consume little to no potassium. Higher potassium intake in those countries is associated with lower blood pressure[1305,1306]. Eating more fruit and vegetables, which have a lot of potassium and virtually no sodium, is well established to be linked with lower blood pressure[1307,1308,1309,1310]. The American Heart Association suggests that **increasing one's potassium intake could reduce hypertension by 17% and extend lifespan by 5.1 years**[1311].

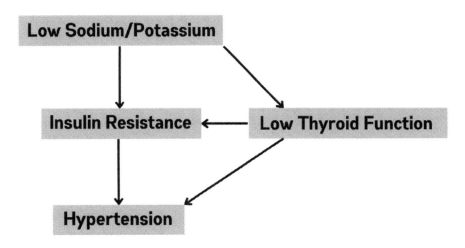

The RDA for potassium set by the Food and Nutritional Board of the Institute of Medicine is 4,700 mg/d[1312]. However, the World Health Organization recommends a potassium intake of 3,150 mg/d[1313]. For hypertension prevention, it's recommended to get over 3,500 mg/d[1314]. **The adequate intake of potassium**

has been set at **3,000-3,400 mg/d for adult men and 2,300-2,600 mg/d for adult women**[1315]. An average person in the U.S. gets less than 2,800 mg/d of potassium[1316], which is why potassium is considered a "nutrient of public health concern" in the U.S. Dietary Guidelines[1317]. Even still, getting only 700-1,200 mg/day of more potassium can reduce systolic blood pressure by 2-3 mmHg[1318]. Increasing dietary potassium intake from 2,340 to 3,120 mg/d is linked to a lower risk of death from stroke in adult women[1319]. Similar results have been found with raising potassium intake from 897 mg/d to 2,106 mg/d; from 1,482 mg/d to 2,769 mg/d and from 2,379 mg/d to 6,513 mg/d[1320,1321]. A meta-analysis of 15 studies among 247,510 people found that increasing potassium intake by 1,640 mg/d was associated with a 21% lower risk of stroke[1322]. Another meta-analysis discovered that higher potassium intake reduces risk of stroke by 24%[1323].

Here are the highest potassium-rich foods[1324,1325,1326,1327]:

Food	Mg of Potassium per Serving	% of RDA
Carrot, dehydrated, 1 cup	1880 mg	47%
Apricots, dried, ½ cups	1,101 mg	23%
Potato, baked, 1 medium	1,000 mg	23%
Swiss Chard, 1 cup	961 mg	20%
Acorn Squash, 1 cup	896 mg	18%
Lentils, cooked, 1 cup	731 mg	16%
Prune Juice, 1 cup	707 mg	16%
Prunes, dried, ½ cup	699 mg	15%
Carrot Juice, 1 cup	689 mg	15%
Passion-Fruit Juice, 1 cup	687 mg	15%

Edamame, 1 cup	676 mg	14%
Tomato Paste, canned, ¼ cup	669 mg	14%
Pomegranate, 1 medium	666 mg	14%
Beet Greens, cooked, ½ cup	654 mg	14%
Squash, mashed, 1 cup	644 mg	14%
Raisins, ½ cups	618 mg	13%
Adzuki Beans, cooked, ½ cup	612 mg	13%
Kidney Beans, canned, 1 cup	607 mg	13%
Coconut Water, 1 cup	600 mg	13%
White Beans, canned, ½ cup	595 mg	13%
Butternut Squash, 1 cup	582 mg	13%
Parsnips, 1 cup	572 mg	13%
Tomato Puree, ½ cup	549 mg	12%
Sweet Potato, 1 medium	541 mg	12%
Spinach, 1 cup	540 mg	12%
Salmon, wild, 3 oz	534 mg	12%
Clams, canned, 3 oz	534 mg	12%
Pomegranate Juice, 1 cup	534 mg	12%
Tomato Juice, 1 cup	527 mg	12%
Beetroot, boiled, 1 cup	518 mg	11%

Baking Powder, 1 tsp	505 mg	11%
Orange Juice, 1 cup	496 mg	11%
Cream of Tartar, 1 tsp	495 mg	11%
Swiss Chard, cooked, ½ cups	481 mg	11%

Human hunter-gatherers have been predicted to obtain somewhere from 5,850-11,310 mg of potassium a day[1328,1329]. However, other more recent studies have suggested that our ancestors consumed mainly megafauna (that are now extinct) and large elephants[1330]. There is thus a strong case that our ancestors primarily consumed meat and hence our potassium intake would likely have been more around 3,000-4,000 mg per day range. Sodium intake has been estimated to be at 1,131-2,500 mg/d; however, these studies do not consider the sodium obtained from blood, interstitial fluids, brackish water, and salt licks[1331,1332]. Thus, **human ancestors probably consumed at least 3,000 mg of sodium per day and their potassium to sodium ratio was likely more around 1:1. People in industrialized societies who eat a lot of processed foods get only 2,100-2,730 mg of potassium and 3,400 mg of sodium a day, which is a potassium to sodium ratio of 0.7:1**[1333,1334,1335]. On a highly pre-packaged and ultra-processed food diet, you may be getting upwards of 7-10,000 mg of sodium, which on top of a low potassium intake is certainly not a good thing. The way to achieve the optimal potassium to sodium ratio of 2-1:1 is to eat a lot of meat, fresh fruits, and vegetables in addition to your other food groups and to season your food with natural sea or rock salt. Try to minimize processed food consumption that has a lot of added sodium.

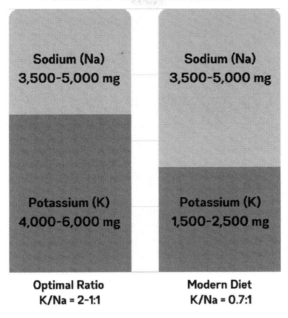

Optimal Dietary Potassium to Sodium Ratio

Optimal Ratio	Modern Diet
Sodium (Na) 3,500-5,000 mg	Sodium (Na) 3,500-5,000 mg
Potassium (K) 4,000-6,000 mg	Potassium (K) 1,500-2,500 mg
Optimal Ratio K/Na = 2-1:1	Modern Diet K/Na = 0.7:1

Maintaining an Optimal Electrolyte Balance

Besides sodium and potassium, there are several other electrolytes needed for maintaining optimal blood pressure. Electrolytes are essentially charged minerals inside your body that help to maintain normal fluid levels within the cells, outside of cells and in the blood[1336]. The main ones are sodium, potassium, magnesium, phosphate, calcium, chloride, and bicarbonate, but others include zinc, copper, iron, manganese, molybdenum, and chromium. Kidneys are the organs that help to maintain electrolyte balance and fluid levels by filtering and reabsorbing electrolytes. In so doing, the body actively adjusts its fluid levels.

An imbalance in electrolytes can have fatal consequences on your health, such as heart failure, hypertension, insulin resistance, arrythmias and even death[1337,1338]. This occurs when you have either too high or too low levels of certain electrolytes in the blood. Most often, electrolyte imbalance is caused by dehydration, prolonged sweatting, vomitting, diarrhea, malabsorption and nutrient deficiencies[1339]. Certain medical conditions can promote this, such as kidney disease[1340], anorexia nervosa[1341] and medical burns[1342]. Some symptoms of electrolyte imbalance are fatigue, irregular heartbeat, high blood pressure, sleeping problems, muscle weakness and cramps, headaches and numbness[1343].

Here are the reference ranges for electrolytes in blood:

- Calcium: 5–5.5 mEq/L

- Chloride: 97–107 mEq/L

- Potassium: 5–5.3 mEq/L

- Magnesium: 1.5-2.5 mEq/L

- Sodium: 136–145 mEq/L

Moving sodium and potassium across cell membranes involves an enzyme called the Sodium Potassium Pump also known as the Na^+/K^+-ATPase. The ATPase transports sodium ions out and potassium ions into the cell. This process is powered primarily by magnesium and ATP[1344]. However, not enough sodium can cause a magnesium deficiency[1345,1346,1347], as can a lack of selenium or vitamin B6[1348]. Thus, salt, vitamin B6 and selenium control your body's electrolyte balance indirectly via the sodium potassium pump because of how they control magnesium in the body. A magnesium deficiency causes the accumulation of sodium and calcium inside the cell, which promotes hypertension and cardiomyopathy[1349]. Magnesium also protects against potassium loss and potassium levels in the muscles won't normalize until magnesium status is restored even when serum potassium levels increase[1350,1351,1352].

Overall, your body needs different minerals for optimal insulin sensitivity and glucose regulation. Deficiencies in almost any mineral but especially magnesium, chromium, iodine, sodium, or potassium can impair insulin sensitivity. This results in high blood sugar, high insulin, hypertension and eventually either diabetes or cardiovascular disease. Insulin resistance is still at the root of all of this, but it's not always caused by an excess consumption of sugary foods. It can also be due to not getting enough salt or other micronutrients.

Hyperglycemia, Nitric Oxide and Blood Pressure Regulation

In addition to electrolytes, one important signaling molecule that regulates blood pressure and cardiovascular disease risk is nitric oxide (NO). It suppresses platelet aggregation[1353], lowers blood pressure[1354], reduces blood clot formation[1355], prevents blood vessel inflammation[1356] and improves the transport of lipids and cholesterol[1357]. In therapeutic settings, nitric oxide boosters are also used to treat erectile dysfunction by promoting blood flow[1358]. NO mediates penile erection and relaxes the smooth muscles of the penis[1359]. That's why hypertension and heart disease are very closely linked to sexual dysfunction[1360]. Nitric oxide's blood flow promoting effects happen through vasodilation of the arteries.

Reduced nitric oxide availability is implicated in hypertension and atherosclerosis[1361]. In hypertensive patients, a single oral lozenge that helps to raise nitric oxide levels in the oral cavity has been found to restore endothelial function, reduce blood pressure and improve vascular compliance[1362]. Lower nitric oxide and higher oxidative stress contribute to pulmonary hypertension[1363].

Here are the nutrients needed for nitric oxide production[1364]

- **Citrulline/arginine** – Arginine and citrulline are the primary amino acids needed to produce nitric oxide. L-citrulline supplementation has been shown to improve arterial stiffness, independent of blood pressure levels, in middle-aged men[1365]. Citrulline also increases blood flow during exercise and improves erectile function[1366,1367]. Supplementing arginine on its own has been found to be unreliable in increasing nitric oxide[1368]. Citrulline is absorbed more readily than arginine and can raise blood arginine levels twice as much as arginine[1369]. Combining citrulline with arginine will elevate nitric oxide levels even more because citrulline reduces the breakdown of arginine in the liver and intestines. Taking extra glutathione or n-acetylcysteine with citrulline may promote nitric oxide synthesis and stabilize it better[1370]. Some cells can't make nitric oxide without glutathione[1371].

- **Calcium** – Endothelial NO synthase (eNOS) and neuronal NO synthase (nNOS), specifically, are controlled by intracellular calcium[1372]. Raising intracellular calcium with glutamate stimulates nNOS to produce nitric oxide[1373]. Calcium also initiates the electron flow in the NO synthase reaction.

- **Eicosapentaenoic acid (EPA)** – the omega-3 fatty acid, has been shown to increase nitric oxide synthesis by increasing intracellular calcium[1374].

- **Iron** – Heme, the oxygen carrying substance, that contains iron is essential for NO synthase. A deficiency in iron has been shown to reduce nNOS in rats[1375,1376].

- **Zinc** – Zinc is bound to all isoforms of NO synthase, making it necessary for NOS activity[1377]. In high amounts, zinc inhibits eNOS and nNOS[1378].

- **Magnesium** – Magnesium increases eNOS gene expression by activating vitamin D[1379]. In healthy humans, magnesium ions also directly enhance endothelial NO production in a dose-dependent manner[1380]. Magnesium deficiency decreases nitric oxide synthesis, whereas magnesium supplementation restores endothelium-dependent vasodilation[1381].

Glucose metabolism is one of the main sources of NADPH, which is needed for nitric oxide synthesis[1382]. That makes NO synthesis very much glucose dependent. However, **hyperglycemia impairs nitric oxide-mediated endothelial function**[1383] and promotes vascular dysfunction in patients with diabetes[1384]. **A deficiency in copper, magnesium and chromium can cause hyperglycemia**[1385,1386,1387], **which lowers nitric oxide contributing to hypertension**. In rats, fructose depletes copper and magnesium[1388,1389], which impairs vascular relaxation and causes hypertension[1390]. Thus, maintaining normal blood sugar levels are vital for healthy blood pressure.

Chapter 8: Artificial Sweeteners and Sugar Substitutes

Most people have a sweet tooth. Sweetness is one of the five primary taste elements (sweet, salty, sour, bitter and umami). Evolutionarily, **it's thought that tasting something sweet helps the organism detect readily available glucose in fruit or honey, which would indicate the presence of energy**[1391]. Many obligate carnivores and some birds have lost their sweet taste, suggesting that the perception of sweetness has evolved to detect sugar primarily from plants[1392,1393]. A bitter taste, on the other hand, indicates potential toxicity or the presence of a high amount of polyphenolic compounds that trigger small stress reactions inside the body that increase antioxidant enzymes like glutathione or superoxide dismutase. That's why many animals, including humans, consume various bitter plants and leaves for medicinal purposes[1394].

By default, most humans, including newborns, react positively to sugar – i.e., they want more of it[1395]. In rodents and humans, sweet substances act as an analgesic that reduces pain perception[1396,1397]. The reason for that has to do with the release of endogenous opioids and the endocannabinoid system[1398]. **It's been shown that sweet tasting substances, including sugar and artificial sweeteners like aspartame, interact with sweet tasting receptors T1R2 + T1R3 dimer on the tongue**[1399,1400,1401]. Disabling the T1R2 + T1R3 dimer sweet receptor with gene editing in mice makes them unable to detect the sweetness of non-sugar artificial sweeteners but not glucose or sorbitol itself[1402,1403]. This has led to the hypothesis that there is an additional peripheral way to detect sweetness and the discovery that sugar transporters inside sweet taste cells can detect glucose and other sugars[1404].

Due to the taste preference towards sweetness that humans tend to exhibit, many people find it hard to give up sugar. That's why over the past decades there has been a large increase in the consumption of artificial sweeteners and other non-nutritive sugar substitutes. They can be derived from natural plant extracts, like stevia, or through chemical synthesis, such as aspartame or acesulfame K. There is a lot of controversy surrounding the health effects of these sweeteners. In this chapter, we're going to cover how artificial and natural sweeteners affect insulin resistance and blood glucose control.

History of Artificial Sweeteners

The first artificial sweetener to be invented was saccharin in 1879 by Constantin Fahlberg at Johns Hopkins University (Baltimore)[1405]. Fahlberg was working with benzoic sulfimide, which is a coal tar derivative, when he tasted something sweet on his hand[1406]. He figured the sweetness was due to the compound on his hands, which he named saccharin, and later synthesized saccharin from o-sulfamoylbenzoic acid. The word saccharin is derived from the word *saccharine* or *sugary*, describing something overly sweet. Saccharin has no nutritional value and contains no calories.

In the mid-1880s, Fahlberg began manufacturing saccharine in Germany, which created a lot of controversy even back then. In 1907, the organization preceding the FDA, The Bureau of Chemistry stated that saccharin was an illegal substitute for sugar[1407]. However, Theodore Roosevelt answered the Director of The Bureau of Chemistry saying that: *"Anybody who says saccharin is injurious to health is an idiot,"* ending the Director's career.

During World War I, saccharin was very popular because of sugar shortages. It was cheaper to produce than sugar. But after World War II, sugar substitutes began to be promoted for weight loss. **In 1977, the FDA discovered saccharin was associated with bladder cancer in rats and demanded products with the sweetener have a warning label. However, in 2000, it was discovered that humans metabolize saccharin completely differently and over 30 human studies show saccharin is safe for human consumption**[1408,1409]. Thus, the warning label requirement was lifted. Saccharin isn't on the list of carcinogenic compounds either. Today, the European Food Safety Authority has stated that consuming artificial sweeteners within the acceptable daily intake (ADI) doesn't cause cancer or other health problems and is safe for humans[1410,1411]. We will be covering the ADIs of different sweeteners later in this chapter.

The FDA has approved 6 artificial sweeteners as food additives: saccharin, sucralose, aspartame, advantame, acesulfame-K and neotame[1412]. The European Union Scientific Committee on Food has approved additionally cyclamate, aspartame-acesulfame salt and neohesperidin dihydrochalcone[1413,1414,1415]. There are more natural sweeteners like stevia glycosides, monk fruit and thaumatin that the FDA has granted the Generally Recognized as Safe (GRAS) status as well[1416,1417].

Artificial sweeteners themselves are classified into nutritive and non-nutritive sweeteners, depending on whether or not they have calories. Nutritive sweeteners include monosaccharide polyols, such as xylitol, mannitol and sorbitol as well as disaccharide polyols like lactitol and maltitol. They're also considered sugar alcohols or polyols. Non-nutritive sweeteners are the commonly known artificial sweeteners without caloric value and they're metabolized differently than regular sweeteners or sugar. All of them have different properties, taste, sweetness and metabolic effects[1418]. Thus, not all of the sweeteners are the same and they have to be looked at individually.

Are Artificial Sweeteners Safe?

In the U.S., around 25% of children and > 41% of adults were consuming artificial sweeteners between 2009-2012, which is a 200% increase among children and a 54% increase among adults compared to 1999-2000[1419]. It's hard to say what epidemiological impact artificial sweeteners specifically have had on the rise in obesity and diabetes in the United States over the past few decades. People might be consuming more artificial sweeteners than before but the same applies to many other foods: sugar, total calories, refined carbs and added oils have all increased, while physical movement has decreased. Thus, the increased consumption of artificial sweeteners is just a drop in the bucket of all the other much more evident reasons to the rise in diabetes and obesity, such as the ones just mentioned.

Artificial sweeteners and non-nutritive sweeteners are considered safe to consume and to help in weight loss and diet adherence[1420,1421,1422]. Observational studies appear to link artificial sweetener consumption to weight gain but randomized clinical trials show the opposite – weight loss[1423,1424,1425]. The association between weight gain and higher artificial sweetener intake is probably due to the fact that many people who end up choosing these diet drinks with artificial sweeteners tend to compensate with higher calorie foods[1426,1427,1428] (i.e. taking a larger calorie dish or an extra serving of fries because they opted for the diet coke). Overall the data suggests that replacing sugar with artificial sweeteners has either a neutral or beneficial effect on weight loss and weight management[1429,1430,1431]. However, just because they are better than full calorie sugar sweetened beverages doesn't necessarily make them healthy.

Some studies have concluded that artificial sweeteners don't appear to raise blood sugar levels[1432]. However, certain artificial sweeteners, such as saccharin and sucralose in humans, as well as saccharin, sucralose and aspartame in animals, have been shown to worsen glycemic responses[1433,1434]. However, stevia and aspartame in one randomized controlled trial did not significantly impair glycemic response[1435]. Aspartame has its own issues and there are many anecdotes of it being associated with headaches and other health issues. Thus, the safest non-nutritive (non-caloric) sweeteners, at least based on the current evidence, would be stevia and monk fruit, as they do not appear to worsen glucose tolerance.

Artificial sweeteners may raise insulin, although significantly less than regular table sugar[1436]. Artificial sweeteners do upregulate intestinal glucose absorption via sodium-glucose cotransporter-1 (SGLT1) and glucose transporter 2 (GLUT2)[1437,1438], but the rate doesn't differ from regular sugar[1439]. Thus, it may be wise to avoid consuming carbs/sugars alongside artificial sweeteners. The **overconsumption of artificially sweetened beverages has been associated with an increased risk of developing diabetes in some observational studies**[1440]. Most scientists agree that we need more research to ascertain the long term health implications of consuming artificial sweeteners[1441]. Even though the evidence is limited, clinical studies suggest that humans should avoid or minimize the intake of saccharin and sucralose. Using more natural non-nutritive sweeteners, like stevia or monk fruit, is more advisable, as they do not appear to come with the worsening of glucose risk and may help to lower daily calorie and sugar intake.

A 2022 systematic review on 21 common sweeteners looking at 5 different healthy human gut microbiome profiles found that only 7 sweeteners altered the gut microbiome: xylitol, mannitol, isomalt, maltitol, lactitol, sorbitol, and hydrogenated starch hydrolysis[1442]. Carbohydrate sweeteners like sorbitol, mannitol, lactitol, maltitol, isomaltitol, and hydrogenated starch hydrolysis had a prebiotic effect on species that may improve blood sugar control[1443]. Thus, the authors concluded that the alcohol-type sweeteners as mentioned could have prebiotic effects. Another review discovered that isomalt, maltitol, lactitol and xylitol can reach the large bowel and promote the number of *Bifidobacteria* in humans, which are linked to health benefits[1444,1445]. However, **both reviews found that saccharin and sucralose shift the gut more towards dysbiosis, which could have harmful effects.**

Some of the changes in the microbiome caused by artificial sweeteners might cause endotoxemia and inflammation in rodents[1446,1447]. That metabolic endotoxemia might promote glucose intolerance and insulin resistance[1448,1449,1450]. Endotoxins can interfere with insulin production and insulin-stimulated glucose uptake[1451]. Compared to other non-nutritive sweeteners, stevia appears to have anti-inflammatory effects on the microbiome by attenuating LPS-induced inflammation[1452,1453].

Artificial sweeteners are perceived by the same taste receptors T1R2 and T1R3 as regular sugars but they bind to different sites[1454,1455]. Thus, **artificial sweeteners generate weaker responses in terms of reward and satisfaction than regular sugars as shown by fMRI images**[1456,1457]. Artificial sweeteners aren't strong stimulators of glucagon-like peptide-1 (GLP-1), peptide YY (PYY) and glucose-dependent insulinotropic peptide (GIP)[1458,1459,1460], which regular sugars stimulate upon ingestion[1461]. GLP-1, PYY and GIP cross the blood-brain barrier and reach the hypothalamus to reduce food intake and appetite[1462]. Most of the artificial sweeteners get metabolized too fast before being able to bind to sweet taste receptors. Because of that reason, human studies show that artificial sweeteners don't increase appetite[1463,1464]. However, **when sucralose is consumed with carbohydrates**, but not alone, **it impairs insulin sensitivity**[1465].

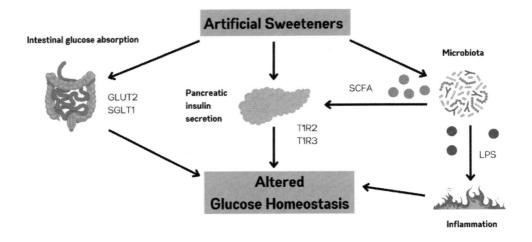

Overall, the data suggests that it's best to avoid artificial sweetners (especially saccharin and sucralose) and to stick to the natural non-nutritive sweeteners such as stevia and monk fruit.

Types of Sugar Substitutes

Here's an overview of the most common sugar substitutes and their impact on your health:

Artificial Sweeteners

- **Aspartame** – most diet beverages are based on aspartame. It's 180-200 times sweeter than sugar. Brands include Equal®, NutraSweet®, and others. Aspartame has had a long track record of being claimed to be unsafe, but that's based on very high doses in animals. Regardless, it may not be tolerated by many people. While it's considered safe for human consumption by over 100 regulatory agencies we need long term studies in humans to know for sure[1466,1467]. The acceptable daily intake (ADI) of aspartame is 50 mg/kg/day. A single can of diet coke contains about 180 mg of aspartame, which means you'd need to consume up to 16 cans of diet coke to exceed the ADI[1468].

- o Aspartame gets fully broken down into aspartic acid and phenylalanine in the gut – 2 amino acids you can obtain in much larger amounts from many whole foods like meat, milk and vegetables[1469]. High amounts of phenylalanine are dangerous to a rare inherited disease called phenylketonuria (PKU) but not for others. Aspartame is quickly broken down into its metabolites and is not found in the blood even after very large doses[1470]. Part of aspartame that gets broken down is methanol, which gets metabolized by the liver.

- o Clinical trials have found that using aspartame instead of sugar helps to reduce calorie intake and bodyweight[1471,1472]. Long-term use of aspartame hasn't been shown to significantly affect A1c or glucose levels in both diabetics and non-diabetics[1473,1474,1475,1476,1477,1478,1479].

- **Sucralose or Splenda** is the world's most commonly used artificial sweetener[1480]. It's 600 times sweeter than table sugar. Unlike other artificial sweeteners, sucralose is much more heat stable and can thus be used in baking[1481]. The FDA approved sucralose for general purposes in foods in 1999[1482,1483,1484]. Only about 11-27% of the sucralose ingested gets metabolized by the body and the rest passes through unmetabolized[1485,1486]. The acceptable daily intake (ADI) of sucralose is deemed to be 5 mg/kg of bodyweight per day and most consumers are getting 1.6 mg/kg[1487].

o In humans and mice, sucralose consumption compared to water, placebo or controls, hasn't been seen to have any effect on bodyweight gain or loss[1488,1489].

o **Sucralose has been found to possibly alter the gut microbiome in a way that impairs glycemic response and insulin secretion in some humans**[1490,1491]. Sucralose can affect the microbiome because it stays in the colon longer than other sweeteners like aspartame[1492,1493]. To be fair, while some human studies show sucralose impairs glycemic responses, other studies in healthy individuals as well as diabetes patients do not show a worsening in glucose, insulin, or A1c levels[1494,1495,1496,1497,1498,1499]. All studies to date are relatively short and hence we need long term studies to fully ascertain the health effects of artificial sweeteners.

o High dose sucralose consumption for 7 days in healthy individuals hasn't been shown to alter glycemic control, insulin resistance or gut microbiome[1500]. In healthy subjects, sucralose enhances GLP-1 release and lowers blood glucose in the presence of carbohydrates but not in newly diagnosed type 2 diabetic patients[1501].

o In healthy individuals, most of the randomized controlled-trials show no difference between sucralose consumption and water, sucrose, glucose or placebo on circulating insulin levels[1502,1503,1504]. However, a few studies have found that short term intakes of sucralose (48-200 mg/day for up to 4 weeks) increases insulin levels[1505,1506,1507].

• **Acesulfame-K or acesulfame-potassium** is a white crystalline powder that's about 200 times sweeter than sucrose[1508]. Because of the intense taste, it's commonly used in beverages and diet drinks. Despite containing potassium, acesulfame-K doesn't affect potassium levels in the body nor is it metabolized by the body in any way[1509].

- After ingestion, acesulfame-K is absorbed entirely and distributed into circulation after which 99% gets excreted by the kidneys and 1% in the feces[1510,1511]. Because of its fast absorption, acesulfame-K doesn't reach the lower GI tract and is unlikely to disrupt the microbiome[1512].

- In mice, consuming the acceptable daily intake (ADI) of 15 mg/kg/day of acesulfame-K for 8 weeks hasn't been found to increase bodyweight, but exceeding the ADI 2-fold (37.5 mg/kg/day) for 4 weeks has been shown to increase bodyweight gain[1513,1514].

- **Saccharin** is 300 times sweeter than sugar and the oldest of artificial sweeteners[1515]. About 85-95% of saccharin gets excreted by the kidneys in urine and 5-15% is eliminated unchanged in the feces[1516,1517]. Thus, a small amount of saccharin that isn't immediately absorbed can affect the microbiome[1518]. The ADI for saccharin is 15 mg/kg/d.

Sugar alcohols

- **Sugar alcohols or polyols** include sorbitol, xylitol, mannitol, erythritol and lactitol, which are used in chewing gum and in foods as as sugar substitute[1519]. They're much less sweet than sugar and artificial sweeteners and don't spike blood sugar levels. Because they are structurally similar to alcohol (although they don't contain ethanol) sugar alcohols don't get metabolized by the body and thus they can cause gastrointestinal distress, bloating and diarrhea.

o **Erythritol** is a common sugar substitute sweetener but your body also produces it via the pentose phosphate pathway (PPP), which is a parallel pathway to glycolysis[1520]. The PPP has been found to be involved with diabetes, cancer and cardiovascular disease[1521]. There is a connection between insulin resistance and the pentose phosphate pathway[1522,1523], which is why your body produces erythritol when under oxidative stress and various metabolic issues. A 2023, study claimed that higher erythritol levels were associated with major adverse cardiovascular disease risk[1524]. However, that's a reverse causation – that the individuals with higher erythritol levels were already metabolically sick and with insulin resistance, which made their bodies produce erythritol through the pentose phosphate pathway. In other studies, erythritol as a sweetener has been shown to lower postprandial blood glucose[1525] and improve endothelial function by reducing arterial stiffness[1526]. Thus, erythritol seems safe to consume for people with diabetes and it's certainly a safer alternative than regular sugar or other artificial sweeteners.

Natural non-nutritive sweeteners

- **Stevia or steviol glycoside** is produced from the South American plant *Stevia rebaudiana*, which makes it a natural sweetener[1527]. Stevia is around 300 times sweeter than sucrose[1528]. The acceptable daily intake (ADI) for steviol equivalents is 4 mg/kg/day or 12 mg/kg/day for stevia extracts[1529].

  o Digestive enzymes and acids in the upper GI tract can't metabolize steviol glycoside but Bacteroides in the colon can[1530,1531]. Thus, stevia can affect the microbiome. Steviol glycoside is broken down into steviol, glycoside and glucoronide[1532,1533]. There is also some glucose that gets formed and it gets metabolized, whereas steviol is glucoronidated in the liver and excreted through urine[1534,1535]. Metabolization of steviol is quite slow by the colonic bacteria[1536].

- o Steviol glycoside consumption has been found to have a positive impact on systolic blood pressure, but no effect on BMI, diastolic blood pressure, fasting glucose, A1c, total cholesterol and HDL-C compared to placebo[1537].

- **Monk fruit or mogrosides** is a sweetener extracted from monk fruit. Since 2017, monk fruit isn't allowed in the EU as a sweetener due to insufficient evidence of its safety[1538], but it's allowed in products as flavoring in concentrations where it doesn't function as a sweetener. In the U.S., monk fruit is deemed safe by the FDA[1539]. Monk fruit doesn't have a determined acceptable daily intake (ADI).

  - o Monk fruit is 150-250 times sweeter than sugar but it has been found to have some antioxidant and anti-glycation effects in animal studies[1540,1541]. Those effects appear to be mediated by the anti-inflammatory properties of mogrosides[1542].

The general advice is that if you can go without sugar alternatives then that's perfectly fine as there doesn't appear to be any health benefits beyond what you couldn't achieve with dietary changes. However, if you're struggling to give up sugar or just like to have something sweet, then certain sugar alternatives can make sense (i.e. stevia and monk fruit). If you consume a small amount of artificial sweeteners, like a can of diet soda, or a bit as a sugar substitute in baking or desserts, then it's likely there will be little to no harm to your health. Diet drinks and artificial sweeteners appear to help with diet adherence and weight loss, which itself would have a positive effect on glycemic control as well. They're obviously not health-promoting products but in small amounts they have a neglible effect on your metabolic health.

Honey and Natural Sweeteners

Fortunately, there are some natural sweeteners as well we can use to satisfy that sweet tooth or help with diet adherence. They're not zero calories, unfortunately, but they can be healthier than regular table sugar. Here's a list of the some natural sugars and sweeteners:

- **Inulin** is a polysaccharide made by plants that's often used as a sweetener in various foods[1543]. As a sweetener, it's most often extracted from chicory[1544]. Other foods that contain inulin include onions, wheat, agave, garlic, bananas, asparagus and artichoke. Inulin isn't digested by the upper GI tract, which reduces its caloric value, and it promotes the growth of *Bifidobacteria,* making it a pre-biotic[1545,1546,1547]. Because inulin doesn't get reabsorbed, it's used to determine the glomerular filtration rate of kidneys[1548].

  o **Inulin-type fructans have been shown to improve cholesterol levels in all populations but the improvement in glucose control is observed only in Type 2 diabetics**[1549,1550,1551,1552,1553]. Inulin-enriched pasta in young healthy men can increase HDL cholesterol by 35.9% and lower triglycerdies by 23.4%[1554].

  o **Replacing inulin with carbohydrate sugars lowers the postprandial glucose and insulin response quite significantly**[1555]. In elderly Type 2 diabetics, milk powder supplemented with inulin and resistant dextrin lowers blood sugar levels before and after meals and decreases insulin resistance and blood pressure[1556]. Adding 10 grams of inulin to the daily diet of middle-aged men and women for 8 weeks significantly reduces fasting insulin and triglyceride levels[1557].

  o Inulin can also increase calcium and magnesium absorption[1558,1559,1560].

  o **Inulin is considered a FODMAP, because of the prebiotic effects on the colon, which could cause digestive issues and gas in some individuals[1561,1562,1563].** Other side-effects include bloating, diarrhea, belching, swelling or allergies[1564,1565]. Thus, it's not recommended to be consuming very large amounts of inulin every day. The safe daily intake for inulin has been deemed to be 10 grams a day in the U.S. and Europe[1566].

- **Honey** is a sweet-tasting substance made by bees[1567]. The sweetness of honey, which is equal to table sugar, comes from its high amounts of fructose and glucose. Honey is about 38% fructose and 31% glucose with the remaining being water and other sugars, such as maltose and sucrose. Because of its sweetness and calories, honey has been valued by all hunter gatherer groups[1568].

  o Honey has a history in folk medicine that traces back thousands of years. It's been found to have antibacterial, antioxidant, anti-inflammatory, cardioprotective, hepatoprotective and antitumor properties[1569,1570,1571,1572,1573,1574,1575,1576,1577,1578,1579]. In diabetic rats, honey has been shown to enhance the effectiveness of metformin on oxidative stress and lipid peroxidation[1580,1581].

  o **Despite the high carbohydrate content of honey, people with and without impaired glucose tolerance show a high tolerance**

to honey in terms of glycemic control[1582,1583,1584,1585]. Honey's also been found to even be suitable for Type 1 diabetics[1586,1587]. The reason for this is thought to be the ability of small amounts of fructose to lower blood sugar as well as increase C-peptide that promotes insulin secretion[1588,1589,1590,1591].

- o People getting 70 grams of honey a day compared to 70 grams of sucrose for 30 days have been found to lose 1.3% body weight and 1.1% body fat, have a 3% lower total cholesterol, 11% lower triglycerides, 4.2% lower fasting blood glucose and 3.2% lower c-reactive proteiin (CRP) in subjects with normal cardiovascular disease markers, and 3.3% lower total cholesterol, 19% lower triglycerides and 3.3% lower CRP in subjects with elevated risk factors[1592]. However, **a 8-week randomized clinical trial on 48 Type 2 diabetics found that consuming honey resulted in higher A1c levels alongside a drop in bodyweight and lipids**[1593]. Thus, it's not recommended to be consuming very large amounts of honey, especially if you have diabetes or glucose intolerance, and instead we recommend to stick to a maximum amount of 1-2 tablespoons of honey per day (but up to 4 tablespoons in heatlhy active individuals).

- o **Honey might also improve diabetic wound healing**[1594,1595] by fighting the microorganisms and lowering the infection in the wound[1596,1597]. It also increases nitric oxide, which speeds up healing[1598,1599]. There's several human studies showing how honey can be effective in the treatment of diabetic ulcers and wounds[1600,1601,1602].

o Honey should not be consumed by infants as it can cause botulism[1603]. It is considered safe to give honey to children after the age of one.

- **Maple syrup** comes from the sap of maple trees that grow in colder climates. It's often used as a condiment on desserts like pancakes, waffles, etc. Maple syrup contains primarily sucrose and water with a little bit of fructose and glucose[1604]. It's quite low in other micronutrients but it does contain some chromium and manganese[1605].

  o Studies show maple syrup has a lower glycemic index than table sugar and can help to balance blood sugar better than regular sucrose[1606,1607,1608]. In mice, maple syrup rich in polyphenols also alleviates dyslipidemia[1609]. Thus, it's the same as with honey – it's better than sugar but it needs to be consumed in small amounts to avoid large glucose excursions.

As you can see, there are some good alternatives to artificial sweeteners in terms of the potential side effects. Granted, honey and maple syrup still raise your blood sugar, which warrants caution. The safest sweeteners appears to be inulin (with the exceptin of the gastrointestinal stress) stevia and monk fruit. You can also use natural substances like glycine and myo-inositol, which can lower blood sugar, but also taste sweet.

How Salt Deficiency Promotes Sugar Cravings

Sugar cravings may also be partly caused by salt deficiency[1610]. Getting depleted of salt due to exercise, diuretics or a low salt diet promotes the appetite for salt by activating dopamine reward centers in the brain[1611,1612,1613]. Without this response, we wouldn't be motivated to seek out this essential nutrient[1614]. Unfortunately, **salt deficiency does not only sensitize the brain to salt, but it also increases the addictive potential of many drugs like cocaine and medications, such as Adderall and opiates through cross-sensitization**[1615,1616,1617,1618]. Thus, sodium depletion not only increases cravings for salt, but it also makes dopaminergic substances like sugar and drugs more addictive. Furthermore, your body has a 'salt thermostat' that autoregulates your desire for salt, shifting you from 'liking' to 'aversion' once you've gotten enough sodium[1619]. Excess salt intake is possible but usually only if you're overeating hyperpalatable ultra-processed foods that hijack leptin signaling and dopamine.

Salt does enhance the flavor of your food and can promote satiety[1620]. Consuming something salty until satiety eventually reduces its pleasantness because of the saltiness, resulting in cessation of eating, which is a term called sensory-specific satiety[1621,1622]. This phenomenon of sensory-specific satiety applies to all other flavors as well – if you eat something with the same taste profile and flavor it will eventually lead to satiety but if you mix things up, i.e. a crunchy appetizer, salty main course and sweet dessert, you can continue eating[1623,1624]. People say 'there's always room for dessert' and that's true because of this fundamental biological aspect of our bodies. Thus, if you're struggling with appetite and overeating, then try to minimize the range of flavors and taste profiles to reach satiety faster.

Chapter 9: Type 1 Diabetes and Autoimmune Disorders

Without a family history of Type 1 diabetes, the risk of developing it is about 1 out of 250. However, if one of your parents has Type 1 diabetes, your own risk increases from 0.4% to 1-9%. In the case of siblings, if one sibling has Type 1 diabetes, the risk of their brother or sister having Type 1 diabetes is 6-9% and with an identical twin the risk is 30-70%[1625]. Around 50% of the heritable diabetes is due to variations in three Major Histocompatability Complex (MHC) class II genes, which are involved in antigen presenting. They are Human Leukocyte Antigen (HLA)-DRB1, HLA-DQA1 and HLA-DQB1. The variations specifically linked to Type 1 diabetes are HLA-DR3 and HLA-DR4-HLA-DQ8, which are more common in European descendants. HLA-DR15-HLA-DQ6 variation is linked to a reduced risk of Type 1 diabetes. There are still dozens more immune system genes associated with a higher risk of Type 1 diabetes.

In 70-90% of Type 1 diabetes cases, the pancreatic beta cells get destroyed by the person's own immune system, which is called symptomatic Type 1 diabetes[1626]. Many months, or even years before this happens, the body starts producing beta-cell targeting antibodies. Individuals with more antibodies or who develop them earlier in life are at a higher risk of Type 1 diabetes. The trigger for these antibodies is not fully clear and it's hypothesized to be caused by environmental and genetic factors[1627]. In the remaining 10-30% of cases, the beta cells get destroyed without any signs of autoimmunity, which is called idiopathic Type 1 diabetes. **After the detection of hyperglycemia, Type 1 diabetes is diagnosed by the presence of autoantibodies in the blood**[1628]. Most tests detect antibodies for glutamic acid decarboxylase, the beta cell cytoplasm or insulin, which are targeted in 80% of Type 1 diabetes cases. Very low C-peptide levels are also indicative of Type 1 diabetes as C-peptide is a marker of insulin release (less insulin gets released as more beta cells are destroyed).

In this chapter, we're going to discuss the connection between autoimmune disorders and Type 1 diabetes. Granted, Type 1 diabetes has a major genetic component that we have not been able to tackle in modern medicine. **Type 1 diabetes is also considered to be irreversible due to the damage to the beta cells**[1629]. So, unfortunately, currently there is no cure for Type 1 diabetes. There are a few clinical trials underway aiming at restoring the body's natural insulin production[1630]. However, it's still possible to manage Type 1 diabetes with the proper lifestyle, diet and insulin pumps. The purpose here is to reveal some insight into the pathology of developing autoimmune disorders and how to manage them to the best of our ability.

What Are Autoimmune Disorders

During the late 19th and early 20th century, it was not considered possible for the immune system to attack itself as we know what happens in autoimmunity[1631]. However, in 1904, Ernest Witebrsky demonstrated that autoimmunity is an actual phenomenon by finding that the red blood cells of paroxysmal cold hemoglobinuria patients reacted with another substance in serum[1632]. Today, it's known that autoimmunity is an innate quality of the immune systems of vertebrates, which is named natural autoimmunity[1633].

Your immune system is one of the most important things for your overall health and longevity as it directly protects you from different pathogens, bacteria, and viruses daily. 'Immunity' comes from the Latin word *'immunis',* meaning 'exempt'. Without a robust and active immune system, you would be constantly sick and potentially die to any random infection. At the same time, **it's as vital**

for the body to differentiate itself from the foreign intruders. This is the essence of autoimmunity – the immune system attacking its own body. Small amounts of autoimmunity have a protective effect by rapidly recognizing unknown antibodies during early infection[1634]. The immune system's helper T cells remember that information and gain a head start against novel viruses that the body hasn't encountered before. This process creates a little bit of collateral damage to the body but in moderation it's not harmful. However, when the immune system can't recognize the difference between self vs non-self, then it can become a problem. At that point, various autoimmune diseases can set in. There are over 100 autoimmune diseases, including Type 1 diabetes, Celiac disease, Graves' disease, multiple sclerosis (MS), inflammatory bowel disease (IBD), rheumatoid arthritis (RA), Hashimoto's disease, lupus and psoriasis to name a few. In the U.S. up to 50 million people are affected by autoimmune disorders[1635].

There are genetic factors that promote autoimmunity but the main reason for its onset is the failed regulation in immune system responses, which creates an imbalance between effector immune cells[1636]. The underlying mechanism to autoimmune responses is the defective removal of self-reactive lymphocytes, like B cells (antibody producers), T cells (killer/helper cells) and natural killer (NK) cells[1637]. Self-antigen abnormalities appear to also be involved, which activates unconventional T cells with pathogenic potential[1638]. Dendritic cells (DCs) are phagocytes that keep T cells in balance and hold autoimmunity at bay[1639,1640] by deleting T cells or generating regulatory T cells[1641]. **In essence, during any immune response the body mounts a certain amount of damaging killer cells to deal with the potential pathogens and the regulatory cells keep them in check to make sure they don't get out of hand. If an imbalance gets created with too many killer cells in relation to**

regulatory cells, autoimmune damage begins to set in, which over time leads to a full-blown autoimmune disorder.

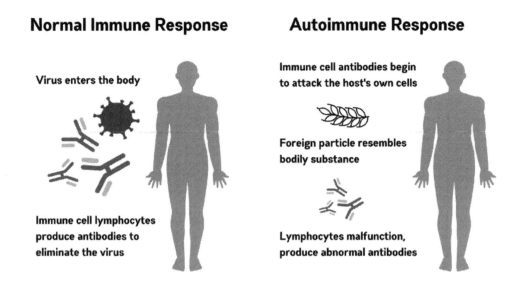

Adapted From: Roberts (2023) 'What Are Autoimmune Disorders?', Very well Health, Dotdash Media, Inc., Accessed Online March 8th 2023: https://www.verywellhealth.com/autoimmune-diseases-overview-3232654

The immune system is divided into the innate immune system (IIS), which is the one you're born with[1642], and the adaptive immune system (AIS), which is what you build throughout your lifetime from exposure to different pathogens[1643]. Autoimmunity can be the result of disorders in both. Autoimmune disorders have been rapidly rising in developed countries since the 1980s. In 1989, the 'hygiene hypothesis' was introduced, which questions whether the higher use of antibiotics, antiseptics, vaccines and sterilized environments play a role in the rise of autoimmunity in children[1644]. Early-life use of antibiotics is linked with inflammatory bowel disease[1645]. **It's been shown that children who aren't exposed to microbes early in life are much more likely to get some sort of**

autoimmune disease[1646]. Infants born via C-section are also more prone to chronic diseases like diabetes, obesity and asthma, which is thought to be due to not coming out of the womb through the mother's vagina that would encoat the child with her vaginal microbiome[1647]. A reduction in bacterial infections, or a decrease in the intake of micronutrients (think vitamin A and D), have been suggested as potential contributors to the rise in Type 1 diabetes[1648]. Obesity, which is considered to be a nutritional disease (overfed but undernourished), is a risk factor for developing autoimmunity as well[1649].

Despite all the different types of autoimmune diseases, they all seem to follow 3 main stages: initiation, propagation, and in some cases resolution[1650]. Here is an overview of them:

1. **Initiation.** This is when autoimmunity officially begins but the disease starts developing well before any visible symptoms, which makes it hard to pin point the exact timing of this stage. There are both genetic and environmental factors that trigger initiation of an autoimmune response.

    a. **Genetic polymorphisms linked to autoimmune diseases** are related to the major histocompatibility complex (MHC), T cell receptors and immunoglobulins[1651]. For example, PTPN22 in humans is linked to type 1 diabetes, rheumatoid arthritis, lupus, Hashimoto's thyroiditis, Graves' disease, multiple sclerosis, and Addison's disease[1652,1653,1654,1655,1656].

        i. Risk alleles in CD25 (rs2104286), which is a protein that assembles Interleukin-2's receptor, are associated with multiple sclerosis and Type 1 diabetes[1657].

        ii. HLA DR (Human Leukocyte Antigen – DR isotype) is an MHC class II cell surface receptor encoded by the HLA complex on chromosome6 region 6p21.31. HLA DR2 is positively correlated with systemic lupus, narcolepsy, and multiple sclerosis[1658]. HLA DR3 is correlated with Type 1 diabetes and Sjogren syndrome[1659,1660]. HLA DR4 is correlated with rheumatoid arthritis, Type 1 diabetes, and pemphigus vulgaris[1661,1662].

b. **Environmental factors that can trigger autoimmunity** include infections, food particles, stress, man-made chemicals, UV radiation-induced programmed cell death and heavy metal exposure[1663,1664,1665]. A lot of foods can also promote autoimmune diseases through intestinal permeability, such as gluten, grains, nightshade, lectins, dairy, sugar, and others[1666,1667,1668,1669]. Certain foods can 'cross-react' and create a similar autoimmune response to gluten in susceptible individuals, such as milk, coffee, corn, rice, and millet[1670].

2. **Propagation.** When the initial inflammation and tissue damage creates a vicious loop of more inflammation. The most common mediators of this inflammation are tumor necrosis factor alpha (TNF-alpha), NLRP3 inflammasome, nuclear factor kB (NF-kB), interleukin-12, interleukin-17A and interleukin-23[1671,1672]. A higher ratio of killer T cells to regulatory T cells also drives autoimmunity[1673].

3. **Resolution.** If the inflammation gets put out, autoimmunity may resolve. This is achieved mainly by limiting killer cell activity and promoting regulatory mechanisms. Regulatory T cells (Tregs) are responsible for controlling the immune response to self and foreign particles (antigens). Tregs are produced by the thymus and secondary lymph organs. Autoimmune inflammation activates Tregs, which starts to control

inflammation and develop immunological memory[1674]. There are other inhibitory receptors that inhibit autoimmune reactions as well, such as CTLA-4 and PD-1[1675].

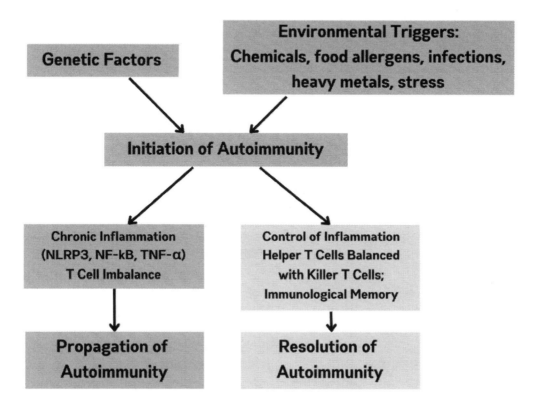

There are certain medications that damage the beta cells or suppress insulin production, resulting in something similar to Type 1 diabetes[1676,1677]. These negative side effects occur in a small amount of people, usually 5-10%. Here are the pharmaceuticals linked with medication-induced diabetes and their hypothetical mechanisms for that[1678]:

Insulin Resistance and Deficiency	Insulin Resistance	Insulin Deficiency
Atypical antipsychotics	Beta-blockers	Beta-blockers
Glucocorticoids	Growth hormone	Calcineurin inhibitors
Nicotinic acid	Megestrol	Diazoxide
Protease inhibitors (first generation)	Thiazide diuretics	Didanosine
Statins		Diphenylhydantoin
		Gatifloxicin
		L-asparaginase
		Pentamidine

Managing Autoimmune Responses and Disorders

Historically, autoimmune disorders are treated with immunosuppressive, anti-inflammatory, and palliative medicine. The most important thing for resolving autoimmunity appears to be lowering inflammation and thus suppressing the flames of autoimmune reactions[1679]. That's why the Standard American Diet, containing a lot of processed carbs, sugar, and seed oils can promote autoimmunity due to its inflammatory effect[1680]. Being obese also undermines cellular immunity to infections and creates a state of chronic low-grade inflammation[1681]. Thus, the key to managing autoimmune reactions is managing inflammation.

There is a direct link between inflammation in the body and the gut microbiome[1682]. In fact, up to 70% of your immune system is located in the gut[1683]. The microbiome helps to identify pathogens and differentiate them from host cells, which plays a vital role in both innate and adaptive immunity[1684]. It's been found that microbiota maturation through early-life nutrition shapes life-long immunity and reduces the risk of many chronic diseases[1685]. An imbalance in the microbiome, also known as a dysbiosis, promotes inflammation and increases the risk of illness, including autoimmune disorders[1686,1687,1688]. The primary way we can interface and interact with our microbiome is through diet and what we eat.

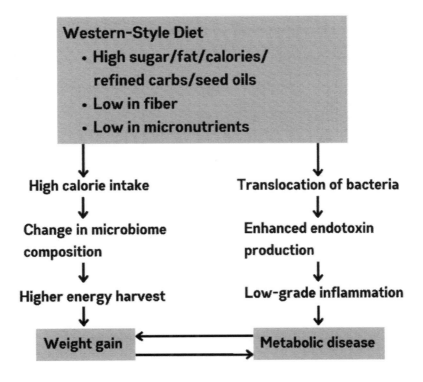

Adapted From: Bischoff et al (2014)

Research has implicated the microbiome with autoimmunity as well with Type 1 diabetes being associated with lower microbial diversity[1689,1690,1691,1692]. Children with Type 1 diabetes have higher levels of certain bacteria like *Globicatella sanguinis, Dialister invisus* and *Bifidobacterium longum[1693]* and less *Bifidobacterium pseudocatenulatum* and *Bifidobacterium adolescentis,* as opposed to healthy controls[1694]. A lower amount of *Akkermansia, Faecalibacterium*, and *Bifidobacterium* can increase the risk of allergies via modulation of T cells[1695]. *Lactobacilli* modulate pro-inflammatory signaling factors like TNF-alpha[1696]. You can get *Lactobacillus* from sauerkraut, yogurt, tempeh, miso, natto, kimchi, and other fermented foods.

An elimination diet can be another potential solution for managing autoimmunity symptoms. If some foods are constantly triggering your immune system, then eliminating them can be the solution. Many people don't fully understand what foods trigger an allergic reaction in them due to never having taken the time to look into it. The most common food allergens include gluten, eggs, fish, nightshade like potatoes and tomatoes, shellfish, peanuts, soy, grains, rye, dairy, etc. Start by eliminating one food item at a time for a few weeks from your diet. If your allergic condition gets better then you have found your answer. You can always ask your doctor to do an allergy test as well.

Why you may be getting allergic and autoimmune reactions to certain foods might have to do with intestinal permeability also called leaky gut syndrome[1697,1698]. **Intestinal permeability or leaky gut is associated with autoimmune disesases and the development of several inflammatory diseases, including Type 1 diabetes**[1699,1700,1701]. In rats, increased intestinal permeability is an early sign of diabetes[1702]. Many things can promote intestinal permeability, such as food allergens, chronic stress, high sugar intake, excessive alcohol consumpion, and inflammation[1703,1704,1705,1706,1707]. **Long-term use of non-steroidal anti-inflammatory drugs (NSAIDS) like aspirin and ibuprofen**

have also been found to increase intestinal permeability[1708]. One of the best known markers of intestinal permeability is a protein called zonulin[1709,1710]. In one study on 339 type 1 diabetics, 42% had elevated zonulin levels[1711]. You want to prevent leaky gut by managing stress and consuming foods that heal the gut lining. Bone broth, tendons, and ligaments have collagen and glutamine and glycine can promote tissue repair. Butyrate is also essential for feeding the colon. It's the main energy source for cells in the large intestine. You can get butyrate primarily from the fermentation of fiber, beans, and legumes but also ghee and butter. An antioxidant called quercetin can also strengthen intestinal tight junctions and repair the gut[1712], which you can obtain from onions and vegetables.

Low vitamin D levels are associated with a higher risk of developing autoimmune diseases[1713]. Vitamin D acts on natural killer cells and T cells[1714]. Most cells, especially immune cells, have vitamin D receptors, which regulate the immune system[1715]. These receptors, however, are stimulated by active vitamin D (called calcitriol), which requires magnesium. Thus, to have adequate vitamin D levels, you also need magnesium. Mutations in the vitamin D3 gene *CYP27B1* are correlated with an increased risk of Type 1 diabetes[1716], Addison's disease[1717], Hashimoto's thyroiditis and Graves' disease[1718].

- Exposure to little sunlight and higher latitude living are thought to increase multiple sclerosis risk[1719]. Seasonality and the corresponding decline in UV light has been seen to increase multiple sclerosis activity[1720,1721]. Data from over 321 European studies have found a correlation between low UV light exposure and a 100-fold increase in the risk of multiple sclerosis[1722]. Additionally, childhood and occupational sunlight exposure is inversely correlated with multiple sclerosis risk and mortality[1723,1724].

- Low exposure to sunlight and low UV irradiation are also considered to be a major component of Type 1 diabetes risk[1725]. Type 1 diabetes onset peaks between the months of October and January and reaches its lowest point during the summer in the northern hemisphere, whereas in the southern hemisphere the opposite pattern occurs[1726]. Supplementing with vitamin D3 in children correlates with an 88% reduction in the risk of Type 1 diabetes[1727]. In Type 1 diabetes, CD4+ T lymphocytes turn pathological and auto-reactive, which damages healthy tissue[1728]. The same thing happens in multiple sclerosis[1729].

Given the strong link between vitamin D, UV light and autoimmune disease risk, sunlight should be considered an important environmental factor for autoimmunity[1730]. The current guidelines show that vitamin D levels below 30 nmol/L is characterized as deficiency, 30-50 nmol/L as insufficient, and above 50 nmol/L as sufficient[1731]. However, the appropriate ranges for autoimmunity are not known. Reaching a vitamin D blood level of 75 nmol/L from supplementing 2,000 IU/day of vitamin D has been shown to maintain intestinal permeability, improve life quality and reduce markers of disease in people with Crohn's disease compared to those below 75 nmol/L[1732]. Thus, the recommended vitamin D ranges are between 50-150 nmol/L.

Vitamin D deficiency is extremely common, especially in regions where the winters are long without a lot of sun. Obese people have 50% less bioavailable vitamin D compared to non-obese individuals and are 3x more likely to be deficient in vitamin D[1733]. This has to do with the fat-soluble vitamin D being stored in the adipose tissue instead of circulating in the bloodstream. Here are someguidelines for managing your vitamin D levels:

- **Check your vitamin D levels.** The optimal range is between 100-150 nmol/L or 40-60 ng/ml. If you're under 30-40 ng/ml, then consider supplementing with vitamin D3.

- **Eat vitamin D rich foods**. Such as egg yolks, cod liver oil, fatty fish especially wild salmon and sardines, liver and salmon roe. Omega-3 fatty acids have also been shown to help with autoimmune conditions, such as rheumatoid arthritis, inflammatory bowel disease, asthma and psoriasis[1734].

- **Supplement vitamin D3 as needed**. How much should you take depends on your current blood vitamin D levels and degree of deficiency.

  - If you're under 20 ng/ml or 50 nmol/L, then you will likely need 6,000-10,000 IU daily for a few weeks until you reach a level of 30-50 ng/ml or 70-125 nmol/L. After that, a daily dose of 2,000-4,000 IU is needed to maintain adequate levels.

  - If you're between 20-29 ng/ml or 50-75 nmol/L, then you will likely need 4,000-6,000 IUs every day for a few weeks to reach 30 ng/ml or 75 nmol/L and above.

  - If you're between 30-50 ng/ml or 75-125 nmol/L, then stick to a maintenance dose of 2,000-4,000 IUs daily.

  - If you're over 50 ng/ml or 125 nmol/L, then you don't need to supplement vitamin D, but should still continue eating vitamin D rich foods and getting natural sunlight.

  - Vitamin D toxicity is rare and tends to happen only if supplementing with extremely high doses (> 10,000 IU) for many months[1735].

- **Spend more time being outside.** Supplementing vitamin D isn't enough – you also need the other health benefits of UV radiation from sunlight. As long as you avoid getting sunburnt, the sun can provide a lot of improvements to your health, especially a rise in nitric oxide, which helps to lower blood pressure.

- **During the winter months, if you live up north, then you need more vitamin D.** A good maintenance dose for vitamin D-sufficient individuals is 2,000-4,000 IU/day, but someone who's vitamiin D insufficient may need up to 7,500-10,000 IUs a day for several weeks. During the summer, you need less vitamin D, perhaps 1,000-2,000 IUs a day.

- **Other fat soluble vitamins like A, K and E help to optimize vitamin D status**[1736]. Eat foods like organ meat (liver) for the vitamin A and K and fatty fish and nuts for vitamin E. Extra virgin olive oil is another anti-inflammatory fat that's been shown to lower pro-inflammatory genes in patients with metabolic syndrome due to its high polyphenol content[1737].

- **Get magnesium.** Most adults should get at least 400 mg a of magnesium a day to maintain optimal magnesium status and activate vitamin D.

Zinc is another essential nutrient for the immune system[1738]. A zinc deficiency creates a pro-inflammatory environment and weakens immunity because it governs over 300 enzymatic reactions[1739]. Since the 1970s, zinc deficiency has been found to be linked to different autoimmune disorders, such as Type 1 diabetes, rheumatoid arthritis, multiple sclerosis, systemic lupus, hepatitis, Celiac's disease and Hashimoto's thyroiditis[1740]. **A zinc deficiency creates an imbalance between killer and regulatory T cells, Th1 and Th2 cells and reduces natural killer cell function**[1741]. This can weaken your overall immune system against foreign pathogens but also make the immune system more likely to cause friendly fire against host cells. Zinc supplementation or eating more high zinc foods can fix these imbalances[1742]. The highest zinc foods are meat and fish.

Consuming antioxidants, however, hasn't been found to have a significant impact on the onset of Type 1 diabetes[1743]. At the same time, polyphenols, which are compounds in certain foods with anti-inflammatory properties, have been found to be linked to lower rates of inflammatory diseases and reduced all-cause mortality[1744]. Polyphenols are high in plants that are environmentally challenged with heat, cold or dehydration and they're found the most in dark pigmented vegetables, berries and fruits, such as broccoli, artichoke, leafy greens, raspberries, blueberries, pomegranate, olives, coffee and beans. A 2010 study showed that the highest polyphenol content can be found in cloves, peppermint, star anise, cocoa powder and oregano[1745].

There are many polyphenolic compounds with a track record of improving inflammatory and autoimmune conditions. Ginger supplementation has been shown to improve symptoms of rheumatoid arthritis by lowering inflammation[1746]. Naringenin, which is a compound found in citrus fruits, inhibits defective T cells, and supports T cell homeostasis restoration[1747]. In mice, naringenin has been found to alleviate autoimmune encephalomyelitis by regulating autoimmune inflammatory responses[1748]. EGCG, the main polyphenol in green tea, increases regulatory T cells and helps maintain an optimal T cell balance[1749]. Curcumin or turmeric has been shown to decrease the symptoms of rheumatoid arthritis, multiple sclerosis, psoriasis and inflammatory bowel disease by regulating NF-kB signaling and inflammatory cytokines[1750]. Some individuals may react negatively to different polyphenols due to issues with their gut microbiome. Thus, everyone should approach their diet and supplementation individually.

How Hyperglycemia Exacerbates Inflammation

There is another pro-inflammatory molecule that gets activated during an infection called HMGB1 (high mobility group box 1). HMGB1 is a damage-associated molecular pattern (DAMP) protein and it binds to chromosomal DNA, toll-like receptor 3 (TLR3), TLR4 and the receptor for advanced glycation end products (RAGE), activating pro-inflammatory inflammasomes NF-kB and NLRP-3[1751,1752]. Many conditions of low-grade inflammation have been found to be involved with HMGB1 activity, such as obesity[1753], insulin resistance, diabetes[1754], thrombosis-related diseases[1755] and polycystic ovary disease[1756].

Plasma HMGB1 levels have been found to be significantly correlated with Type 1 diabetes by impairing regulatory T cell function[1757] and Type 2 diabetes via inflammation and insulin resistance[1758,1759,1760,1761]. Plasma HMGB1 levels were found to be positively correlated with a higher waist to hip ratio, blood pressure, HOMA-IR, and triglycerides as well. During the progression of Type 1 diabetes, damaged beta cells and immune cells can continuously release HMGB1 as an innate alarmin[1762]. In mice, blocking HMGB1 secretion delays diabetes onset[1763] and can attenuate diabetic neuropathy[1764]. Anti-HMGB1 therapy has also been shown to prevent autoimmunity after pancreatic islet transplantation in mice and humans[1765,1766,1767].

Both hyperglycemia/diabetes and HMGB1 increase expression of the receptor for advanced glycation end products (RAGE)[1768,1769]. As the name suggests, RAGE enables more advanced glycation end products (AGEs) to attach to cell surfaces, which exacerbates inflammation and diabetic complications[1770]. Advanced Glycation End Products (AGEs) are proteins that become glycated after exposed to sugar through what's called the Maillard reaction[1771]. The biggest source of AGEs tends to be diet because of the quality of ingredients and cooking methods used. Low levels of AGEs are generally fine and are not an issue because the body has defense mechanisms and antioxidant systems to eliminate them. Chronic AGE accumulation, however, will promote inflammation and cellular damage[1772].

The chronic inflammation from RAGE-induced glycation is thought to cause organ damage and even organ failure[1773]. RAGE mediates sepsis-triggered amyloid-β accumulation, which promotes neurodegeneration and cognitive impairment[1774]. RAGE has been found to be involved with arthritis[1775] and atherosclerosis[1776]. AGEs are found in the progression of many age-related diseases, such as Alzheimer's[1777], cardiovascular disease[1778], renal dysfunction[1779], diabetes, insulin resistance, and stroke[1780]. AGEs directly directly cross-link certain proteins like collagen to promote vascular stiffness and thus affect vascular structure negatively[1781]. AGEs also cause glycation of LDL cholesterol, which promotes its oxidation[1782]. Oxidized LDL is a major risk factor in atherosclerosis[1783]. Furthermore, **circulating levels of AGEs and RAGE isoforms are associated with all-cause mortality and cardiovascular disease complications in Type 2 diabetes[1784].**

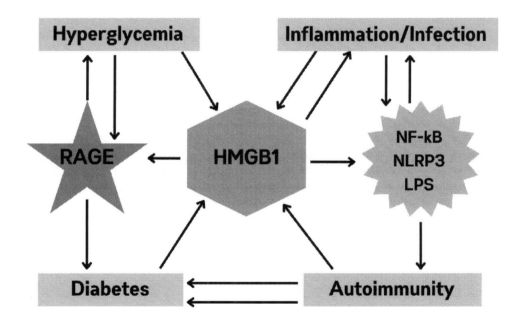

Foods high in fat and protein are more suspectible to AGE formation during cooking, especially when broiled, deep fryed or grilled at high temperatures[1785]. **However, you absorb only a very small amount of AGEs from diet and directly from food sources.** It's also been found that vegetarians have higher concentrations of AGEs compared to non-vegetarians[1786]. Therefore, AGEs you get externally aren't nearly as important as the ones you create internally. The *'fructositis'* hypothesis states that a higher fructose to glucose ratio promotes an intestinal environment that promotes the formation of AGEs and other proinflammatory cytokines internally. Glycation of fructose in early research was also drastically underestimated because of inaccurate measuring techniques[1787].

A diet high in AGEs is considered to start above 15,000 kilo units of AGEs per day[1788]. Here's a list of the amount of AGEs in common foods:

- Almonds (30g): 1642 kU

- Avocado (30g): 473 kU

- Cashews (30g): 2019 kU

- Peanut Butter (30g): 2255 kU

- Beef (90g): 1468 kU

- Chicken, boiled in water (90g): 1011 kU

- Chicken, roasted then BBQ (90g): 7922 kU

- Fried Bacon (13g): 11905 kU

- Raw Lamb (90g): 743 kU

- Raw Salmon (90g): 472 kU

- Broiled Salmon (90g): 3012 kU

- White Cheese (30g): 2603 kU

- 1 fried egg: 1,237 kU

- Whole Wheat Bread (30g): 16 kU

- 1 tablespoon of cream: 325 kU

- ¼ cup (59 ml) of whole milk: 3 kU

- Celery (100g): 43 kU

- Grilled Vegetables (100g): 226 kU

It's been found that following a low AGE diet for 4 weeks improves insulin sensitivity in overweight women[1789]. An isocaloric and macronutrient-matched low AGE diet for 2 weeks improves insulin sensitivity in overweight men compared to a high AGE diet[1790]. **Low AGE diets can improve cardiometabolic parameters in people with and without Type 2 diabetes**[1791]. The improvements in insulin resistance and total systemic AGE load on low AGE diets occur in healthy and diseased individuals independent of physical activity, calorie intake and adiposity[1792]. Thus, it's worthwhile to consider your cooking methods and how you prepare your foods, especially if they're high in AGEs.

Calorie restriction has been shown to reduce AGE formation[1793,1794,1795]. It's also one of the few interventions shown to reverse biomarkers of actual biological aging in humans[1796,1797]. The reason why restricting calories inhibits AGE formation has to do with how it increases the body's antioxidant defences like glutathione[1798]. Type 2 diabetics have lower glutathione status and higher amount of AGEs[1799]. With increased glutathione, the body has more ability to counteract glycation and oxidation, whereas with low glutathione the susceptibility for glycation is much higher[1800,1801]. Thus, when in a calorie deficit, even the foods with more AGEs have less of a harmful effect on the body. In a calorie surplus, the body's antioxidant capacity gets exceeded, leaving you more vulnerable to oxidative stress and AGE damage.

Dietary AGEs in excess could be problematic and certainly won't make things better. However, they still have a limited effect on your glycemic control and metabolic health. The far worse contributor to the adverse consequences of AGEs is already existing inflammation and elevated blood sugar levels. This is where we have to focus on the environment or the internal milieu of the body in which these foods are being consumed.

Inhibiting RAGE and improving glycemic control reduces the expression of HMGB1 and its pro-inflammatory effects[1802]. Thus, controlling levels of AGEs, RAGE and HMGB1 can have therapeutic value for diabetes and its related conditions. HMGB1 is already considered a drug option for hyperinflammatory conditions[1803]. Blocking HMGB1 expression can extinguish excess inflammation and slow down the progression of disease. Additionally, inhibiting the other receptors that HMGB1 binds to like lipopolysaccharides (LPS), TLR2, TLR4 and interleukins should also be considered.

Endotoxins also known as lipopolysaccharides (LPS) are large molecules made of lipids and polysaccharides found in the outer membrane of gram-negative bacteria[1804]. They activate innate immunity, via pro-inflammatory cytokines[1805,1806], and can promote sepsis, intra-vascular coagulation and organ failure[1807,1808]. Endotoxemia is thought to originate from small intestine bacterial overgrowth (SIBO) and increased intestinal permeability[1809]. **Epidemiological studies link increased endotoxemia with obesity and insulin resistance**[1810]. It might be more so the result of poor dietary habits and just eating junk rather than the cause. However, in germ-free mice, injecting purified endotoxin from E. coli induces obesity and insulin resistance[1811]. So, there is likely a direct causal role as well.

Endotoxins are linked to certain pathogens like *Salmonella, E. coli, Haemophilus influenzae, and Vibrio cholerae*[1812]. Sugar and artificial sweeteners lower the body's reaction to endotoxin and promote its spread[1813]. Raw sugar contains 100 mg of E. coli endotoxin per gram whereas beet sugar has less than 1 ng/g[1814]. Thus, sugar from whole foods like fruit, tubers and vegetables is neglible. In fact, the indigestible fiber and phenolic compounds in carrots prevent the absorption of endotoxins in the intestine[1815]. Slicing some carrots into your food or having them as a snack on an empty stomach is great for lowering endotoxemia. **Magnesium deficiency increases NF-kB and HMGB1 secretion from LPS-infected macrophages[1816].**

These pro-glycation and pro-inflammatory molecules – HMGB1, TLR4, LPS, NLRP3, AGEs, RAGE and KF-kB - all interact with each other and exacerbate each other's harmful effects on diabetes and autoimmunity. Here are some nutraceuticals that can inhibit these inflammasomes and thus lower inflammation:

- **Pyridoxamine**, which is a naturally occurring isoform of vitamin B6, can also scavenge reactive oxygen species and inhibit AGE formation[1817]. Oral pyridoxamine has shown some promise in phase II clinical trials on diabetic neuropathy[1818].

- **Rosemary and other spices like cinnamon, cloves, marjoram and tarragon** have been found to inhibit and protect against advanced glycation end-products (AGEs)[1819,1820]. Their protective effects are mediated by their large polyphenol content[1821]. Rosemary also lowers fasting glucose, cholesterol, and triglycerides[1822]. Whenever you're cooking something at high temperatures, especially meat or starchy carbs, you should add some rosemary to them as it can protect against some of the oxidation and glycation. Other phenolic compounds that show pro-inhibiting effects on AGE formation include blueberry extract and various flavonoids like quercetin, lutein and rutin[1823,1824].

- **Glycine** is an amazing amino acid for protecting against AGEs and hyperglycemia because it suppresses AGE formation, boosts glutathione, supports collagen synthesis and lowers blood sugar levels[1825,1826]. Supplemental GlyNAC (Glycine and N-acetylcysteine) at a dose of 100 mg/kg/day of both glycine and NAC has been found to lower insulin resistance by 22% after just 14 days in Type 2 diabetics[1827].

- **Carnosine** is an amino acid that has inhibitory effects on AGE formation and has antioxidant properties[1828,1829]. In Type 2 diabetics, 500 mg of L-carnosine lowers fasting glucose, triglycerides, AGEs, and TNF-alpha[1830]. Taking carnosine as a supplement isn't that effective at raising carnosine levels in the body, but **beta-alanine, another amino acid, does increase carnosine levels**[1831]. Beta-alanine, as well as L-histidine (the other amino acid making up carnosine), have been shown to lower AGEs as well[1832].

- **Alpha-lipoic acid (ALA) has also been shown to inhibit AGE glycation through increased glutathione**[1833,1834].

- **Glycyrrhizin** is a HMGB1 antagonist that lowers its expression[1835,1836]. Glycyrrhizin is the primary sweet-tasting compound of licorice root. It also has inhibitory effects on LPS-induced inflammation[1837,1838]. In mice, glycyrrhizin showed anti-inflammatory and protective effects on LPS-induced acute lung injury[1839]. Glycyrrhizin has also been seen to inhibit LPS-induced inflammatory response in mouse endometrial epithelial cells by inhibiting TLR4 signaling pathway[1840].

- **Ferulic acid**, a plant phenolic compound, has been shown to decrease HMGB1, IL-6, IL-8 and LPS[1841,1842,1843]. In mice, ferulic acid protects against LPS-induced kidney injury by suppressing inflammation and upregulating antioxidants[1844]. Ferulic acid can also have protective effects against high glucose-induced protein glycation and lipid peroxidation[1845]. Foods with ferulic acid are vegetables, the bran of cereal grains, barley, flaxseed, legumes, and beans[1846,1847]. Flaxseed lignans can also decrease HMGB1 and several pro-inflammatory cytokines[1848].

- **Ginseng** reduces LPS-induced release of HMGB1[1849]. *Angelica sinensis* (also called dong quai or female ginseng) protects mice against lethal endotoxemia and sepsis by decreasing HMGB1[1850]. Korean red ginseng reduces HMGB1 by suppressing pro-inflammatory cytokines[1851]. Using ginger extract in root canals has been shown to eliminate[1852].

- **Green tea** might decrease LPS-induced release of HMGB1 and other pro-inflammatory cytokines in patients of sepsis[1853]. Supplemental green tea extract inhibits HMGB1 release in rats exposed to cigarette smoke[1854]. EGCG, the main polyphenol in green tea, reduces HMGB1/RAGE expression and alleviates lung injury in PM 2.5-exposed asthmatic rats[1855]. EGCG also stimulates autophagy, the clearance of cell particles, and reduces HMGB1 in endotoxin-stimulated macrophages[1856].

- **Coffee** intake lowers AGE formation[1857]. The reason has to do with coffee's high polyphenol content (mainly chlorogenic acid and its transformation into ferulic acid)[1858]. Black coffee alone contains very few AGEs as well but adding milk and sugar increases its AGE content[1859].

- **Probiotics like *Lactobacillus rhamnosus* and *Bifidobacterium Breve*** inhibit HMGB1 and pro-inflammatory cytokines on macrophages exposed to cigarette smoke[1860]. You can get them from foods like kefir, yogurt, kimchi, sauerkraut, miso, natto and tempeh.

- **DHA (docosahexaenoic acid)** supplementation can lower HMGB1 and prevent LPS-induced accumulation of macrophages[1861]. DHA can also suppress pro-inflammatory mediators produced by LPS[1862]. Dietary omega-3 fatty acids also decrease TLR4 receptor recruitment, which suppresses pro-inflammatory pathways[1863,1864].

- **Chloroquine, dexamethasone, and gold sodium thiomalate** block extracellular release of HMGB1 in a dose-dependent way[1865]. In mice, chloroquine inhibits HMGB1 inflammatory signaling and protects against lethal sepsis[1866].

- **Quercetin** hampers HMGB1 release and pro-inflammatory function by LPS[1867]. In mice, quercetin mitigates liver fibrosis through HMGB1/TLR2/TLR4/NF-kB signaling[1868].

- **Vitamin D** deficiency is linked with higher inflammation in coronary arteries caused by HMGB1[1869]. In asthmatic mice, the HMGB1/TLR4/NF-κB signaling pathway has a major role in asthma pathogenesis and vitamin D has a regulatory effect on this pathway[1870]. Supplementing vitamin D for 12 weeks combined with Nordic walking training has been seen to reduce HMGB1 and IL-6 in elderly women[1871]. Vitamin D and vitamin D receptor signaling inhibits LPS-induced inflammation in the oral epithelia[1872].

- **Riboflavin (vitamin B2) deficiency** triggers a pathological activation of macrophages, which promotes excessive HMGB1 and TNF-alpha[1873]. Foods high in riboflavin are liver, eggs, dairy, salmon, mushrooms, meat, spinach, and almonds.

Exercise also lowers HMGB1 and leads to a lower baseline level of inflammation. In healthy young men, high-intensity training releases alarmins like HMGB1 and S100A8/A9[1874]. Don't be scared by this, intense physical exertion is supposed to release these danger molecules and damage-associated molecular patterns (DAMPs) like HMGB1 and others. This is supposed to signal the body that it needs to adapt and recover. After a period of rest, all these biomarkers would normalize and the body is stronger than before, which is the phenomenon of hormesis. **If your body is exposed to certain types of stressors in moderate amounts, then it will learn how to deal with them better in the future.** That's how working out works. It has even been shown that pretreatment with exogenous HMGB1 protects against hepatic ischemia/reperfusion injury[1875]. HMGB1 can also support the migration and proliferation of regenerative cells at the sites of injury[1876]. Thus, the dose makes the poison. Regular exercise raises inflammation and other damage molecules acutely but over the long term they will be lower at baseline.

Heat exposure and sauna also work by hormesis use via regulating heat-shock proteins. Administration of exogenous heat-shock protein 70 (HSP-70) 18 hours before injection of endotoxins increases the resilience against an endotoxin challenge[1877]. Heat-shock protein 72 (HSP-72) is protective against LPS-induced oxidative stress and TNF stimulation[1878,1879]. Heat-shock protein 27 (HSP-27) blocks HMGB1 translocation and protects against inflammation[1880]. Pre-treatment with heat in cultured human periodontal ligament cells, lowers HMGB1 and other pro-inflammatory cytokines in response to mechanical stress you'd experience from exercise[1881].

In conclusion, autoimmune disorders are very complicated with a lot of uncontrollable factors, such as certain genetic predispositions. However, there are many controllable variables as well, such as diet, lifestyle, and environment. The purpose of this chapter wasn't to provide a cure for Type 1 diabetes and as of now there is no cure for this condition. Instead, we intended to provide options for managing the inflammatory storm of autoimmunity by supporting the immune system and helping to prevent the onset of chronic inflammatory conditions that exacerbate autoimmune disorders.

Chapter 10: Circadian Rhythms and Glucose Control

Metabolic syndrome and obesity are often thought to be diseases caused by poor diet, overeating, and not exercising. As we've shown throughout this book, those factors are one of the biggest determinants of gaining weight and poor glucose control. However, there is a growing body of research that implicates circadian rhythms and sleeping patterns in the development of diabetes and other chronic ailments as well.

Circadian rhythms are diurnal rhythms connected to the day and night cycles of the environment found in all animals, plants, cyanobacteria and even fungi[1882]. It's been discovered that every cell and organ inside the body has its own circadian clock that connects and corresponds with the master circadian clock inside the brain's hypothalamus called the suprachiasmatic nucleus (SCN)[1883]. The SCN regulates virtually all physiological processes inside the body, including timing of hormone release, metabolism, digestion, and sleep-wakefulness cycles.

Being in synch with our body's natural circadian rhythms maintains optimal cellular functioning and homeostasis, whereas being misaligned promotes disease. **Disruptions in circadian rhythms have been linked to diabetes, cardiovascular disease, obesity, Alzheimer's, and cancer**[1884,1885,1886]. The World Health Organization considers night shift work, which is a form of circadian disruption, a carcinogen because of the way it disrupts the body's natural diurnal rhythms[1887]. Shift work is associated with other diseases, including cardiovascular disease, Alzheimer's, weight gain and diabetes[1888]. Diabetics who work the night shift have a worse glycemic control and higher

HbA1c levels[1889,1890]. Circadian rhythms affect longevity and aging as well by regulating antioxidant systems like Nrf2[1891,1892,1893].

In this chapter, we're going to look at all the ways circadian rhythms affect blood sugar regulation, insulin sensitivity, leptin sensitivity and overall metabolism. We will be also covering information about fixing your circadian rhythms, improving sleep and practicing time-restricted eating, which is also a concept originating from the circadian rhythm research.

The Link Between Circadian Rhythms and Glucose Regulation

The term '*circadian*' was first composed in 1959 by Franz Halberg who derived the word from the Latin words '*circa*' (about) and '*dies*' (day)[1894]. In 1977, the International Committee on Nomenclature of the International Society for Chronobiology created a more official definition, with the word '*circadian*': *relating to biologic variations or rhythms with a frequency of 1 cycle in 24 ± 4-h; circa (about, approximately) and dies (day or 24 h)*[1895].

Early research thought that the daily human circadian rhythm was closer to 25 hours[1896]. However, that was because the participants were exposed to artificial light, which disrupts the natural circadian rhythm. **A 1999 Harvard study showed that the daily circadian rhythm in humans lasts roughly 24 hours and 11 minutes, which mimics the length of the solar day**[1897]. If an organism's circadian clock corresponds with the day and night cycles of the environment, then they're *entrained* and synchronized. That rhythm would persist even without outside signals i.e., being isolated in a bunker without light.

The main circadian rhythm in the human body is the diurnal cortisol-melatonin rhythm. These 2 hormones control your wakefulness as well as sleep wakefulness cycles, thus being the overarching hormones that regulate processes linked to either rest and recovery or physical action.

- **In the morning, cortisol rises to wake you up, increase wakefulness, alertness and give you energy by mobilizing fatty acids and raising blood sugar into the blood stream.** Cortisol, well known as a stress hormone, often gets a bad reputation because stress has a negative connotation. It's true that chronically elevated cortisol can induce insulin resistance and downregulate glucose transporters like GLUT4[1898,1899]. However, from a circadian rhythm perspective, it's vital for optimal health to produce adequate amounts of cortisol in the morning[1900]. **Blunting the morning cortisol response has been associated with insulin resistance and Type 2 diabetes**[1901]. Thus, it's natural and healthy to see a rise in cortisol in the morning. Cortisol starts rising before dawn around 4-6 AM and peaks at 8 AM and then it goes back low and stays low throughout the day[1902].

- **In the evening, however, melatonin production starts to rise, preparing your body for sleep**[1903]. Melatonin is often thought to be the sleep hormone, but it also governs many other important processes, such as reducing inflammation, improving vascular endothelial function, managing the immune system, supporting bone development, protecting against macular degeneration, and regulating longevity pathways, such as sirtuins and autophagy, which makes melatonin quite powerful as an anti-aging hormone[1904,1905,1906,1907,1908,1909,1910,1911,1912]. **Suppression of melatonin at night is linked with obesity, metabolic syndrome, cardiovascular disease, depression, and cancer**[1913,1914,1915,1916].

Melatonin production starts to occur soon after the onset of darkness and reaches its peak from midnight to 2-4 AM[1917].

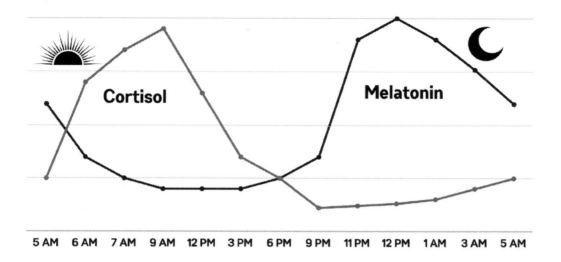

Adapted From: Selmaoui and Touitou (2003)

Naturally, your body is the most insulin sensitive in the earlier part of the day[1918,1919,1920,1921,1922,1923,1924]. It's been found that insulin sensitivity in skeletal muscle peaks during the morning and reduces progressively in the evening independent of training status[1925]. The variation in morning and evening glucose response can be quite significant with pre-diabetic adults showing 40 mg/dl higher oral glucose tolerance test results at 7 PM compared to 7 AM[1926]. These circadian fluctuations of insulin sensitivity are independent of fasting duration[1927]. However, fasting blood sugar levels are typically lower in the afternoon and evening than in the early morning because cortisol is higher in the morning, which mobilizes more glucose into the bloodstream[1928,1929].

Beta-cell responsiveness and the subsequent insulin secretion is higher in the morning than at other times of the day[1930,1931]. However, insulin secretion in response to a meal appears to peak between 12-6 PM[1932,1933]. Total insulin secretion is 16-51% higher in the afternoon or early evening than in the morning[1934]. That rhythmicity contributes to diurnal glucose control. In normal weight individuals, insulin sensitivity is impaired by 34% in the evening compared to the morning[1935]. This difference is explained by other factors, such as circulating free fatty acids, growth hormone and cortisol that inhibit insulin secretion[1936,1937,1938,1939,1940,1941].

Interestingly, the diurnal rhythms in glucose tolerance and insulin sensitivity are either delayed or absent in obese or older individuals[1942,1943]. **People with diabetes have these rhythms delayed by several hours or are absent completely**[1944,1945]. Diabetics lack a diurnal rhythm in peripheral insulin sensitivity and muscle glycogen storage, but they have a clear rhythm in hepatic glucose storage and hepatic insulin sensitivity[1946,1947]. As a result, diabetics have the lowest insulin sensitivity in the morning, making their blood sugar levels rise higher after waking up, and the highest insulin sensitivity around 7 hours after waking up[1948].

Adipose tissue insulin sensitivity is 54% higher at noontime than at midnight[1949]. Thus, it's not recommended to be eating very *large* amounts of carbohydrates later in the day, especially before bed and especially in individuals with already existing diabetes or aspects of insulin resistance. Overall, in healthy individuals, glucose tolerance decreases in the evening and at night.

Lipids and cholesterol metabolism are regulated by the circadian rhythms in several rate-limiting steps[1950,1951]. Cholesterol synthesis peaks at 10 PM in conjunction with melatonin and autophagy, exhibiting a 109% amplitude[1952,1953]. However, there are some discrepancies in the timing of the peak in cholesterol synthesis, depending on meal timing[1954]. Postprandial triglyceride levels have been reported to be higher, and total cholesterol and LDL-C levels lower, after a single meal eaten at night compared to daytime[1955]. Among European Caucasians, LDL and cholesterol circadian rhythm amplitudes by about 10%[1956,1957], whereas in Spanish and Indians it can amplitude up to 20-30%[1958,1959]. Men appear to have a greater amplitude in triglyceride levels than women (36% in men vs 24% in women) and serum triglycerides can rise 2-fold higher after a meal in men than in women due to differences in estrogen levels[1960]. Insulin resistance partly mitigates this gender-specific difference in fasting and postprandial triglycerides[1961].

Circadian Alignment

Peripheral Clocks

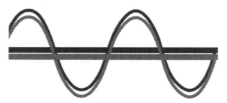

Central Clocks

- Cortisol-melatonin rhythmicity
- Fluctuations in insulin/glucose
- Optimal insulin sensitivity
- Optimal glucose tolerance

Circadian Misalignment

Peripheral Clocks

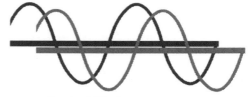

Central Clocks

- Cortisol-melatonin irregularity
- Absence of fluctuations in insulin/glucose
- Insulin resistance
- Glucose intolerance

How to Achieve Circadian Rhythm Alignment

Circadian rhythms are supposed to prepare an organism for the challenges of the environment, specifically the day and night. **The signaling cues that regulate the circadian rhythms include light, temperature, magnetism, movement and food**[1962,1963,1964,1965]. Most of the circadian signaling happens through the eyes via the light that reaches the suprachiasmatic nucleus (SCN)[1966]. Differences between light and darkness is what directly determines melatonin production as melatonin production begins in the absence of blue and green wavelengths of light[1967]. That's why melatonin is also called 'the hormone of darkness'. However, **bright light exposure during the day increases melatonin secretion at night**, which makes getting daylight exposure an important determinant of circadian rhythm alignment[1968]. In fact, morning bright light exposure is the number one way to realign and synchronize your body with the day and night cycle of the environment you're in. Elderly individuals who don't get exposed to enough sunlight show diminished melatonin secretion[1969]. With age, melatonin production already begins to decrease, which is why it's thought that older people don't sleep as much as younger people[1970]. A decrease in melatonin production is why seniors wake up more frequently, fall asleep slower, and spend less time in deep and REM sleep[1971,1972,1973]. Aging also diminishes the transmission of light to the SCN via the retinas, causing age-related circadian rhythm mismatch[1974].

Observational studies have shown a correlation between exposure to light at night with obesity and Type 2 diabetes[1975,1976]. Sleeping in 18–38 lux light increases the prevalence of diabetes by 51%[1977]. It's been found that unfavorable factors to sleep and circadian rhythm alignment, light and noise exposure are associated with poorer glycemic control in Type 2 diabetes patients[1978,1979,1980]. **One prospective study on elderly people over the course of 10 years found that exposure to night light (≥3 lux) increased BMI gain by 10%**[1981] and elevated triglycerides and cholesterol compared to sleeping in less than 3 lux light[1982]. That's because artificial light, specifically blue and green light between the wavelengths of 380-500 nanometers, inhibits melatonin production and results in circadian rhythm mismatch[1983,1984]. LED lights are five times more powerful at blocking melatonin production than incandescent light bulbs[1985]. On the flip side, moderate amber and red light in the evening will also promote melatonin production, thus resulting in more autophagy during sleep[1986]. Blue light at night has the opposite effect. Using blue light blocking glasses can protect against the melatonin-suppressing effects of artificial light[1987,1988]. Wearing blue light blocking glasses before bed has been shown to improve total sleep time and sleep quality in people with insomnia[1989].

However, **you don't want to avoid blue light during the daytime and morning as it helps to produce melatonin at night** by increasing a protein in the brain called POMC (Proopiomelanocortin)[1990]. UV light hitting your skin activates a gene called p53, which upregulates the gene encoding POMC[1991]. Exposure to sunlight also increases brain-derived neurotrophic factor (BDNF) levels, which is like fertilizer for the brain, as it plays an important role in neuronal survival and growth[1992,1993]. Getting exposed to bright lights in the morning or early afternoon for 3-20 weeks reduces markers of insulin resistance[1994,1995], body fat[1996], and appetite[1997]. Light regulates leptin and ghrelin – the 2 hormones that control appetite and food intake[1998,1999]. Thus, getting a little sunlight in the morning or early afternoon can help set your circadian rhythms and improve your sleep and metabolic health. At night, however, you want to avoid artificial blue and green light and sleep in as dark of an environment as possible.

Natural Light Cycle of the Human Circadian Rhythm

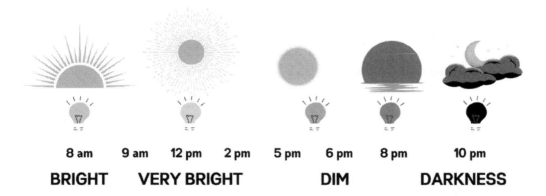

8 am	9 am	12 pm	2 pm	5 pm	6 pm	8 pm	10 pm
BRIGHT	**VERY BRIGHT**				**DIM**		**DARKNESS**

Besides light, temperature can also affect sleep quality and circadian rhythms. **A drop in body temperature is a signal for melatonin production**[2000] as naturally ambient temperature would go down after the sun had set. It's been noted that sleeping in a slightly colder room improves sleep onset, time spent in deep sleep and overall sleep satisfaction[2001]. Sleeping at higher temperatures also decreases REM and deep sleep[2002]. Individuals with an elevated core temperature report having troubles staying asleep[2003]. According to the National Sleep Foundation, the optimal temperature for sleep is 60–67°F or 15.5–19.4°C[2004]. Temperatures above 71°F (21.7°C) or below 53°F (11.7°C) are more likely to reduce sleep quality. Thus, both too hot as well as too cold temperatures can be detrimental for sleep. You have to find out what works best for you.

To set your circadian rhythms, you have to follow a consistent sleep and wake up time. **It's been shown that going to bed and waking up around the same time improves sleep onset, overall sleep quality and recovery**[2005]. A consistent bedtime is associated with weight loss and better health in young adult women[2006]. If you can control one thing, then it should be the time you go to bed as that's arguably more important for health and circadian rhythm alignment. Waking up can vary based on the season and time of sunrise. However, going to bed consistently around the same time embeds your sleep into the natural melatonin rise that occurs around sunset. We understand that this is not always possible, especially in people who are doing some sort of shift work or who travel a lot. In that case, taking naps at a convenient time and trying to stick to a natural rhythm on the off days can help to realign the optimal rhythm. There are also a few supplements that can counteract sleep loss, such as creatine[2007,2008,2009] and caffeine after waking up[2010,2011] as well as taking melatonin before bed[2012,2013]. In those who are shift workers, making your 'daytime' as bright as possible and your 'nighttime' as dark as possible is the best way to set your circadian rhythms.

Whenever you've experienced circadian rhythm mismatch due to a night shift, traveling or just going to bed too late, the most effective way to realign these rhythms is to get exposed to morning daylight, preferably from the sun. This is going to immediately synchronize your inner clocks with the environment and facilitates melatonin production at night. You essentially want a big signal in the morning that tells your body its daytime. That includes bright light exposure upon waking, moving your body in the morning ideally with exercise and eating breakfast. Caffeine can also be a powerful tool for getting energized and becoming awake in the morning if needed. However, you do want to wait 1-2 hours after waking up until the body's natural cortisol production has peaked. Otherwise, you might crash and feel tired in the afternoon. The half life of caffeine is also 5.7 hours[2014], which means that if you drink coffee at 12 PM, then 50% of it will still be in your system at 6 PM. Thus, stop consuming caffeine ideally before 12 PM.

Melatonin Supplementation

There's evidence showing that melatonin supplementation before bed can help you to fall asleep faster and get more deep sleep[2015,2016,2017]. Melatonin supplements are considered safer and with fewer side effects than sleeping pills and other drugs[2018]. Typical doses of melatonin supplements range from 0.1-10 mg/day. More isn't always better and a lot of people report feeling tired taking more than 1 mg. **The human body only makes around 0.1-0.3 mg of melatonin before bed**[2019]. Up to 80% of the melatonin is produced at night with serum levels being around 80-120 pg/ml[2020]. During daytime when you're exposed to light, melatonin levels are quite low at 10-20 pg/ml[2021].

Studies find that melatonin supplements don't interfere with your body's melatonin production even at doses of 50 mg/day[2022,2023]. So, it's perfectly safe and it can be a reliable sleep aid with no dependency or negative feedback loop. However, melatonin at very large doses of 75 mg and above acts as a contraceptive[2024]. That's why women have minimal melatonin production around ovulation when their body is primed to get pregnant, whereas peak melatonin production is at the beginning of their cycle when the likelihood of pregnancy is low[2025]. Current smokers also have lower melatonin levels than non-smokers[2026].

Diabetic patients have been shown to have lower melatonin production at night than non-diabetics[2027]. Melatonin supplementation with doses ranging from 2-10 mg/d can alleviate diabetic complications, improve glycemic control, reduce HbA1c and improve response to metformin treatment[2028,2029,2030,2031]. Supplemental melatonin has even been shown to significantly decrease triglycerides and total cholesterol (at doses $\geq$ 8 mg/d for $\geq$ 8 weeks)[2032] and improve insulin sensitivity and inflammatory markers (3 mg/d) in obese patients[2033]. Melatonin can counteract the oxidative stress and inflammation on the beta cells, heart and other vital organs caused by diabetes[2034,2035,2036].

People with poor glycemic control and lipids might see an improvement in their biomarkers with melatonin supplementation due to the better quality sleep and the antioxidant effects. Regardless, you should facilitate natural melatonin production as much as possible by controlling your light environment, getting daylight exposure, reducing bright light before bed and consuming foods that help with melatonin production.

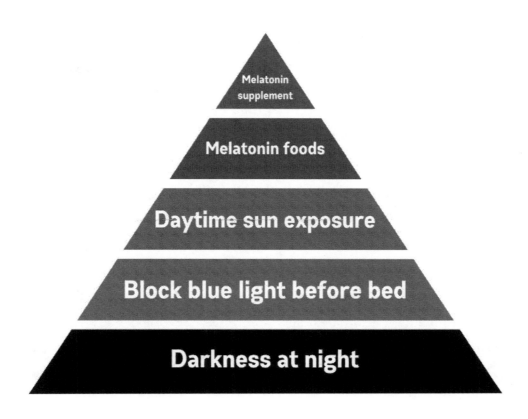

Adapted From: Minich et al (2022)

Melatonin is produced by serotonin in the brain. To make serotonin, you need to get the amino acid tryptophan into the brain[2037]. You can get tryptophan from protein, such as poultry, meat, eggs, seeds, cheese, and some carbohydrate sources like squash. The problem is that tryptophan competes with other amino acids to cross the blood-brain barrier. If you have a lot of other aminos circulating the blood at the same time, then tryptophan will have a much harder time getting into the brain[2038]. However, carbohydrates can enable that tryptophan to reach the brain by raising insulin that would clear the bloodstream from those other amino acids[2039]. This is perhaps why certain people report sleeping better if they have some carbohydrates in the evening. To make the serotonin and then melatonin, you need to get tryptophan into the brain only once a day. So, it doesn't have to be in the evening.

There are also certain foods that contain melatonin and have been shown to raise circulating melatonin levels[2040,2041]. They include cherries, tart cherry juice[2042], almonds, pistachios[2043], eggs[2044] and milk[2045]. How much melatonin a food has depends on the amount of sunlight that plant or animal has been exposed to[2046]. There are also certain phytonutrients like lutein, zeaxanthin, and beta-carotene, which you can get from carrots, salmon and eggs, that can protect the eyes against the harmful effects of excess blue light[2047,2048,2049]. Kiwis have been shown to improve sleep onset, duration, and efficiency thanks to their ability to raise serotonin[2050]. Carbohydrates like white rice or potatoes can also raise serotonin thanks to insulin[2051]. The bioavailability of oral melatonin supplementation is quite low (about 15-37%)[2052,2053], which is why you want to focus on producing most of it naturally through the tryptophan-serotonin conversion. Numerous vitamins and minerals are also needed to convert serotonin into melatonin (particularly b-vitamins and magnesium).

Time-Restricted Eating

Another critical component to circadian rhythms we need to discuss is food intake and meal timing[2054]. **The master clock inside the brain is connected to nutrient-sensing pathways that detect the presence of calories**[2055]. It turns out that when you eat is a lot more important to your health than previously thought. In most animals, eating is confined within a certain time, leaving a short period of fasting that coincides with sleep. During that extended fasting period, the body has a chance to go through various self-maintenance and repair processes, such as autophagy[2056]. Hepatic autophagy is suppressed in the presence of hyperinsulinemia[2057], which means constantly eating with insulin resistance makes it virtually impossible for the body to eliminate dysfunctional cell components that would occur during autophagy. The average American consumes their food over a 15-hour period,[2058,2059] which is another form of circadian disruption in addition to light exposure.

Disrupted eating affects the expression of the molecular clock in peripheral tissues[2060] and uncouples it from the SCN[2061]. For instance, restricting food intake solely to the light phase in mice (their natural sleep time) completely reverses the phase of the circadian clock in the liver, stomach, intestines, heart, pancreas, and kidneys, without affecting the phase in the SCN[2062]. Just delaying meals by 4 hours has also been found to result in a phase shift in the circadian clock in mouse liver[2063]. Conversely, studies find that rhythmic feeding is sufficient to maintain circadian rhythms of clock genes in peripheral tissues during constant light or darkness or after lesions to the SCN[2064,2065,2066]. This suggests that fasting-feeding cues can be just as powerful in entraining the peripheral clocks located in the body's organs than the light and dark cycles[2067].

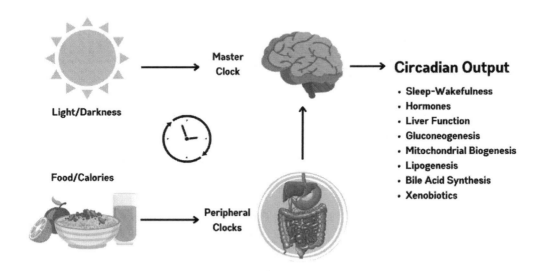

Adapted From: Tahara and Shibata (2016)

197

Time-restricted eating (TRE) refers to confining one's daily calorie intake within a certain timeframe. Intermittent fasting is a more commonly known colloquial term for time-restricted eating. They're essentially the same thing although with some minor differences. Typical TRE windows are 16/8, where you eat within 8 hours and fast for 16 hours, one meal a day (OMAD) and 20/4, where you eat within 4 hours and fast for 20 hours. There are longer intermittent fasting schedules, like alternate day fasting (ADF), extended fasting for several days and the fasting mimicking diet (consuming around 500-600 calories per day).

It has been found that TRE restores circadian rhythms and provides multiple restorative, as well as preventative, metabolic health benefits[2068,2069,2070,2071,2072,2073]. Mice fed a fattening diet are protected against obesity, hypertension, and inflammation if they are doing time-restricted eating during overfeeding[2074]. The mice eating without time restrictions get obese and sick fast. In human studies, TRE does result in lower fasting insulin and blood sugar[2075], better lipid profile[2076], weight loss[2077] and activation of longevity factors like sirtuins and autopahgy[2078]. A study on pre-diabetic men showed that eating the same amount of food within 6 hours of TRE, improved glycemic control, insulin sensitivity, blood pressure, and oxidative stress compared to eating that same food within a 12-hour window[2079].

In humans, time restricted eating results in modest weight loss and fat reduction[2080,2081,2082]. **It also reduces plasma triglycerides, inflammatory markers, blood pressure and atherogenic lipids**[2083,2084,2085]. Most of these studies observe a decrease in self-reported calorie intake, which mediates a lot of the health benefits. It's much easier to subconsciously eat fewer calories and thus lose weight when you are eating in a shorter window. In 2015, a study tested how eating an entire day's caloric intake within 10-11 hours affect overweight individuals[2086]. Essentially, their eating window ended around 8 PM. They lost about 4% body weight in 16 weeks and retained it for up to a year. This was accompanied by a spontaneous 20% reduction in calories just from skipping out random snacks or alcohol late at night. The participants also reported improved sleep and higher alertness during the day.

However, a tightly controlled, cross-over feeding trial, found that 5 weeks of early TRE (last meal of the day before 3 PM) increased insulin sensitivity and beta-cell responsiveness and reduced oxidative stress compared to controls even without energy restriction or weight loss[2087]. Four days of early-TRE (8 AM to 2 PM) has also been shown to decrease fasting and post-prandial glucose and increase daytime energy expenditure, SIRT1 expression, clock genes and autophagy genes[2088,2089]. Another study on resistance-trained men on the same lifting routine put one group on a 12-hour eating window and the other one on the 16/8 method with 8 hours of fasting. Both groups saw small improvements in strength and muscle growth but the 16/8 group lost more body fat (-1.6 kg VS -0.3 kg)[2090]. Their inflammation was also lower.

A 2019 review in The New England Journal of Medicine concluded that both human and animal studies show the benefits of intermittent fasting are not just a result of weight loss, calorie restriction or reduced oxidative stress[2091,2092,2093]. Instead, fasting turns on the body's defense systems and antioxidant pathways, such as autophagy and sirtuins. Autophagy is thought to be a central part of the life-extension effects of calorie restriction in animals. Sirtuins are silent information regulators of genes in the cell[2094]. They promote DNA repair and longevity.

Early Time-Restricted Eating vs Late Time-Restricted Eating

Epidemiology suggests that breakfast skippers are at a higher risk of developing Type 2 diabetes and obesity[2095]. However, this association is due to the fact that breakfast-skippers tend to smoke and engage in other unhealthy habits as well. Skipping breakfast without eating late or overeating calories isn't linked to weight gain or worse metabolic health[2096,2097,2098]. Skipping dinner has been shown to reduce body weight, plasma glucose, and hepatic fat more so than eating six meals spread throughout the day even when calorie intakes were the same[2099].

Regardless, it is more likely that early TRE (eating during the day instead of at night) is more optimal for metabolic health, especially in improving insulin sensitivity and glucose control. Insulin sensitivity and glucose uptake are naturally higher in the beginning of the active phase[2100,2101,2102]. Thus, eating at night is not ideal. **Having to digest a lot of food before bed may also takes energy away from the repair and restorative processes that occur in your sleep.** Another reason to avoid eating large meals close to bedtime is the increase in acid reflux, which can lead to Barrett's disease and esophageal cancer.

A study done on 11 overweight individuals, showed that early time-restricted feeding (eTRF) between 8 AM and 2 PM improves 24-hour glucose levels, alters lipid metabolism, and circadian clock gene expression in just 4 days compared to a non-fasting group eating between 8 AM and 8 PM[2103]. An 8-hour feeding window between 10 AM to 6 PM has also been shown to reduce blood pressure, lower body fatness, and improve cholesterol profile[2104].

Delaying the first meal and doing late time restricted eating instead (skip breakfast, eat lunch and dinner) isn't that well researched and the metabolic effects aren't that clear. Although, delayed TRE has been found to delay peripheral clocks in metabolic organs and *per* rhythms in adipose tissue[2105]. In athletes engaged in resistance training, late TRE (12-8 PM) reduces fat mass without changing fat-free mass[2106]. However, eating a single large meal only between 5 and 9 PM has been found to impair glucose tolerance the next morning[2107]. In mice, late TRE results in higher bodyweight and delayed clock genes compared to early TRE even when calorie consumption is similar[2108]. To know whether there's any difference between early time-restricted eating vs late time-restricted eating, we must compare the two intermittent fasting schedules. Fortunately, one study did exactly that.

One study (Hutchinson et al April 2019) took 15 obese men and had them eat within a 9-hour window, starting with either breakfast (8 AM–5 PM) or with lunch (12-9 PM). They did one protocol for a week, stopped, and ate normally for 2 weeks to negate the adaptations and tried the second routine for another week. **Regardless of eating earlier or later, the participants showed better glycemic control, no difference in average blood sugar levels, body weight, hunger response, total energy expenditure, sleep duration, gastric emptying rate, gastrointestinal hormones (ghrelin, GLP-1, GIP, amylin, PYY), triglycerides, or free fatty acids[2109].** This study also has a much more scientific and better structure than the previous study we mentioned where the participants were compared to a group who wasn't even doing time-restricted eating.

One 2022 study found that a single meal per day in the evening lowers body weight, increases fat oxidation and results in lower 24-hour blood glucose levels than eucaloric 3 meals a day among 30-year-old lean individuals[2110]. The one meal a day subjects lost more bodyweight (-1.4 ± 0.3 kg) than the 3 meals a day subjects (−0.5 ± 0.3 kg). Among that weight loss, the one meal a day group lost 0.7 kg as fat and 0.7 kg as lean mass, whereas the 3 meals a day one lost 0.1 kg as fat and 0.4 as lean mass. Furthermore, the one meal a day was found to also lower plasma glucose during the second half of the day more than the 3 meals a day. Another 2009 study on a 20/4 eating window vs 3 meals a day without a reduction in calorie intake found that it caused 2 kg more fat loss, whereas lean mass was the same[2111]. The 20/4 group also had lower triglycerides (93 vs 102 mg/dL), higher HDL (62 vs 57 mg/dL), and higher LDL (136 vs 113 mg/dL). In other words, time restricted eating does have benefits even when calorie intake isn't reduced.

Dinners are also the most shared meals of the day whereby friends and family come together. These are the only times for some individuals to bond and engage in social communication. Group eating and food sharing are found to be one of the best ways to strengthen family and community relationships[2112]. Thus, early TRE can be challenging both socially and biologically. Skipping dinner when the rest of the group is eating can have unwanted consequences on the individuals social and emotional health.

Independent of all other factors, you would be more insulin sensitive and glucose tolerant during the earlier parts of the day because it fits the human diurnal rhythm. However, your subjective insulin sensitivity depends on your physical activity, muscle mass, and general metabolic flexibility. **In truth, your body is the most insulin sensitive and glucose tolerant after intense physical exercise.** That's why people who do resistance training are healthier, leaner, and can get away with eating more carbohydrates because their body just shuttles glucose into the skeletal muscle and stores it as glycogen.

Strength training increases insulin-mediated glucose uptake, GLUT4 content, and insulin signaling in skeletal muscle in patients with Type 2 diabetes[2113]. Even if you tend to practice intermittent fasting or eat later in the day, you can still mitigate the reduced responsiveness to carbs if you compensate for it with resistance training and muscle building. At that point, that glucose may improve your health by replenishing glycogen stores.

Overall: It doesn't matter whether you eat breakfast and lunch, lunch and dinner, brunch, and an early dinner, or just one meal a day, as long as you confine the eating window. A smaller eating window is still the most important variable when it comes to the benefits of fasted physiology. Compared to regular eating with 3 meals a day and snacks, any form of time-restricted eating is better even if you're eating later in the day. As your eating window gets smaller, you can get away with more because the body spends more time in a fasted state. You're not going to miss out on the benefits of fasting if you eat later in the day.

Chapter 11: Improving Insulin Sensitivity

Throughout the book, we've shown that a lot of the pathology and development of diabetes has to do with hyperglycemia and hyperinsulinemia, which over the long term either leads to, or is the result of, insulin resistance. The threshold at which this happens can vary, depending on a person's personal fat threshold and genetics. However, **a person's biomarkers, specifically lipids, blood sugar and insulin, play a major role in the onset and severity of insulin resistance.** What's more, after insulin resistance has set in, the way you reverse it is through improving those same biomarkers, such as fasting blood sugar, post-prandial (after a meal) blood sugar, fasting insulin, A1c (3-month average blood sugar level) and triglycerides.

Recall the 2 landmark trials in 1993 and 1998 that showed how maintaining a tight control on glycemic responses and overall insulin dynamics resulted in a significant reduction in diabetic complications and lower markers of diabetes[2114]. **In both studies, the intensive group (use of insulin and hypoglycemic agents) resulted in 1-2% lower A1C and 70-80 mg/dl lower blood sugar levels compared to the conventional therapy group (only diet and pharmaceuticals as needed)**[2115,2116]. The intensive group who had Type 1 diabetes also had a 57% reduced risk of non-fatal myocardial infarction, stroke or death from cardiovascular disease compared to the conventional therapy group[2117].

Granted, these individuals were using pharmaceutical insulin and other hypoglycemic drugs, but it goes to show the power of better management of glycemic control. We're not in any position to advise for or against the use of insulin or any other pharmaceuticals – that is between you and your doctor. However, what we can do is talk about the fundamentals of managing one's diet and lifestyle in a way that yields favorable results in the key biomarkers related to insulin resistance and diabetes.

Exercise is Key to Insulin Sensitivity

One of the cornerstones of Type 2 diabetes prevention is prevention of insulin resistance – the cell's inability to respond to insulin. The opposite of that condition is insulin sensitivity – whereby normal amounts of insulin are able to shuttle glucose from the bloodstream into the cells and store it as glycogen. Homeostatic Model Assessment for Insulin Resistance (HOMA-IR) is a test used to measure the level of insulin resistance[2118]. HOMA-IR calculators can take blood glucose and insulin to calculate insulin sensitivity. Optimal HOMA-IR seems to sit around 0.8-1.3 but some data consider normal HOMA-IR ranges for healthy individuals at 1.4-1.6, whereas above 2.0 indicates insulin resistance[2119,2120,2121]. Having a HOMA-IR < 1.6 is associated with optimal glycemic control, whereas risk of insulin resistance begins to increase above 1.6[2122]. A HOMA-IR of 1.82 or higher has been associated with prediabetes[2123]. Thus, you want HOMA-IR below 1.6 and ideally < 1.3.

The main way to improve insulin resistance is through exercise and weight loss[2124]. There is an inverse relationship between physical activity and development of diabetes[2125]. It has been shown that engaging in at least 150 minutes of physical activity per week and losing weight can reduce the incidence of diabetes by 58%, whereas just taking metformin can reduce the incidence of diabetes by 31% compared to placebo[2126]. **Doing vigorous exercise at least once a week can decrease the risk of diabetes by 46%**[2127]. A 6-year randomized controlled trial showed that exercise resulted in a 46% reduction in the incidence of diabetes in patients with impaired glucose tolerance[2128].

Physical activity and exercise increase your insulin sensitivity by activating glucose transporters like GLUT4, depleting muscle glycogen stores, lowering blood sugar levels in the bloodstream and activating fuel sensors such as AMPK that reflect increased energy demand. As a result, the body has no other option but to start absorbing glucose at a higher rate because it's needed for fueling the muscles. During lower intensity exercise, such as cardio, your body is burning predominantly fatty acids with a subsequent drop in both blood lipids and blood sugar levels[2129]. **Acute aerobic exercise increases muscle glucose uptake 5-fold, which can remain elevated up to 48 hours, depending on the duration of exercise**[2130,2131]. In Type 1 diabetes, aerobic exercise improves insulin resistance and lipid levels[2132]. At higher intensities, which for most people means crossing the 65-75% VO2 max threshold, you start burning more muscle glycogen and less fat for fuel. **High intensity interval training (HIIT) promotes skeletal muscle insulin sensitivity and glycemic control in Type 2 diabetic adults**. Thus, it is important to engage in both low intensities, i.e., jogging or cycling, as well as high intensity aerobic exercise i.e., sprinting or interval training[2133,2134]. In Type 1 diabetes, high intensity training does not lead to harmful effects on glycemic control i.e., hyperglycemia or hypoglycemia[2135,2136,2137].

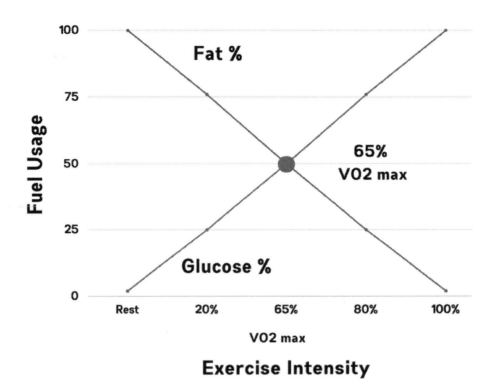

Resistance training, such as lifting free weights or machine weights, increases insulin sensitivity and glucose disposal more than cardio[2138,2139,2140,2141], as there is a greater depletion of muscle glycogen stores[2142,2143]. Insulin resistance due to obesity decreases glucose disposal specifically in skeletal muscle[2144]. Near-maximum muscle contractions activate GLUT4 more so than cardio, leading to superior glucose disposal in the short term[2145]. **When you activate GLUT4 receptors you can clear the bloodstream of glucose better even if you have insulin resistance, which makes it especially powerful for people with diabetes and glucose intolerance.** Thus, high intensity training with resistance training is one of the most impactful ways to override insulin resistance wherein the cells are not responding to insulin. It enables the body to work as if it has normal insulin sensitivity and glucose tolerance in that moment thanks to the activation of GLUT4. Resistance training in Type 2 diabetics improves glycemic control and metabolic health[2146]. However, in the long term, you should also do cardiovascular training, as that improves cardiovascular health, your body's ability to burn fat for fuel, and improves blood lipids. Additionally, cardio helps lower blood pressure even in hypertension patients resistant to blood pressure lowering medication[2147].

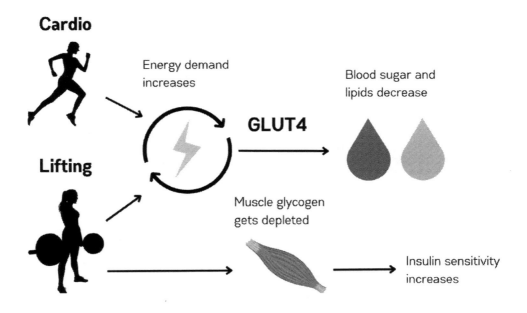

Diabetes is an independent risk factor for low muscle strength and lower exercise tolerance[2148]. It also accelerates the decline in muscle and strength that already naturally occurs with age[2149,2150]. Low muscle mass also increases the risk of insulin resistance, weight gain and diabetes due to lower glucose disposal[2151]. **The muscle atrophy that occurs in diabetes is due to inflammation that activates muscle breakdown pathways and insulin resistance that reduces the storage of muscle glycogen**[2152,2153]. Type 2 diabetics have higher levels of inflammatory cytokines, such as c-reactive protein, TNF-alpha and IL-6[2154,2155,2156]. In Type 2 diabetes, there is also decreased muscle protein synthesis and lower activation of the mammalian target of rapamycin (mTOR) pathway that regulates muscle growth[2157,2158]. Insulin resistance even in non-diabetic patients increases protein degradation[2159]. Reversing the insulin resistance even with insulin-sensitizing drugs like rosiglitazone (Avandia) can recover impaired protein synthesis[2160].

Regular exercise, both aerobic and resistance training, can lower systemic and muscle inflammation in Type 2 diabetes patients even without changes in fat mass[2161,2162,2163,2164,2165]. Resistance training is the most powerful way to attenuate muscle atrophy as well under different atrophic circumstances, such as aging, bed rest, chronic kidney disease or diabetes[2166,2167,2168]. **Just 6-12 weeks of resistance training 3x a week at 70-80% of 1 repetition maximum is enough to improve muscle strength and size in Type 2 diabetes patients**[2169,2170,2171,2172]. Resistance training is also the only way to counteract anabolic resistance seen in diabetes where insulin can't activate mTOR, which is needed for muscle growth[2173,2174,2175]. Mechanical stimulus from lifting weights is the primary activator of the mTOR complex that stimulates muscle growth and protein synthesis[2176,2177,2178].

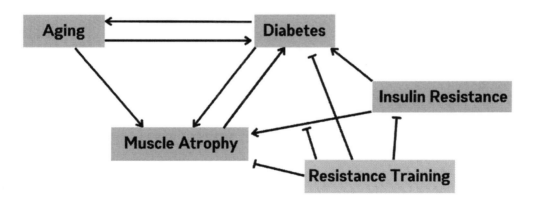

There are many methods of training and different workout plans. **For muscle hypertrophy, you need to be training at an intensity of 60-80% of your 1 repetition maximum**[2179], **which would translate into doing sets of 5-12 reps (where the last 1-3 reps are difficult) for 3-5 sets.** However, it's been shown that blood flow restriction training can yield similar responses even at 20-30% of 1 rep max[2180]. Training a muscle group like legs, shoulders, back or chest twice a week yields superior gains than once a week[2181]. A 2010, paper summarized the current most evidence-based recommendations for training with weights for muscle hypertrophy:

> *"Current research suggests that maximum gains in muscle hypertrophy are achieved by training regimens that produce significant metabolic stress while maintaining a moderate degree of muscle tension.*
>
> ***A hypertrophy-oriented program should employ a repetition range of 6–12 reps per set with rest intervals of 60–90 seconds between sets.*** *Exercises should be varied in a multiplanar, multiangled fashion to ensure maximal stimulation of all muscle fibers.*
>
> *Multiple sets should be employed in the context of a split training routine to heighten the anabolic milieu.* ***At least some of the sets should be carried out to the point of concentric muscular failure, perhaps alternating micro cycles of sets to failure with those not performed to failure to minimize the potential for overtraining.*** *Concentric repetitions should be performed at fast to moderate speeds (1–3 seconds) while eccentric repetitions should be performed at slightly slower speeds (2–4 seconds).*
>
> *Training should be periodized so that the hypertrophy phase culminates in a brief period of higher volume overreaching followed by a taper to allow for optimal supercompensation of muscle tissue."*[2182]

For someone who's completely sedentary and insulin resistant, any form of physical activity would improve their condition. Even walking every day can reduce the risk of diabetes and manage glycemic control[2183,2184]. **Getting around 10,000 steps a day appears to yield the lowest risk of all-cause mortality in adults with prediabetes or diabetes**[2185]. Fast walking speed is also associated with a lower incidence of diabetes in older people[2186]. Gait speed is a strong predictor of survival in older subjects with those walking 0.1 meters/second faster being linked to 12% increased survival[2187]. Going for a short 10–15-minute walk after eating can be a very powerful tool for managing the postprandial blood sugar rise[2188]. **Long periods of sitting are associated with poorer glycemic control in people with Type 2 diabetes**[2189,2190]. Breaking up prolonged sitting with brief bouts of standing for less than 5 minutes[2191,2192] or light walking every 20-30 minutes improves glycemic control in sedentary overweight individuals and in women with impaired glucose tolerance[2193,2194,2195]. Walking for 15 minutes after eating also improves the postprandial glucose response and glycemic control[2196]. In fact, **a 15-minute walk after a meal appears to be better at lowering the postprandial glycemic response than walking before a meal or no exercise at all in Type 2 diabetics**[2197].

Making Your Fat More Insulin Sensitive

Another major determinant of insulin sensitivity is the composition of your adipose tissue. A certain amount of body fat is beneficial for evolutionary reasons – it's your mobile pantry for calories to withdraw from during times of food scarcity. All excess calories, whether they come from carbs, protein, or fat, end up as triglycerides in the adipose tissue. The process of converting carbs into triglycerides and storing them as body fat is quite a labor-intensive process and burns up to 7% of the calories from the carbs. When you're in a calorie deficit, you mobilize those same triglycerides to burn for energy. **In addition to the difference between visceral and subcutaneous fat, there is also a difference between brown adipose tissue (BAT) and white adipose tissue (WAT)**[2198].

- **Brown Adipose Tissue (BAT) also called brown fat helps with thermoregulation and heat production**[2199]. BAT generates heat through shivering and non-shivering thermogenesis[2200]. That's why newborn babies and hibernating animals like bears have a lot of brown fat[2201], but adults have it as well to a certain degree[2202,2203]. Because of increasing energy expenditure and insulin sensitivity, brown fat is much more beneficial for metabolic health and body composition[2204,2205]. It's thought to be helpful in treating obesity and diabetes[2206]. Activating brown adipose tissue improves insulin sensitivity, glucose tolerance, weight loss, triglycerides, and cholesterol levels[2207,2208,2209,2210]. In fact, the amount of brown adipose tissue is inversely correlated with body-mass index, especially in older people[2211]. With age, brown fat decreases[2212].

- **White Adipose Tissue (WAT) also called white fat is predominantly used for energy storage**. It also acts as a thermal insulator. Both visceral and subcutaneous fat are comprised of white adipose tissue. White fat makes leptin, the satiety hormone, and asprosin, which is a protein that releases glucose into the blood[2213,2214]. Obese individuals have higher levels of asprosin, which is thought to contribute to insulin resistance and metabolic syndrome[2215,2216]. Weight loss through bariatric surgery lowers asprosin levels[2217]. Thus, too much white fat in relation to brown fat can promote obesity and diabetes.

- **You can convert white adipose tissue into beige adipose tissue, which resembles both brown and white fat**[2218]. This process can be achieved via stimulation of the sympathetic nervous system and adrenaline.

Asprosin reduces browning-related genes and proteins that would help this conversion[2219].

The biggest difference between brown and white fat cells is the number of mitochondria in them. **White fat cells contain very little mitochondria and a large lipid droplet, whereas brown fat cells have a lot of mitochondria and few small lipid droplets**[2220]. Beige fat cells have a number of mitochondria somewhere in the middle of brown and white fat, which is why they look beige or light brown[2221]. Thus, the more mitochondria, the browner the fat cell becomes. This is the reason why brown fat increases energy expenditure more than white fat – they have more mitochondria. Brown fat also contains more capillaries that can oxygenate the tissues better. Brown adipose tissue is located around the spinal cord, trachea, upper chest, neck, scapula, kidneys, and the pancreas[2222]. White and beige fat is spread throughout the entire body.

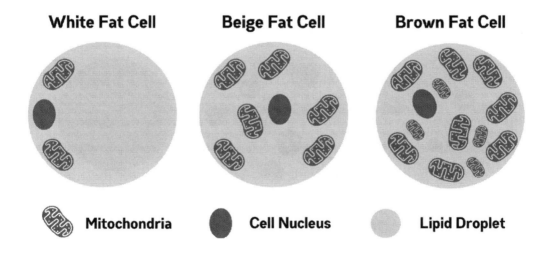

Redrawn From: Cedikova et al (2016)

Cold exposure is the fastest way to activate brown adipose tissue and promote the browning of white fat into beige fat[2223,2224,2225]. Shivering through cold exposure increases metabolic rate, thermoregulation, fat oxidation and burning of white fat[2226]. Some of the mechanisms by which cold exposure increases brown fat is through changing the gut microbiome[2227]. People with more brown fat may burn 15% more calories than those without it[2228]. **Cold also raises adiponectin levels, which is a protein that helps to regulate blood sugar and glucose uptake via GLUT4 activation**[2229,2230]. Thus, brown fat helps with weight loss and improving glucose levels. Cold exposure also reduces inflammation[2231]. In diet-induced obese mice, cold resolves obesity-induced inflammation and insulin resistance, which improves glucose tolerance[2232].

One hour of immersion in 57.2°F or 14°C water raises metabolic rate by 350%[2233]**!** Being immersed in 68°F (20°C) water for 1 hour increases metabolic rate by 93%, whereas 90°F or 32°C water does not. Thus, being exposed to cold water at a temperature of 68°F or 20°C is going to burn a lot of calories to keep you warm. This process is dependent on brown fat. Going into a freezing cold ice bath or lake is not very comfortable and can be hard to accomplish for a lot of people. Fortunately, it doesn't have to be that extreme and you can get some benefits of brown fat activation just from the seasonal fluctuations in temperature. **It's been shown that the average metabolic rate can be ~9% higher at a temperature of 59°F or 15°C compared to 71.6°F or 22°C while wearing regular clothes**[2234]. In a 2013 study, people who were exposed to 62.6°F or 17°C for 2 hours a day for 6 weeks showed higher amounts of brown fat, non-shivering thermogenesis and about a 5% lower body fat mass[2235]. A 10-day experiment on obese men found that sitting in a cold room with a temperature of 58°F or 14°C for 6 hours per day increased the metabolic rate by 14%[2236]. In another study, they took 11 already lean men and kept them in a cold room with a temperature of 67°F (19°C) while simultaneously wearing a cooling vest at a temperature of

62°F or 16°C for 90 minutes. After just 30 minutes, their metabolic rate rose by 16.7% and fat burning increased by 72.6%[2237]! **Cold exposure doesn't increase hunger or food intake even when you burn more calories**[2238]. Granted, if you end up going into a calorie deficit due to burning a lot more calories from cold exposure-induced shivering thermogenesis, then it would naturally make you hungrier. At that point, your body is increasing hunger as a natural response to energy restriction. It's not the cold making you hungrier – it's the calorie deficit.

Exercise also promotes white adipose tissue browning[2239,2240]. It can even reverse the decrease in brown fat caused by an obesogenic diet[2241]. Obesity decreases blood vessel formation and capillary density in the adipose tissue, which results in a state of low tissue oxygenation[2242], leading to increased inflammation and insulin resistance[2243]. With less blood flow, it becomes harder to burn the fat cells. Exercise prevents this and promotes capillary density[2244]. During exercise, brown adipose tissue takes up less glucose than white fat and increases circulating levels of a lipid called lipokine, which increases energy expenditure[2245]. Exercise mimicks shivering, which stimulates irisin secretion and promotes the creation of brown fat[2246]. Irisin is a myokine or muscle hormone that drives browning of white fat and thermogenesis (the burning of calories through the release of heat)[2247].

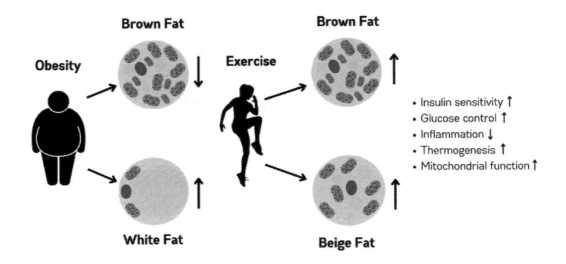

Redrawn From: Garritson 2021

Melatonin – the sleep hormone – can also affect brown fat. In one study, diabetic rats who had higher melatonin also had more activated brown fat[2248]. This can be connected to sleep quality and duration as sleep restriction reduces leptin levels[2249,2250]. Sleep loss reduces the diurnal rhythm amplitude of leptin in healthy men[2251,2252]. Chronic sleep deprivation attenuates leptin receptor-mediated signaling pathways[2253]. Circadian rhythms and light are intrinsically connected to leptin signaling as well as subcutaneous white fat cells have a light-sensitive pathway mediated by melanopsin[2254]. Morning red and green light but not blue light exposure can decrease ghrelin (the hunger hormone)[2255]. This makes it important to get full spectrum sunlight as it comes with all the wavelengths, instead of artificial light that only has blue light.

Chapter 12: Lowering Glucose Spikes and Postprandial Triglycerides

What you eat has the most immediate impact on your blood sugar levels. Recall the glycemic index – if you take a teaspoon of pure glucose your blood sugar would rise exponentially, whereas if you eat the equivalent amount of calories from salad, meat or pure butter it would yield a completely different result.

Granted, **everyone's reaction to any type of food depends greatly on their current metabolic health and insulin sensitivity.** Other factors include whether you exercised, just woke up, or the time of the day – all of which have a major influence as well. If your GLUT4 receptors are fully activated and your muscle glycogen is depleted from a 60-minute hard workout, then even a soda or juice with pure sugar and no fiber could result in an insignificant rise in blood sugar if you're already very insulin sensitive and with optimal metabolic health. On the other hand, someone with Type 2 diabetes and obesity would see their postprandial blood sugar rise above what's normal even after eating a piece of fruit. Thus, **just because one food is low glycemic on paper for one person, it might not be so for someone else and the same applies to high glycemic foods.**

Regardless, for disease prevention and insulin sensitivity, it's worthwhile to minimize large surges in blood sugar and insulin for optimal metabolic health. That's what we'll be discussing in this chapter – how to manage hyperglycemia, hyperinsulinemia, hyperlipidemia, and post-prandial blood sugar levels.

Lowering Glucose Spikes Before and After Meals

Postprandial hyperglycemia and hyperlipidemia also called postprandial dysmetabolism are a risk factor for cardiovascular disease and atherosclerosis[2256]. Prolonged periods of elevated glucose and triglycerides in the blood after eating promote inflammation, endothelial dysfunction (damage to blood vessels) and sympathetic hyperactivity[2257]. Over time this can lead to insulin resistance, paving the road to diabetes. Type 2 diabetics have a high prevalence of postprandial hyperglycemia[2258].

A significant number of adults have a fasting blood sugar in the non-diabetic range (<126 mg/dl), but after eating a meal or taking an oral glucose tolerance test, they show hyperglycemia characteristic of impaired glucose tolerance (>140 mg/dl) or full diabetes (>200 mg/dl) [2259,2260,2261]. There is a linear relationship between glucose levels after taking an oral glucose tolerance test and the risk of cardiovascular death and all-cause mortality[2262]. Starting at 87 mg/dl, the risk for cardiovascular disease begins to increase and by 140 mg/dl the risk is already 58% higher[2263,2264]! At a post-prandial glucose level of < 87 mg/dl, there is coronary atherosclerosis regression, whereas above that there is coronary atherosclerosis progression. Prediabetes and diabetes are diagnosed when plasma glucose is ≥140 mg/dl and ≥ 200mg/dl, respectively, 2-hours after drinking 75 grams of sugar (known as the oral glucose tolerance test). [2265,2266].

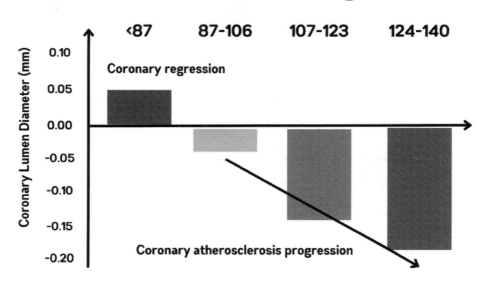

2-Hour Glucose (mg/dl)

Adapted From: O'Keefe et al (2008)

The glycemic index (GI) and load are a major determinant of postprandial glycemia with higher GI foods increasing the risk of hyperglycemia[2267]. High GI and low fiber foods independently increase the risk of cardiovascular disease and Type 2 diabetes[2268,2269]. Minimally processed foods that have fiber, such as vegetables, fruits, nuts, seeds, and whole grains raise postprandial glucose and triglycerides to a much lesser extent than refined foods[2270]. Dietary antioxidants and polyphenols found in berries, dark leafy greens, dark chocolate, tea and dark-pigmented vegetables like broccoli and cabbage can also lower postprandial inflammation and oxidative stress[2271]. Thus, it's important to include these foods with every meal, especially when eating higher GI foods. Eating carbohydrates after protein and fiber, instead of carbohydrates first, can also result in lower postprandial glycemia[2272]. Berries help reduce the post-prandial glucose response to sugar[2273] and the post-prandial insulin response to bread[2274]. Other studies have corroborated these findings showing that berries reduce the post-prandial glucose/insulin response to sugar and prevent the late hypoglycemic effect and compensatory free fatty acid rebound[2275,2276]. Essentially, eating berries delays the absorption of sugar. Thus, one of the easiest ways to lower the glucose/insulin response from a carbohydrate or sugar load, is to consume berries[2277].

Restricting refined carbohydrates, such as wheat and cereal, improves postprandial glucose and reduces intra-abdominal fat, especially in those with insulin resistance[2278]. **However, you don't have to be on a low carb diet to avoid postprandial glucose excursions.** In fact, a high carb/high fiber plant-based diet can lower postprandial glucose and lipids even better than a high monounsaturated fat low carb diet[2279]. It's thought the reason for this is the higher fiber content that (1) slows down glucose responses of meals and (2) binds to the fats and reduces their absorption[2280]. A low-fat high carb plant-based diet has also been shown to result in up to 700 fewer calories consumed per day than an animal-based ketogenic diet on an ad libitum energy intake[2281]. The reason has to do with primarily the lower calorie content of plants. This is likely why many people see good initial benefits with plant-based diets, but typically see their health decline if they stay on them for a long period of time due to the lack of bioavailable nutrients. Thus, for acute weight loss, some people do find that eating a higher fiber plant-based diet can help.

The glycemic index of a food however should not be taken at face value, as most people do not eat single foods by themselves. Thus, blood sugar responses after a meal are determined by the overall macronutrient composition of the meal and are lower with the addition of fat and protein. Also, the dose makes the poison. For example, small amounts of high glycemic carbs like white rice or white potatoes have a much smaller effect on postprandial glucose compared to larger quantities[2282]. **Ultra-processed foods, especially, that are high in calories and with quickly absorbable carbohydrates can lead to exaggerated postprandial**

surges in blood sugar and triglycerides[2283,2284]. That's due to a disrupted Randle cycle that causes insulin resistance and oxidative stress[2285,2286]. Even non-diabetic individuals see increased free radical stress from hyperglycemia when they're given intravenous glucose[2287]. On the other hand, more traditional diets low in processed foods, such as the Mediterranean and Okinawan diet that are lower in refined carbs, with no added sugars, and high in antioxidant rich fibers improve postprandial glucose and lipids[2288].

Here are some things that you can add to your meal to lower the postprandial rise in glucose:

- **Ceylon Cinnamon** can significantly reduce postprandial glucose by slowing gastric emptying[2289]. Consumption of cinnamon is associated with lower fasting plasma glucose, total cholesterol, LDL-C and triglycerides[2290]. However, you must be careful with the type of cinnamon you consume as the conventional cinnamon is cassia cinnamon that contains high amounts of coumarin that may cause liver damage[2291]. **The correct cinnamon is Ceylon cinnamon**. If the label doesn't say it's Ceylon specifically, then it's probably cassia cinnamon.

  o You can also use cinnamon as tea, which has been found to reduce blood sugar levels in response to a meal[2292,2293]. Taking 3-6 grams of a cinnamon for 40 days has been shown to lower *pre*-meal glucose levels in healthy adults[2294]. Giving 5 grams of cinnamon immediately before an oral glucose tolerance test or 12 hours before it has been shown to lower glucose area under the curve in response to the glucose test by 13% and 10%, respectively, compared to placebo[2295]. Ingesting 3 grams of cinnamon every day for 2 weeks has been shown to reduce the glucose response to an oral glucose tolerance test on day 1 (-13.1%) as well as on the 14th day (-5.5%) and improve insulin sensitivity in healthy adults[2296]. Thus, long-term intake of cinnamon with meals can provide continuous benefit to lowering the glucose area under the curve and improve insulin sensitivity.

- **Vinegar (white vinegar and apple cider vinegar)** significantly reduces postprandial glycemia and insulin thanks to its acetic acid content that slows down gastric emptying and carbohydrate absorption[2297,2298]. **Apple cider vinegar** is one of the most well-known types of vinegar with a lot of evidence that it can reduce blood sugar levels and A1c significantly[2299,2300,2301].

  o Vinegar contains many bioactive compounds that have antidiabetic, antioxidant, anti-obesity, and cholesterol-lowering effects, such as acetic acid, gallic acid, catechin, epicatechin, chlorogenic acid, caffeic acid, p-coumaric acid, and ferulic acid[2302]. In Type 2 diabetics, apple cider vinegar ingestion can improve whole-body insulin sensitivity by 19% and by 34% in subjects with insulin resistance compared to placebo[2303].

  o Consuming apple cider vinegar with a bagel and juice meal can lower the 60-minute glucose response by 55%[2304]. Taking 1-2 tablespoons of white vinegar when eating white rice or white bread can reduce postprandial glucose by 25-35% and increase post-meal satiety 2-fold in healthy subjects[2305]. Adding just 1 gram of acetic acid from vinegar, an amount you'd use for salad dressing, can lower the glucose response after eating bread by 31.4%[2306].

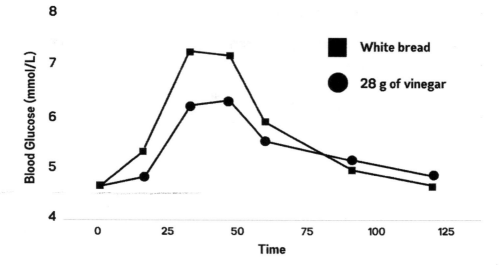

Adapted From: Östman et al (2005)

o Vinegar helps with weight loss and satiety as well, in addition to lowering glucose, and people who take vinegar with their meals typically eat 200-275 fewer calories for the rest of the day[2307,2308]. Taking either 15 ml or 30 ml of "apple vinegar" a day for 12 weeks has been shown to significantly reduce visceral fat, waist circumference and triglycerides compared to placebo[2309]. Unless using something like balsamic vinegar on a salad, apple cider vinegar should be diluted in around 8 oz. of water.

o Vinegars have anti-bacterial properties that help to eliminate various pathogens, such as *E. coli* and *Candida*[2310,2311,2312]. This can prevent the onset of microbial dysbiosis that would jeopardize your glucose tolerance and insulin sensitivity[2313].

o **To get the required amount of acetic acid for blood sugar regulation, you need to dilute 1-2 tablespoons of apple cider vinegar in 8 ounces of water.** Apple cider vinegar is 5-6% acetic acid, whereas regular vinegar is significantly higher[2314].

223

Remember that acetic acid can be harmful to your throat and teeth when consumed alone[2315]. It can cause throat burns in children[2316] and when applied to the skin can cause skin burns[2317]. Thus, it's better to either mix it with olive oil in salad dressing or consume with water.

- **Protein** is an important addition to any meal because of its importance in exercise recovery and muscle growth[2318], but also because it can significantly lower the glycemic load of a meal. High fat proteins, like bacon, cheese and sausages may worsen postprandial dysmetabolism due to their high saturated fat content, especially when eaten together with high glycemic carbohydrates[2319,2320]. Leaner proteins like fish, chicken, steak, and pork, on the other hand, reduce glucose excursions and improve insulin sensitivity[2321]. A high protein meal at breakfast has been shown to reduce the glucose response at lunch[2322]. Adding whey protein to a pure glucose drink lowers the postprandial glucose area under the curve by 56% and increases insulin response by up to 60%[2323]. Protein also has the highest thermic effect of food (20-30%) compared to the 7-15% of carbohydrates and 2-4% of fat, which refers to how many calories get spent on digestion[2324,2325]. For most healthy people, a recommended amount of protein per meal is around 30-50 grams, the higher end being for those with greater muscle mass.

- **Olive oil** is considered one of the healthiest fats in the world thanks to its favorable effects on lipids and cholesterol[2326]. Extra virgin olive oil reduces the postprandial glycemic response to a high GI meal[2327]. Olive oil increases postprandial GLP-1 secretion, reduces glucose absorption, and lowers cholesterol[2328,2329,2330]. Compared to linoleic acid-rich sunflower oil, oleic acid-rich olive oil lowers fasting glucose and insulin, and plasma cholesterol and LDL levels[2331]. Olive oil with vinegar is the primary salad dressing in the Mediterranean diet, which probably contributes to the benefits of the diet.

- **Nuts** like almonds can lower postprandial glucose and insulinemia[2332]. Adding 90 grams of almonds to a high glycemic meal has been shown to reduce postprandial glucose area under the curve by 58%[2333]. Eating nuts at least 5 times a week is associated with a 50% lower diabetes risk and 20% lower coronary artery disease risk[2334]. Dried fruits have a lower GI than refined carbs and thus also reduce the glycemic response to high GI foods[2335]. However, dried fruits can also be high in calories, which is why they should be eaten in moderation and should not substitute fresh fruit.

- **Exercising** either before or after eating within 2 hours of a meal shown lowers postprandial glucose and triglycerides by 50%[2336]! Instead of sitting on the couch after a meal, which would be one of the worst things for your glucose levels, go for a short walk. Cumulative daily physical activity is associated with lower 2-hour glucose challenge scores in a dose-dependent manner, meaning the more you stay active the lower your results will be, whereas cumulative sedentary time is associated with higher scores in a dose-specific manner[2337]. After a low glycemic meal, the body will prefer to burn fatty acids instead of glucose for fuel compared to a high glycemic meal[2338].

- **Tea** at small doses can lower postprandial glucose in healthy individuals[2339]. This effect is probably due to the high polyphenol and catechin content of tea that enhance insulin action. Adding milk to the tea, however, decreases the insulin-potentiating activity in a dose-specific manner[2340]. Habitual tea consumption is linked to a lower risk of diabetes[2341].

- Green tea consumption has been found to reduce the risk of diabetes thanks to its high amount of antioxidants and ability to control postprandial glucose and lipids[2342,2343,2344,2345]. In diabetic rats, green tea lowers hyperglycemia by activating muscle GLUT4[2346]. Drinking green tea daily can also lower A1c and inflammation[2347,2348]. In Japan, people who drink 6 cups of green tea a day have been found to have a 33% lower risk of developing Type 2 diabetes compared to drinking one cup a week[2349]. EGCG, the main catechin in green tea, inhibits fat cell proliferation, increases antioxidant defence and blocks lipid formation[2350,2351,2352,2353]. There appears to be an inverse relationship between habitual tea consumption and body fat % and body fat distribution[2354].

- Black tea also lowers postprandial glucose levels in both normal and pre-diabetic individuals[2355]. It contains antioxidant compounds called theaflavins and thearubigins that lower cholesterol and glucose[2356]. **You do need to be a somewhat careful with consuming green and black tea as both can inhibit the absorption of thiamine**[2357].

- Hibiscus tea is another tea that has been shown to lower insulin resistance, hyperglycemia and dyslipidemia[2358,2359]. It also reduces AGE formation and glycation-induced oxidative stress[2360].

- Chamomile tea is a common herbal tea that has many health benefits but it can also lower blood sugar levels. In an 8-week study, drinking 5 ounces (150 ml) of tea made with 3 grams of chamomile 3 times a day after every meal resulted in significant reductions in A1c and insulin levels compared to the control group[2361].

- o **Lemon balm** is another herbal tea that has essential oils that can help promote cellular glucose uptake[2362]. Taking 700 mg of lemon balm extract capsules for 12 weeks has been found to significantly lower fasting blood glucose, A1c, blood pressure, triglycerides and inflammation compared to a control group[2363].

- **Coffee** consumption is associated with a lower risk of diabetes and a reduced incidence of diabetic retinopathy[2364,2365,2366]. That association is lowest among those who drink black coffee with no added ingredients like sugar or milk[2367]. But even in the presence of those ingredients, coffee consumption appears to have a protective effect on diabetes, it's just smaller compared to black coffee alone. **Drinking both caffeinated and decaffeinated coffee may lower diabetes risk[2368], which is probably more so due to the high polyphenol and antioxidant content of coffee than the caffeine**[2369,2370]. Similar to black and green tea however, coffee can inhibit thiamine absorption[2371].

  - o In a 2014 study on 100,000 people over the course of 20 years those who increased their coffee consumption by over 1 cup a day over a 4 year periood saw an 11% reduction in Type 2 diabetes risk, whereas those who reduced their coffee consumption by over 1 cup a day had a 17% higher risk of Type 2 diabetes[2372]. It's been observed that consuming 1-2 cups of coffee per day is associated with the lowest risk of all-cause mortality compared to no coffee consumption at all[2373].

  - o **Caffeine alone** could have negative effects on glucose control as taking caffeine pills before eating results in higher postprandial glucose and markers of insulin resistance[2374,2375]. There is also a genetic component to this, depending if someone is a fast metabolizer or slow metabolizer of caffeine[2376]. People with the homozygous CYP1A2*1A allele are fast caffeine metabolizers, whereas those with CYP1A2*1F are slow caffeine metabolizers. Slow metabolizers have a higher risk of getting non-fatal heart attacks and hypertension from caffeine ingestion[2377,2378].

- **Turmeric and its main bioactive compound curcumin** intake can reduce blood sugar and lipid levels[2379]. Curcumin has glucose lowering and insulin-sensitizing effects[2380]. Supplementing curcumin for 9 months lowers the number of prediabetic individuals developing full diabetes[2381]. Ingesting 750 mg twice daily of a turmeric extract for 6 months in a study of 213 Type 2 diabetic patients significantly reduced total body fat, viseral fat, waist circumference, triglycerides and insulin resistance[2382]. The antioxidants in curcumin, as well as cinnamon, ginger, cloves and red chili, can have beneficial effects against obesity, inflammation and insulin resistance[2383]. Curcumin scavenges reactive oxygen species and boosts the body's antioxidant enzymes[2384].

  - The amount of curcumin in turmeric powder isn't very high – around 3.14% by weight[2385]. Thus, from one teaspoon of turmeric powder, you get about 0.15 grams of curcumin, which is around the amount people in India consume daily[2386]. In curry powder, the amounts of curcumin is even less because curry contains other ingredients like coriander, cumin, and chili. Curcumin isn't very bioavailable and is poorly absorbed but consuming it with black pepper, which contains piperine, enhances curcumin's absorption by 2000%[2387].

- **Garlic** can improve insulin sensitivity and metabolic syndrome in fructose-fed rats[2388]. Historically, garlic has been recommended for managing high cholesterol and triglycerides[2389]. Indeed, a meta-analysis of 29 studies found that garlic consumption reduces total cholesterol and triglycerides[2390]. In subjects with metabolic syndrome, consuming aged garlic for 12 weeks raised adiponectin levels[2391]. Eating 1-2 garlic cloves a day is likely enough to get most of the health benefits[2392].

  - **Garlic also benefits diabetes as it can lower blood glucose levels in addition to cholesterol and triglycerides**[2393,2394,2395,2396]. Most of the therapeutic effects of garlic are mediated by allicin, which is the main bioactive compound in garlic[2397]. To activate allicin, you need to crush the garlic and let it sit for a while. In one study, swallowing whole garlic had no effect on serum lipid levels but crushed garlic reduced cholesterol and triglycerides[2398]. Heating, pickling or boiling garlic significantly reduces allicin content[2399,2400].

This may look like a long list of things to do for lowering your glucose levels but even incoporating just 1 or 2 of these will likely have a significant impact on your glucose levels. Thus, make sure to monitor your glucose levels closely, especially if you are on medications, and make sure to talk with your doctor before changing your diet or supplement regimen. To specifically target glucose levels after a meal, you have to make sure you get enough protein and fiber in your meal that will lower the blood sugar response. Opting for lower glycemic foods is also important, especially if you have poor glucose control and existing insulin resistance. Adding vinegar and olive oil to vegetables or a salad makes the dish tastier while lowering the postprandial rise in glucose. For seasonings, use turmeric and ceylon cinnamon.

Supplements and Pharmaceuticals for Diabetes

There are also some anti-diabetic supplements and pharmaceuticals that could help with blood sugar regulation and diabetes:

o **Metformin is the most prescribed anti-diabetic drug that lowers blood sugar by inhibiting gluconeogenesis and improving insulin sensitivity**[2401,2402]. It also suppresses the mTOR pathway[2403]. Metformin is also associated with a reduction in cardiovascular disease mortality, cancer, diabetes, and overall mortality[2404,2405,2406]. Additionally, metformin is associated with a reduced risk of diabetes-related deaths and all-cause mortality in overweight subjects[2407].

  o However, **metformin may blunt whole-body insulin sensitivity and skeletal muscle mitochondrial function in response to aerobic exercise in older individuals**[2408]. Thus, it is not ideal for periods of building muscle and training hard. Metformin may be preferable for populations with co-morbidities or immobility that force them into a sedentary lifestyle, but everyone else should focus on regular exercise.

  o Metformin has become a popular longevity supplement due to its blood sugar lowering effects that many recreational longevity enthusiasts have started to use. It's been found that diabetics taking metformin have an 18% increased median all-cause survival compared to the rest of the population not taking metformin, despite diabetes patients having higher mortality[2409,2410,2411]. Thus, it might seem like taking metformin increases longevity. However, a large meta-analysis didn't replicate these findings[2412]. Metformin is a prescription drug used for the purpose of managing diabetes and insulin resistance. Thus, unless your doctor prescribes you metformin, it's not advisable to take it recreationally.

- **GLP-1 Receptor Agonists (GLP-1-RA)** are a class of diabetic drugs that lower blood sugar levels quite significantly by mimicking the actions of GLP-1 (glucagon-like peptide-1) they increase insulin production, decrease glucose production by the liver and slow gastric emptying[2413,2414,2415]. It's been found that GLP-1-RA in Type 2 diabetics lowers all-cause mortality by up to 12% and improves cardiovascular disease outcomes[2416]. They also appear to decrease stroke risk[2417]. GLP-1 receptor agonists are prescription drugs that you would need to discuss with your doctor whether you would benefit from taking them or not.

  - **Semaglutide** is one of the GLP-1-RA made in 2017 that's received a lot of press due to effective weight loss studies over the past few years[2418,2419,2420]. It's been found to be more effective than previous weight loss drugs but not more effective than bariatric surgery[2421]. Semaglutide works by mimicking GLP-1, which increases insulin production and thus lowers blood sugar levels, as well as inhibits glucagon, which results in additional blood sugar reduction[2422]. It also promotes the growth of pancreatic beta cells, making it a possible intervention for improving individuals with pancreatic beta cell damage[2423,2424]. The weight loss effects of semaglutide come from appetite suppression and reduced food intake[2425,2426,2427]. However, individuals who stop taking semaglutide tend to regain at least some of the weight they lost with the drug.

- **Sulfonylureas** are the oldest diabetes drugs that have been used for over 50 years[2428]. They work by making the pancreas produce more insulin as well as suppress glucagon[2429,2430,2431]. Sulfonylureas are well-tolerated, but the main side-effect is hypoglycemia[2432]. In clinical practice, sulfonylureas are often combined with metformin to improve glycemic control rapidly[2433,2434]. Sulfonylureas are a prescription drug that are recommended to be used only for a few months in patients with diabetes to achieve better glycemic results before incorporating insulin. Many doctors are starting to shy away from prescribing them due to the risk of low blood glucose levels.

- **Berberine** also called natural metformin is an alkaloid found in barberry and other plants[2435]. It has anti-diabetic effects, which is why it's often considered a natural alternative to metformin[2436,2437]. In human studies, berberine has been shown to decrease waist circumference, triglycerides and systolic blood pressure[2438].

- **Glycine** is an amino acid with many important functions – particularly its need in the formation of glutathione, creatine and collagen[2439,2440,2441,2442]. It also improves insulin sensitivity and lowers blood glucose by potentiating insulin's effects[2443,2444,2445,2446,2447]. In diabetics, supplementing 5 grams of glycine 3-4 times a day improves their A1c levels[2448,2449]. **Ingesting glycine with 25 grams of glucose attenuates the glucose response by over 50% compared to ingesting glucose alone**[2450].

  o Glycine can counteract many complications of diabetes by lowering inflammation and inhibiting the AGE pathway, reducing the formation of AGEs and increasing the breakdown of AGE precursors[2451,2452,2453]. Diabetes patients also have glutathione deficiency[2454], which can be restored with glycine and n-acetylcysteine supplementation[2455].

- **Chromium** is a mineral that has very potent blood sugar lowering effects[2456]. Taking anywhere between 200-1,000 mcg of chromium picolinate per day has been shown to improve glucose control and insulin sensitivity in diabetic or prediabetic individuals[2457,2458,2459]. Thus, it can be a good supplement for people with poor glucose control.

Supplementing with inositol has been found to have insulin-sensitizing effects[2460,2461,2462]. Markers of cardiovascular disease, such as cholesterol and lipids have also been shown to get better after supplementation with inositol[2463,2464]. Myo-inositol (the active ingredient in most supplements labeled as inositol) is a carbocyclic sugar that makes up every cell membrane as phosphatidylinositol, making it important for cell membrane structure and function[2465]. It has half the sweetness of table sugar. Inositol isn't considered an essential nutrient, but our bodies don't produce enough for optimal health[2466].

Diabetic animals and humans exhibit depleted intracellular myo-inositol, and they excrete more myo-inositol in the urine[2467,2468,2469,2470]. High blood glucose inhibits myo-inositol uptake by competing with myo-inositol transporters[2471,2472,2473,2474]. Depletion of myo-inositol contributes to the development of diabetic neuropathy[2475]. Thus, diabetes and impaired glucose tolerance promotes myo-inositol depletion, while simultaneously increasing your demand for myo-inositol.

Here are the benefits of myo-inositol[2476,2477,2478,2479,2480,2481,2482,2483,2484]:

- Improves glucose oxidation
- Drives glucose into skeletal muscle
- Improves glycogen synthesis and formation in skeletal muscle
- Drives creatine into skeletal muscle
- Drives calcium into bone
- Maintains cell membrane potential
- Improves insulin signaling
- Breaks down fat and improves cholesterol
- Improves TSH (Thyroid Stimulating Hormone) signaling
- Improves energy - ATP production increases from better glucose utilization for energy and inositol compounds provide the phosphate needed for ATP production
- Improves sleep (deep sleep can increase by 1-3 hours)
- Has a calming effect

Many factors deplete the body of inositol including[2485]:

- Magnesium deficiency
- Manganese deficiency
- Coffee/caffeine
- Elevated glucose levels
- Insulin resistance
- Lack of salt

You can get inositol from foods, such as nuts, seeds, and fruits. In animals and plants, myo-inositol gets stored as inositol-containing phospholipids or as phytic acid, respectively[2486]. All living cells contain inositol phospholipids. Phytic acid is the primary stored form of phosphorus in plant tissues. Thus, nuts, grains and beans are some of the highest food sources of inositol[2487]. Unfortunately, inositol from phytates is not very bioavailable to non-ruminant animals like humans. Luckily, fruits, specifically citrus fruits, and cantaloupe, are also high in inositol. For example, 120 grams of grapefruit juice contains about 470 mg of myo-inositol. In other common foods, the amount of inositol ranges from 225-1,500 mg/d per 1,800 calories consumed[2488].

Food	Myo-Inositol Content mg/100 g
Grapefruit Juice	376
Peanut Butter	300
Bran Flakes	271
Whole Grapefruit	117
Navy Beans	65
Green Beans	55
Brussel Sprouts	40
Whole Wheat Bread	40
Lima Beans	44
Roast Beef	25
Ham	13
Skim Milk	10

Adding inositol-containing foods into your meal can lower the postprandial glucose response as well as improve overall insulin sensitivity[2489]. Supplementing inositol has also been shown to improve overall glucose and insulin levels[2490,2491]. **The optimal amount of myo-inositol per day is 2-4 grams for improving insulin sensitivity**[2492]. However, it can have laxative effects in people who aren't used to it. Thus, those individuals should stick to 500-1,000 mg multiple times a day.

The Blood Sugar Fix Meal Sequence

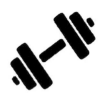

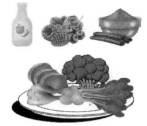

Before the meal
- Exercise before eating
- Eat a high protein breakfast
- Supplement with chromium glycine and inositol
- Supplement with thiamine (thiamine HCL, benfotiamine and/or allithiamine)

During the meal
- Consume 1-2 tbsp apple cider vinegar diluted in 8 oz of water
- Eat protein and vegetables first before carbs
- Add berries or cinnamon to decrease glucose spike

After the meal
- Take a 10-15 min walk after eating

*If you drink tea consume at least 2 hours before or 1 hour after eating to avoid inhibiting thiamine absorption

The Dawn Phenomenon

Your blood sugar levels are supposed to rise naturally in the morning due to waking up and the increase in cortisol. However, **some people get abnormally higher blood sugar between 2 AM and 8 AM, which is called the dawn phenomenon**[2493]. The reason for this, at least in Type 1 diabetics, has to do with an exaggerated production of glucose during the night caused by excessive surges in growth hormone that inhibit insulin's effects, resulting in elevated blood glucose levels[2494]. This response is worse if you have beta cell dysfunction or insulin resistance. Type 2 diabetics get the dawn phenomenon primarily from insulin resistance and obesity[2495,2496]. It's been found that there is a correlation between the dawn phenomenon and obesity and insulin resistance with the frequency of the dawn phenomenon increasing with BMI[2497]. In insulin-dependent diabetics, morning cortisol rise doesn't account for the dawn phenomenon[2498]. The dawn phenomenon is not the same as the Somogyi effect, which is a post-hypoglycemic hyperglycemia rebound that happens during the night. Basically, if you don't eat while sleeping your blood sugar drops and as a result the liver rushes out too much blood glucose to maintain stable blood sugar levels. Although both have similar end results, they have different causes.

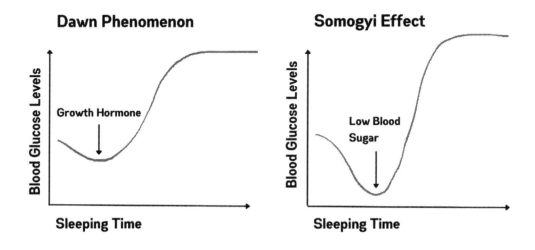

Generally, managing the dawn phenomenon includes overall lifestyle improvements, such as dietary changes, exercise and in the case of diabetics with an A1c above 7% (even after lifestyle interventions) the use of oral diabetic medications or even insulin[2499]. Managing the dawn phenomenon is much more difficult in people with an A1c above 7%[2500]. The dawn phenomenon can extend beyond breakfast if the person is eating a high carb breakfast on top of their already elevated blood sugar levels. Losing postprandial (after meals) glycemic control has been shown to be a first step in developing elevated fasting blood sugar levels[2501]. The second step is high blood sugar in the morning and the third step is hyperglycemia at night. **It's been shown that acute moderate-intensity aerobic exercise before breakfast can reduce the morning rise in blood sugar in Type 2 diabetics**[2502]. Thus, if you do have some excessive hyperglycemia in the mornings, going for a walk or doing other forms of moderate intensity exercise may help. Consuming 2 tablespoons of apple cider vinegar diluted in water at bedtime has also been shown to lower morning glucose levels[2503].

Chapter 13: The Blood Sugar Fix Diet

It's time to talk about implementing all the knowledge we've covered so far. At the end of the day, the needle isn't going to be moving in the right direction, unless you put things into practice. That applies especially to diabetes and glucose problems where you must follow specific routines and habits in terms of exercise, movement, meal timing and food choices. In this chapter, we're going to be talking about **The Blood Sugar Fix diet** – what your diet should look like for various stages of your health.

How Much Protein to Eat

Let's start with the most important macronutrient of them all, even for glucose regulation, protein. Most of your body is made of protein and it's an essential component of building and maintaining muscle[2504]. On this program, the goal is to set yourself up for life by starting to exercise with both weights and cardio because that's the most powerful determinant of your long-term insulin sensitivity and metabolic health. That's why getting enough protein to support this type of exercise routine is important. But protein has more direct benefits for glucose tolerance and insulin resistance as well.

Higher protein diets are always better for weight loss than low protein diets because you burn more calories digesting protein through the thermic effect of food (TEF)[2505,2506]. Protein has a TEF of 20-30%, carbs 7-15% and fat 2-4%[2507]. On a mixed diet, you would spend about 5-15% of your total calories on energy expenditure[2508]. Thus, getting a larger proportion of your daily calories from protein you'll be burning up to 20-30% of those calories just digesting them.

For example, eating a steak that has around 1,000 calories provides you with 700-800 calories after digestion. That helps to create a calorie deficit without any effort, which is important to prevent weight gain, obesity, and insulin resistance.

Protein also tends to be more satiating than carbohydrates or fats, providing longer satiety[2509,2510]. Eating high protein foods for breakfast, such as eggs, promotes satiety and decreases calorie intake in subsequent meals compared to eating cereal or a bagel for breakfast[2511,2512]. At lunch, having an omelet, instead of a jacket potato meal, reduces calorie consumption at dinner[2513]. **Individuals who are allowed to eat as much as they want on a diet comprised of 30% protein, end up eating on average 441 fewer calories a day compared to a diet of 10% protein**[2514]. That's a big difference. A rough estimate is that 1 pound of fat is around 3,500 calories[2515], which would mean that just by switching to a high protein diet without doing anything else you could expect to lose almost a pound of weight per week.

When you're in a calorie deficit, protein helps to mitigate the muscle loss that would naturally occur[2516,2517]. Losing muscle during weight loss is detrimental to long-term weight maintenance because skeletal muscle makes up 15-17% of your resting metabolic rate[2518,2519,2520]. **The number 1 thing to mitigate loss of lean muscle tissue during weight loss is to do resistance training because it signals the body to burn fat and keep muscle instead of the opposite**[2521,2522,2523,2524,2525]. It's been shown that resistance training or high intensity interval training combined with a high protein diet (2.3 g/kg or 35% of total calories) is more effective in lean mass preservation and fat loss than a low protein diet (1 g/kg or 15% of total calories) during a 40% calorie deficit over a 2-week period[2526]. Combining high intensity exercise yields more results for fat loss when combined with a high protein diet of 2.4 g/kg compared to a low protein intake of 1.2 g/kg[2527].

The current Recommended Daily Allowance (RDA) for protein is 0.36 g/lb (0.8 g/kg) of bodyweight[2528]. However, this is deemed to cover only essential physiological requirements[2529]. Many nutrition experts consider this amount to be inadequate[2530], especially for the elderly who may need more to keep their muscle mass with age[2531]. It's been shown that the requirement for optimal muscle growth is 0.7-0.8 g/lb or 1.4-1.6 g/kg of lean body mass[2532]. Going above that doesn't appear to yield any additional benefits. However, during a calorie deficit, getting up to 2.2-3.3 g/kg does provide additional protection against muscle loss[2533,2534,2535,2536,2537]. Eating up to 1.0-1.5 g/kg of protein has been found to improve glycemic control and muscle mass in older adults[2538]. A good general rule is to aim for around 1-1.25 g of protein per pound of lean or ideal bodyweight if you're working on optimizing your body composition and trying to lose weight[2539]. The reason for this is because the higher thermic effect of protein would convert some of the calories you eat into calories lost through digestion.

You might be wondering about the effects of protein on blood sugar and insulin levels. **Historically, higher protein intakes have been considered dangerous to diabetics but today the recommendations have shifted to supporting a protein intake that comprises 20-30% of daily calories for Type 2 diabetes**[2540]. The initial hesitation to recommend more protein is thought to originate from a 1915 study in which eating 6.25 grams of protein produced 3.5 grams of glucose[2541]. However, several studies after that one found that consuming up to 2 grams of protein per kilogram of body weight in a single meal in both diabetics and non-diabetics shows no changes in blood glucose levels[2542,2543]. **Thus, protein doesn't appear to contribute to sustained elevations of glucose, but it does acutely raise insulin (although the spike is not as pronounced as with refined carbs)**[2544]. The insulinotropic effects of protein can improve glucose clearance from the bloodstream in diabetes patients with impaired glucose control[2545,2546,2547]. Adding protein to a meal, especially leaner proteins, reduces the postprandial glucose excursion of that meal and lowers the glycemic response of the next meal[2548,2549].

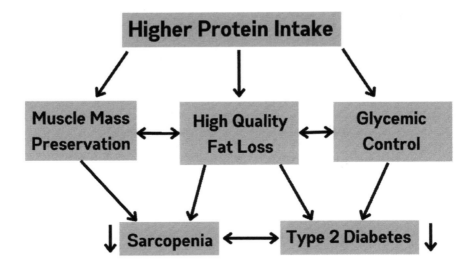

Adapted From: Beaudry and Devries (2019)

To be fair, some observational studies (which can't determine causation) have noted that proteiin from red meat intake is associated with an increased risk of Type 2 diabetes, whereas plant proteins are associated with a reduced risk[2550,2551,2552,2553]. However, there are limited randomized controlled trials to support those claims or that the type of protein would have a significant effect beyond just the total protein content of the diet. One factor that may contribute to these associations is that if animal protein isn't balanced with enough base (whether it be from bicarbonate waters, bicarbonate/citrate supplements, or fruits/vegetables) this can increase the acid load on the body contributing to insulin resistance[2554,2555]. Another potential reason is that red meat (especially grain finished) is higher in calories/fat than plant protein. Losing weight is a major factor that reduces the risk of diabetes and improves glycemic control[2556].

Additionally, animal protein consumption may simply be capturing people who are eating more fast food (burger that also comes with fries and a soft drink). Eating plant proteins that have more fiber will generally result in lower energy intake and higher satiety[2557,2558,2559]. Thus, we recommend eating animal protein with a side of asparagus, broccoli, Brussel's sprouts, etc. Eating foods naturally high in fiber can reduce caloric intake by 700 calories per day[2560]. Thus, if you tolerate it, don't fear foods naturally high in fiber. However, compared to soy protein, whey protein leads to greater lower subsequent food intake and lower postprandial glucose[2561]. Thus, the satiety effect of food is important for controlling caloric intake, which is fundamental to weight loss and diabetes management. Whatever diet and protein enables you to adhere to a smaller calorie deficit, the more suitable it is for you. Regardless, when it comes to meat consumption, choosing leaner proteins, especially when eaten with carbohydrates, is better for glycemic control and insulin sensitivity as high amounts of fats can disrupt glucose regulation and insulin production.

Dairy protein appears to reduce diabetes risk and improve insulin sensitivity[2562,2563]. **Every additional serving of dairy per day is associated with a 9% lower risk of Type 2 diabetes in men, independent of body mass index, physical activity levels and family history of diabetes**[2564]. In women, the risk is 4% lower[2565]. Consuming 4 servings of low-fat dairy milk or yogurt a day has been found to reduce plasma insulin by 9% and improve insulin resistance by 11% in overweight and obese individuals over a 6-month period[2566]. The reason is thought to be partly due to the higher protein content of dairy, its ability to bind and excrete fats and that certain species of probiotics can counteract weight gain and insulin resistance[2567,2568]. **Milk proteins also have insulinotropic properties, which enhance insulin secretion and glucose clearance, while having a low glycemic effect**[2569]. Supplementing with whey protein for 12 weeks reduces fasting plasma insulin by 11% and insulin resistance by 10% in overweight and obese individuals[2570].

You've probably also heard that protein is bad for the kidneys, which is why you should be on a lower protein diet. However, there's no evidence that a higher protein intake would harm kidneys in healthy people[2571,2572]. Too much protein could be bad for those with already existing kidney disease[2573] (although most, if not all of this harm, may actually be due to the acid load and simply balancing the acid load would likely allow for a higher protein intake). Even eating 30% of daily calories from protein hasn't been shown to adversely affect renal function[2574,2575]. A 2-year weight loss trial that compared a high protein diet (30% of calories as protein) to a low protein diet (15% of calories as protein) in 419 Type 2 diabetics saw no difference in renal function or other adverse side-effects[2576]. The American Diabetes Association does recommend a protein intake of 0.8-1.0 g/kg/d for individuals who have early-stage chronic kidney disease (CKD) and 0.8 g/kg/d during later stages of CKD[2577].

You can ask your doctor to assess your kidney health and functioning using the below methods.

- **Blood Pressure** – hypertension damages small blood vessels in the kidneys. Most people are below 140/90. If you have kidney failure, most doctors will say that blood pressure should be lower than 130/80 but 120/80 is considered normal.

- **Protein in Urine** – traces of albumin protein in urine is an early sign of kidney disease. Optimally, you want to have less than 30 mg of albumin per gram of urinary creatinine.

- **Serum Creatinine** – poor kidney functioning leads to the accumulation of creatinine in the blood, typically a waste product. A normal serum creatinine is 0.7-1.3 mg/dL for men and 0.6-1.1 mg/dL for women. However, it can vary, depending on other variables, as having more muscle can increase serum creatinine.

- **Glomerular Filtration Rate (GFR)** – this is a calculation of kidney functioning based on creatinine levels, age, race, gender, etc. A score over 90 is good, 60-89 should be monitored, and less than 60 for three months indicates kidney damage.

- **Cystatin C** – is one of the best ways to estimate kidney function as muscle mass, exercise and creatinine levels will not affect the results, unlike GFR. A normal cystatin C is 0.6-1 mg/L.

To improve kidney health, you want to eat a healthy diet, maintain an active lifestyle, consume an adequate amount of salt, potassium, and magnesium, consume bicarbonate or fruits/vegetables, stay hydrated and avoid refined carbs/sugars/omega-6 seed oils. You should also avoid smoking and excessive alcohol intake.

Overall, a slightly higher protein intake appears to be beneficial for glucose homeostasis and insulin sensitivity. Not only does it help with weight loss and body composition, but it also improves postprandial glucose excursions in many ways. It might be warranted to not eat protein above the 0.8 g/lb of bodyweight for someone with impaired kidney function, but if enough base is consumed in the diet, slightly higher protein intakes may be tolerated, especially if more of that protein comes from plant sources. An intake of 0.7-0.8 g/lb is already close the maximum benefit you get for muscle growth. Eating less than 0.6 g/lb of bodyweight in general is not recommended as that would entail getting more calories from either fats or carbohydrates. Unless someone has severe kidney damage, aiming for 20-30% of daily calories from protein is more optimal, especially for someone who has impaired glucose tolerance and insulin resistance. If you don't have any kidney issues, then ingesting up to 35% of total calories as protein is likely optimal.

Recommended Protein Intakes

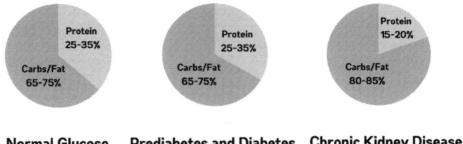

| Normal Glucose Tolerance | Prediabetes and Diabetes Insulin Resistance | Chronic Kidney Disease Renal Dysfunction |

How Many Carbohydrates Should You Eat?

Arguably a more relevant macronutrient for diabetes and glucose regulation are carbohydrates. Consuming high sugar or high glycemic index foods is one of the biggest contributors of insulin resistance and impaired glucose tolerance[2578,2579,2580,2581]. However, **the quality of carbohydrates eaten appears to be much more important than the total quantity of carbohydrates**. It's been shown that diets high in starch and low in fiber are associated with a greater risk of Type 2 diabetes[2582].

A 2009 study found that **among Seventh Day Adventists, those eating a fully vegan high carb diet have half the rate of diabetes than those who are vegetarians or non-vegetarians**[2583]. However, this is likely because they limit refined carbohydrates, sugars, and processed foods, rather than any benefit of eating plants over animal foods. The Seventh Day Adventists are a religious group in California who lean towards an overall healthier lifestyle than the average American. Thus, these types of studies should not be used to support vegan diets, but rather that eliminating ultra-processed foods can have beneficial effects. We know that vegan diets lack many nutrients (bioavailable iron, B2, B12, K2, creatine, carnitine, carnosine, taurine, etc.) and are not ideal for optimal long-term health.

The key differentiating factor is high quality whole plant foods, as those eating less healthy plant-based foods, such as fruit juices, fried potatoes, potato chips, refined grains and vegan desserts have been shown to experience a 16% higher risk of diabetes compared to those eating unprocessed plant-based foods who have a 34% lower risk of diabetes[2584]. Fresh fruit consumption as opposed to fruit juices are associated with lower risk of diabetes and lower risk of death among diabetic individuals[2585]. Whole grain intake but not refined grain intake is linked to reduced Type 2 diabetes risk[2586]. However, this is compared to the Standard American Diet, and should not be taken as whole grains are good to consume for blood glucose control. We believe that avoiding most whole grains (since most are highly refined, particularly whole grain bread/cereal) will improve blood sugar control. Generally, **plant-based dietary patterns and inclusion of whole food plant-based foods are associated with reduced risk of Type 2 diabetes in a dose-specific manner**[2587].

Increases Diabetes Risk	Reduces Diabetes Risk
White bread Whole grains (compared to lean meats, dairy, fruit, and vegetables)	Quinoa and steel cut oats (but they still need to be limited due to their carbohydrate content)
Fruit juices	Whole fruit
Pastries	Oatmeal
Milk chocolate	Dark chocolate
Ice cream	Greek Yogurt
Soda	Milk
Potato chips	Whole potato
Crackers	Vegetables
Candy	Nuts/Seeds
Processed meat	Legumes/Beans (limit due to the carbohydrate content)

A 2017 meta-analysis found that whole grains, fruit, and dairy consumption was linearly associated with a reduced risk of Type 2 diabetes, whereas sugar-sweetened beverages, processed meat and red meat was linked to an increased risk[2588]. The link between sugary drinks is self-explanatory. With processed meat, the increased risk is also mediated by the fact that if you eat processed meat, you are likely eating lower quality ham, sausages, and/or hot dogs. With natural red meat like grass-fed beef, however, the link isn't that clearly defined. In fact, a 2021 prospective study found that there is no association between unprocessed red meat and poultry intake and mortality or cardiovascular disease, whereas the link exists with processed meat intake[2589]. Thus, **the quality of the meat matters as much as the quality of the carbohydrates**. The same way all carbs don't promote diabetes, all meat doesn't do so either.

A lot of low-carb, ketogenic diets that include meat have been found to yield positive effects in treating diabetes and insulin resistance[2590,2591,2592]. Long-term studies on obese patients on a low-carb ketogenic diet see that it's effective for losing weight, lowering BMI, and decreasing markers of metabolic syndrome[2593,2594,2595,2596]. **A 2021 meta-analysis on 23 trials with 14,759 participants found that 6 months of a low carbohydrate diet can result in higher rates of Type 2 diabetes remission than control diets**[2597]. **However, after about a year the differences flatten out.** Similar results are observed in weight loss. It's been shown that the differences between low fat and low carb diets on weight loss also become equal after a year even when low carb diets yield more weight loss in the short term[2598,2599,2600,2601,2602,2603,2604,2605]. That greater short-term weight loss is partly explained by the fact that insulin makes you hold onto more water and when you go on a low carb diet you initially lose a lot of water weight.

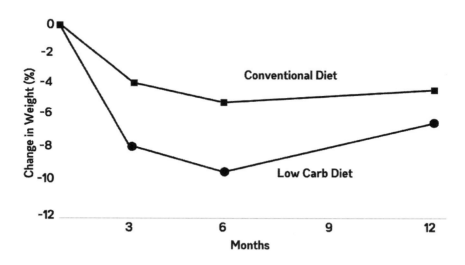

Adapted From: Foster et al (2003)

Low carb diets haven't been found to be metabolically superior to high carb diets if calories are equated for[2606,2607,2608,2609]. When people report anecdotally of being able to lose weight with a low carb ketogenic diet, it's due to reduced subconscious calorie consumption. Removing certain high carb foods and implementing more protein, as is common on low carb diets, can result in greater satiety and less hunger, which enables the person to eat fewer calories. As a result, their biomarkers improve and their insulin resistance gets better because of the weight loss. However, even in studies where both low carb and conventional diets yield weight loss results, the low carb diets generally result in slightly better blood sugar and insulin levels in the short-term but in the long term the results are the same in both diets[2610,2611,2612,2613]. The difference is that the LDL cholesterol on low carb diets almost always increases even with weight loss and drop in glycemia[2614].

Thus, carbohydrate restriction in the short-term can be very effective and fast in improving markers of diabetes and insulin resistance, especially in overweight individuals. However, it's very clearly shown how long-term ketosis and high fat diet causes short-term insulin resistance (essentially carbohydrate intolerance)[2615]. Granted, that insulin resistance is resolved after carbohydrates are introduced back into the diet but staying in ketosis for the rest of your life is not the most optimal way to maintain insulin sensitivity. What's more, it's not necessary to be on a strict low carb ketogenic diet to see improvements in metabolic health, diabetes or weight loss, as even a low fat high carb diet can result in the same effects. The determining variable is adherence to what suits you the most. Many people find restricting carbohydrates to be the most effective way to keep the weight off and blood sugar down. However, others find that being more active and consuming a moderate intake of carbohydrates works best for them. Many times, your activity level and level of lean mass will determine how many carbohydrates are right for you. Additionally, carbohydrate intake should be based on your level of insulin sensitivity.

3 tiers of carbohydrate intake based on your current glycemia and metabolic health:

- **Normal glucose regulation:** If your fasting blood sugar is <5.6 mmol/L (<100 mg/dL) and your A1C is <5.7%, then you're in normal metabolic health in terms of glucose tolerance. Consuming around 100-200 grams of carbohydrates per day (the higher end in those who are more active or with more lean muscle mass)

  - If you're exercising a lot with both weights and cardio, and you're also lean, then you can eat up to ~ 300 grams of carbohydrates on intense workout days. If you start to see that your glucose levels are getting worse, then dial down the carbohydrate intake and adjust as needed. The main goal is that most of your carbohydrate intake comes from whole foods. If you do eat some refined carbohydrates/sugars, ideally that should occur after an intense workout.

  - If you have normal glucose levels, you can also do cyclical carbohydrate restriction, which means eating low carb on some days and incorporating more carbs on other days. Usually, people eat low carb keto for 2-5 days in a row and then have a high carb meal. Or you can eat low carb on non-training days and high carb on training days.

- **Prediabetes:** If your fasting blood sugar is 5.6–7.0 mmol/L (100–125 mg/dL) and your A1C is 5.7-6.4%, then you're in the prediabetic range. In that case, **it's recommended to restrict carbohydrates to < 100**

grams a day in the short-term to bring your glucose levels back to normal.

- ○ You must figure out the reason why you're beginning to show early signs of diabetes. Is it a lack of exercise, micronutrients, sleep deprivation or chronic stress? Whatever the case is, identifying the reason is important. Otherwise, you'll be forced to always be controlled by your carbohydrate intake, because the fact of the matter is that a healthy metabolism should be able to tolerate carbohydrates in reasonable amounts (it's appropriate for our human physiology). The main issue is usually being too sedentary and under muscled. Having more muscle allows you to consume more carbohydrates and get away with it. Carbohydrate restriction is more of a band-aid to the problem, but it doesn't fix the root cause.

- **Diabetes:** If your fasting blood sugar is ≥7.0 mmol/L (≥126 mg/dL) and your A1C is ≥6.5%, then you're in the diabetic range. In that case, for the quickest improvements in your glycemia, **it's recommended to restrict carbohydrates to < 50 grams a day.** However, this should be done gradually as you don't want to go from consuming 300 grams of carbs to 40 grams right away. Going down by 50-100 grams of carbohydrates per week is more sustainable. This will not only begin to improve your insulin sensitivity but also puts out the flame of chronic hyperglycemia that would keep promoting the pathologies and co-morbidities of diabetes, like atherosclerosis and neuropathy.

  - ○ It's very likely that even if you have diabetes, you will be able to eat a reasonable amount of carbohydrates in the future. You just need to improve your insulin sensitivity and glucose tolerance, which may take time. However, in the short-term, it's better to restrict carbs to allow the body to regain some of its normal functions.

Recommended Carbohydrate Intakes

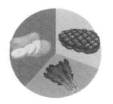

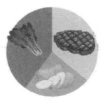

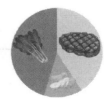

Normal Glucose Tolerance 100-300 g/day

Prediabetes <100 g/day

Diabetes <50 g/day

The way you reintroduce carbohydrates is also very relevant when doing a low carb diet for several months in a row. Within a week, you do not expect the carbohydrate restriction to cause any insulin resistance, but it would develop after a few weeks. **That's why whenever you do plan to have a meal that has more carbs like a potato or bread, you shouldn't consume it by itself or in large quantities after having been in ketosis for several weeks.** That would result in abrupt hyperglycemia. Instead, you must break ketosis with a smaller amount of carbohydrates, preferably low glycemic complex carbohydrates like vegetables or even fruit. The idea is to slowly sensitize the body to carbohydrates again before bombarding it with a large dose of carbs or sugar. Thus, breaking ketosis with pizza and donuts isn't very smart, as you'll promote hyperglycemia and potentially reverse a lot of the work done beforehand. Instead, you should start small and slowly increase your carbohydrate intake.

Being on a very low carbohydrate diet can also backfire in terms of glycemic control and weight loss. For example, you may end up eating too many calories from added fats, which can be equally harmful to weight gain and insulin resistance. Avoiding low calorie plant foods like vegetables, berries and fruits also may lead to a calorie surplus from eating too many high calorie foods, such as cheese, fatty meat and fat bombs like heavy cream or butter. At this point, even having lower levels of insulin and blood sugar aren't going to prevent you from weight gain and developing poor metabolic function. There's a lot of evidence that a higher fiber intake helps with losing weight and keeping it off[2616,2617,2618]. Fiber also decreases the amount of fat you absorb from a meal by binding with fats[2619,2620].

More importantly, fiber reduces postprandial glucose excursions and lowers the glycemic load of a meal[2621,2622,2623,2624,2625,2626]. It's recommended that a diet for diabetics should provide at least 25-50 grams of fiber per day or 15-25 grams of fiber per 1000 calories consumed[2627]. One cup of broccoli (~90 grams) contains around 2.2 grams of fiber[2628]. A single medium-sized apple, however, has 4.4 grams of fiber[2629]. In our opinion, a moderate intake of fiber (10-20 grams per day) is best because if the diet is too high in fiber, it's generally too low in micronutrients.

Here are the highest fiber sources[2630]:

Food Source	Amount of Fiber
Oats, raw, 1 cup	16.5 g
Split peas, 1 cup	16.3 g
Lentils, 1 cup	13.1 g
Chickpeas, 1 cup	12.5 g
Kidney beans, 1 cup	12.2 g
Avocado, 1 cup	10 g
Chia seeds, 1 ounce	9.75 g
Raspberries, 1 cup	8 g
Pear, medium size	5.5 g
Artichoke, 100 grams	5.4 g
Quinoa, 1 cup	5.2 g
Apples, 1 medium	4.4 g
Almonds, 3 tablespoons	4 g
Beetroot, 1 cup	3.8 g
Sweet potato, 1 medium	3.8 g
Carrots, 1 cup	3.6 g
Brussels sprouts, 1 cup	3.3 g
Banana, 1 medium	3.1 g
Dark Chocolate, 70-85%, 1 ounce	3.1 g
Strawberries, 1 cup	3 g

Broccoli, 1 cup	2.4 g

Fibrous carbohydrates with more resistant starch, like cooked and cooled potatoes or resistant starch-fortified muffins even, can lower postprandial glucose area under the curve by 33% and postprandial insulin area under the curve by 38%[2631]. Thus, it's worthwhile to prepare your high glycemic carbs in a way that increases their resistant starch content. For that, you have to lightly cook them and let them cool down in the fridge overnight. After that, you're still allowed to re-heat them without worrying that the resistant starch would be destroyed. Green and yellow-to-green bananas also have significantly more resistant starch and less glucose than yellow and yellow-to-ripe bananas. However, for many people it may be best to simply workout, build muscle and eat a ripe, or slightly green, banana.

How Much Fat to Eat

Once you've figured out how much protein and carbs you're going to eat, then fat would make up the rest of your calories. There is no reason to try to max out on fat or add it beyond what is necessary because after you've covered your physiological needs for fat, then it just becomes an extra source of calories with no additional benefits. A higher fat intake itself isn't going to improve insulin sensitivity or glucose tolerance. The carbohydrate restriction combined with a higher fiber and protein intake will do that. In fact, excessive fat intake can be harmful for long-term insulin sensitivity and glucose tolerance.

The minimum amount of fat per day is recommended to be 15% of total calories[2632]. However, South-East Asia, like Vietnam, live on diets comprising of only 6-7% fat[2633]. Most people will do best on a fat intake between 20-40% of total calories. On a low carb diet, or during a low carb period, your fat % could be up to 60% but any more than that isn't really recommended as you would have to start restricting protein. **If you are on a low carb diet due to blood sugar issues, then your protein intake should already be at least 30-35%.** The lowest carbohydrate intake in that scenario would be 10% because otherwise you're undereating fiber, which isn't optimal for satiety. For those who are active and lean, the optimal macronutrient breakdown will sit somewhere around 20-40% carbohydrates, 25-35% protein, and 25-55% fat. For those on low carbohydrate diets, the macronutrient breakdown will look like this i.e., 5-15% carbohydrates, 25-35% protein and 50-70% fat.

Your fat calories should come predominantly from low inflammatory sources that improve insulin sensitivity and glucose clearance. Namely, omega-3 fatty acids from fish and seafood, saturated fats from dairy like yogurt and cottage cheese, fat from grass-fed meat, and monounsaturated fat from extra virgin olive oil, avocados and a little from nuts and seeds (although many people don't tolerate nuts/seeds). Cooking with omega-6 seed oils like canola oil, corn, sunflower, soybean, and safflower oil will likely worsen insulin resistance and impair glucose tolerance. You should not combine high amounts of saturated fats (sour cream and butter) with high glycemic carbohydrates like rice or potatoes. A little is fine, but don't overdo it.

Fat intake recommendations based on 3 tiers of glucose levels:

- **Normal glucose tolerance:** For most people this will be 20-40% carbohydrates (on hard work out days you could eat a higher carb intake of up to ~ 50% of your daily calories). Ideally, protein should make up around 25-35% of total calories, the higher end being more appropriate for work out days.

- **Prediabetes:** If you have signs of prediabetes, then the first thing to reduce is total carbohydrate intake to 30% or less of daily calories. The protein intake should be somewhat higher around 30-40%, which gives 30-35% of daily calories left for fat.

- **Diabetes:** With diabetes, a low carb diet in the short term is the way to go for fastest improvement in blood glucose and insulin levels. That would mean dropping carbohydrate intake to 20% or lower. Protein should again still be relatively high at 35% or even at 40%, which would give 40-60% of daily calories from fat.

The Blood Sugar Fix Recommended Macros

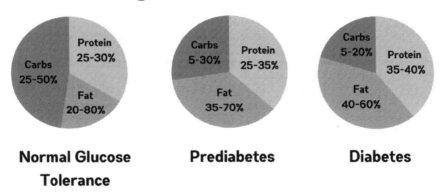

The key in adjusting your fat and carb intake is cycling through periods of higher carb and lower fat or lower carb and higher fat intake. Eating high carb and high fat at the same time promotes obesity and insulin resistance by disrupting the Randle Cycle and increasing total calorie intake. Thus, an intake of 40-45% fat and 40-45% carbs with only 10-20% of your calories coming from protein isn't optimal for weight loss nor glucose tolerance. Ideally, this is what the macronutrient intake should look like

1.) Intense workout days in those who have good glucose tolerance:

- 40-50% carbs, 20% fat, and 30-40% protein

2.) No to low intensity workout days (those who have good glucose tolerance)

- 25-30% carbs, 30-35% fat, and 25-35% protein

3.) Those who are insulin resistant (with normal kidney function):

- 10-15% carbs, 50% fat, and 35-40% protein

Most Americans consume a high carb (40-50%), high fat (40-50%), low protein (10-15%) diet, whereas the ideal diet for weight loss is moderate fat (30-40%), moderate carb (30%), high protein (25-40%). Of course, resistance training and cardio should be performed during the week, which would necessitate protein intake at the higher end of that range (35-40%).

Healthy cooking oils

- Extra virgin olive oil

- Butter

- Ghee

- Tallow

- Coconut oil

Cooking oils to avoid

- Soybean oil

- Sunflower oil

- Safflower oil

- Cottonseed oil

- Canola oil (rapeseed)

- Corn oil

- Grapeseed oil

- Rice bran oil

- Peanut oil

- Sesame oil

Meal Structure

Regardless of your current metabolic health, most of the food you eat in volume should be lean meat, dairy and low glycemic fibrous fruits, and vegetables. Starchy carbohydrates should be more complimentary and adjusted based on the situation. The actual number of calories from animal foods would be greater than from plants because they're higher in calories than vegetables or fruit. Per serving, something like yogurt or meat can have 2-3x the amount of calories than broccoli even when that serving of broccoli is 2-3x larger in size. Thus, fibrous plant foods help to promote quick satiety, reducing hunger, slowing down gastric emptying, and decreasing postprandial glucose spikes. They're also important to be eaten with fattier meals as they bind to some of the fats and reduce their absorption. Dairy improves insulin secretion and thus lowers the glucose response to a meal, which is why it's recommended to eat some dairy with a carbohydrate meal as well. **For someone with impaired glucose tolerance, every meal should be low in refined carbohydrates, 30-50 grams of protein and at least one meal should include dairy.** However, you must be careful with choosing the type of dairy you eat as a lot of the dairy products tend to have a lot of added sugars. So, choose unflavored and no sugar added yogurts and cottage cheeses. For those who have good insulin sensitivity, adding a little honey or maple syrup with some cinnamon is perfectly fine. You can even add chocolate or vanilla whey protein to your yogurt to boost its protein content. Those who are insulin resistant may want to take 1-2 tablespoons of apple cider vinegar diluted in 8 oz. of water prior to or during a meal that contains a fair amount of starchy carbohydrates (like rice or potatoes).

Recommended Plate Reference

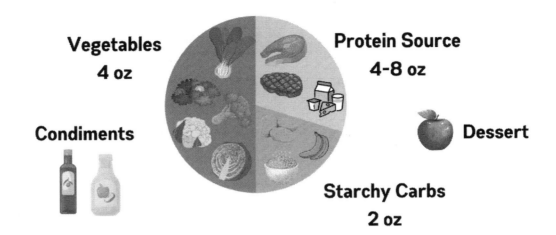

Vegetables
4 oz

Protein Source
4-8 oz

Condiments

Dessert

Starchy Carbs
2 oz

THE BLOOD SUGAR FIX FOOD PYRAMID

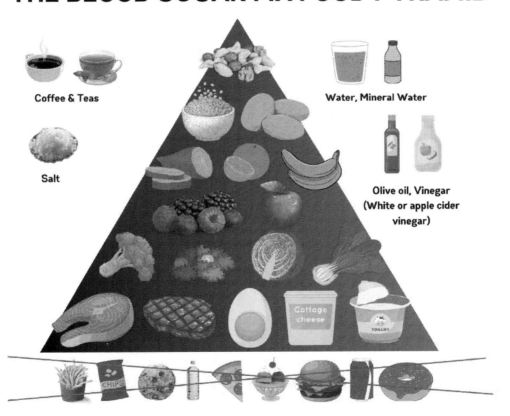

Coffee & Teas

Water, Mineral Water

Salt

Olive oil, Vinegar
(White or apple cider
vinegar)

The Blood Sugar Fix Food Pyramid describes the proportion of calories coming from different foods. If you follow the meal plate reference showed beforehand, it's easy to achieve satiety after every meal with little spikes in glucose. Regardless, you should still go for a 10–15-minute walk after eating even a low glycemic food as it will help with digestion and lowering any rise in blood sugar that would naturally occur.

Overall, it's recommended to practice some time-restricted eating as well to not disrupt your circadian rhythm and help to adhere to a lower calorie intake. Times spent in a purely fasted state with nothing else consumed but coffee, tea or water would help lower your glucose and insulin levels, which is hard to achieve while eating. That's why intermittent fasting can be so powerful for improving insulin sensitivity and glucose tolerance. Generally, **you should stop eating 3 hours before bed.** The two easiest ways to intermittent fast are either 1.) Skip breakfast or 2.) Have an early dinner. Some people prefer the 16/8 method wherein they eat within 8 hours. Whichever window you choose, you don't need any more than 3-4 meals a day and it's better to minimize snacking in between meals. If you do crave a snack, then have a low glycemic piece of fruit (apple or berries), Greek yogurt, or beef jerky for some protein.

Limit or Avoid	Consume to Satiety
Cereal	Greek Yogurt
Juice	Cottage Cheese
Muffins	Pastured Eggs
Waffles	Grass-Fed- Meat, Chicken, Beef, etc.
Bagels	Organic Bacon, Sausages
Donuts	Steel Cut Oats
Toast	Ezekiel Bread with Almond Butter, Bananas, and Cinnamon (snack)
Croissants	Fruit and Berries
McMuffins	Fish, Sardines, Salmon
Sausage Biscuits	Omelet
McGriddles	Cheddar Cheese Stick
Pancakes	Nuts (if tolerated)
Hotcakes	Nut Butters (consume in moderation, ensure there's no seed oils added)
Hash Browns	Celery, Peanut Butter, Raisins (snack)
Hot Dogs or Cheese Dogs	Cheddar Cheese Stick
Cheesecake	Pickles, Olives

Macaroni Salad or Potato Salad	Grass-Fed Jerky (Beef, venison, bison, etc.)

Foods eaten in the Standard American Diet aren't a mandatory part of any human's diet. They're ultra-processed and manufactured to be overconsumed and promote insulin resistance. That's why you shouldn't have any fear of missing out from a health perspective. However, it's obvious that they taste great. Fortunately, there are many healthier alternative foods you can substitute the modern foods with that have a superior effect on your blood glucose levels and metabolic health.

Replace or Limit This	Eat This Instead
Yellow Banana (great post workout however)	Greenish Banana (more fiber)
Wheat Bread	Ezekiel Bread
Ice Cream	Yogurt or Cottage Cheese with Berries
Big Mac	Steak or Bun-less Burger Wrapped in Lettuce
French Fries	Organic Potatoes/Sweet Potatoes
Pizza	Cauliflower Crust Pizza
Sugary Cereal	Greek Yogurt with Nuts and Seeds
American Cheese	Raw Grass-fed Cheese

Salad Dressing	Extra Virgin Olive Oil
Butter and Margarine	Grass-Fed Butter
Eggs	Pastured Eggs
Grain-Fed Meat	Grass-Fed Meat
Milk Chocolate	70%+ Dark Chocolate
Fake Juices	Citrus Fruit (clementine, orange, etc.) or small amounts of 100% fruit juice
Peanut Butter	Almond Butter (small amounts of peanut butter on occasion is fine)
Potato Chips	Nuts with salt or pickles

Conclusion

We hope that The Blood Sugar Fix helps you improve your insulin sensitivity and achieve optimal metabolic health. No matter what your level of glucose tolerance – whether it be normal or diabetic – the information here when put into practice will have a positive effect on your blood sugar levels. As a final summary, here are some of the most important key takeaways and tips to remember from the book.

1. **Eat whole foods predominantly** – 80-90% of the time eat whole foods including meat, fish, eggs, dairy, fruit, vegetables and some nuts and seeds if tolerated. Some processing of food, as in the case of dairy and olive oil, isn't inherently harmful.

2. **Limit ultra-processed food consumption** – this includes pastries, pizza, cookies, chips, milk chocolate, candy, hot dogs, etc. The more processed the food becomes, the higher the likelihood of it raising your blood sugar and making you gain weight. These foods are refined and with added sugar and fat that promote weight gain and insulin resistance.

3. **Stay physically active** – you should do something physical activity every day whether that be lifting weights (3-5 times per week), cardio (3 times per week), hiking, cleaning the house or just going for long walks (every day, if possible, preferably after meals). Movement is one of the biggest determinants of your glucose tolerance and insulin sensitivity.

4. **Sleep enough** – try to get at least 7-8 hours of sleep per night.

5. **Morning daylight exposure** – synchronize your circadian clocks and offset proper cortisol production with exposure to natural sunlight after waking up. If the sun hasn't risen yet you can use indoor lighting.

6. **Time-restricted eating** – don't eat too close to bed and don't snack throughout the day. Have 2-3 solid meals and if you need a snack then have something low glycemic, preferably high protein.

7. **Walk after meals** – go for a 10–15-minute walk after eating to lower the blood sugar spike and improve digestion.

8. **Consume vinegar and/or olive oil with your food** – Consume 1-2 tablespoons of apple cider vinegar in 8 oz. of water. Add extra virgin olive oil to your vegetables.

9. **Eat some dairy with fatty meals** – if you have a meal that has more fats or even carbs, then incorporate some dairy like cottage cheese or yogurt to reduce the amount of fat absorbed.

10. **Drink mineral waters** – drinking mineral waters also helps with lipids and digestion.

11. **Load up on protein and fiber** – most of your plate should comprise of fibrous vegetables with a good amount of protein (~ 30-50 grams of protein per meal).

12. **Opt for lower glycemic carbohydrates** – whenever you can, choose the lower glycemic option. Instead of white bread, or even whole grain bread, choose vegetables. When cooking potatoes, don't overcook them and let them cool down and eat them the next day to increase their resistant starch content.

13. **Dim light at night** – dim down the lights to not disrupt your sleep and promote poor glucose regulation the next day. Using blue blocking glasses enables you to still use your technology that emits artificial blue and green light. But ideally you should also install lights with a dimmer

option or have a salt lamp next to your bed instead of a regular indoor lighting.

14. **Consume Ceylon cinnamon** with carbohydrate meals.

15. **Supplement with chromium** (200-1,000 mcg), **glycine** (2-3 grams) **and inositol** (1-2 grams) before meals.

16. **Supplement with thiamine HCL** (50 mg/day), **benfotiamine** (350 mg 2-3 times/day) **and allithiamine** (50-300 mg/day). Glucose oxidation requires thiamine as a cofactor and supplementing with all 3 forms of thiamine is likely more optimal than just one.

17. **Supplement with magnesium** (100-400 mg/day). Magnesium supplementation has been shown to improve insulin sensitivity.

Diabetes is obviously a very serious and harmful condition. It causes a lot of suffering in many ways. With Type 1 diabetes the situation is unfortunate as there is currently no cure for this condition. You can only manage the symptoms and severity of the disease. It doesn't mean that a Type 1 diabetic can't live a fulfilling life – they absolutely can, especially when taking care of their body and following a physically active lifestyle with proper dietary habits. The same applies to Type 2 diabetes, which is certainly treatable.

The information in this book should not replace professional medical advice. However, it can certainly enhance your results in terms of improving your body composition and glucose tolerance. Medications can only take you so far because they do not fix the root of the problem regarding insulin resistance and glucose intolerance. To solve that, you must fix your diet, exercise, sleep, stress, and your overall lifestyle. That's exactly why we wrote this book. We wish you all the best on your journey to achieving and maintaining optimal metabolic health and glucose tolerance.

References

[1] GBD 2015 Disease and Injury Incidence and Prevalence Collaborators (2016). Global, regional, and national incidence, prevalence, and years lived with disability for 310 diseases and injuries, 1990-2015: a systematic analysis for the Global Burden of Disease Study 2015. Lancet (London, England), 388(10053), 1545–1602. https://doi.org/10.1016/S0140-6736(16)31678-6

[2] Danaei, G., Finucane, M. M., Lu, Y., Singh, G. M., Cowan, M. J., Paciorek, C. J., Lin, J. K., Farzadfar, F., Khang, Y. H., Stevens, G. A., Rao, M., Ali, M. K., Riley, L. M., Robinson, C. A., Ezzati, M., & Global Burden of Metabolic Risk Factors of Chronic Diseases Collaborating Group (Blood Glucose) (2011). National, regional, and global trends in fasting plasma glucose and diabetes prevalence since 1980: systematic analysis of health examination surveys and epidemiological studies with 370 country-years and 2·7 million participants. Lancet (London, England), 378(9785), 31–40. https://doi.org/10.1016/S0140-6736(11)60679-X

[3] De Silva et al (2018). Inequalities in the prevalence of diabetes mellitus and its risk factors in Sri Lanka: a lower middle income country. International journal for equity in health, 17(1), 45.

[4] Menke et al (2015) 'Prevalence of and Trends in Diabetes Among Adults in the United States, 1988-2012', JAMA. 2015;314(10):1021-1029. doi:10.1001/jama.2015.10029

[5] World Health Organization. (1999). Definition, diagnosis and classification of diabetes mellitus and its complications : report of a WHO consultation. Part 1, Diagnosis and classification of diabetes mellitus. World Health Organization. https://apps.who.int/iris/handle/10665/66040

[6] Daneman D. (2006). Type 1 diabetes. Lancet (London, England), 367(9513), 847–858. https://doi.org/10.1016/S0140-6736(06)68341-4

[7] Smyth, S., & Heron, A. (2006). Diabetes and obesity: the twin epidemics. Nature medicine, 12(1), 75–80. https://doi.org/10.1038/nm0106-75

[8] Laforest, S., Labrecque, J., Michaud, A., Cianflone, K., & Tchernof, A. (2015). Adipocyte size as a determinant of metabolic disease and adipose tissue dysfunction. Critical Reviews in Clinical Laboratory Sciences, 52(6), 301–313. doi:10.3109/10408363.2015.1041582

[9] Bergman, R. N., Kim, S. P., Catalano, K. J., Hsu, I. R., Chiu, J. D., Kabir, M. , Hucking, K. and Ader, M. (2006), Why Visceral Fat is Bad: Mechanisms of the Metabolic Syndrome. Obesity, 14: 16S-19S.

[10] Virtue, S., & Vidal-Puig, A. (2010). Adipose tissue expandability, lipotoxicity and the Metabolic Syndrome — An allostatic perspective. Biochimica et Biophysica Acta (BBA) - Molecular and Cell Biology of Lipids, 1801(3), 338–349. doi:10.1016/j.bbalip.2009.12.006

[11] Taylor, R., & Holman, R. R. (2014). Normal weight individuals who develop Type 2 diabetes: the personal fat threshold. Clinical Science, 128(7), 405–410. doi:10.1042/cs20140553

[12] Al-Goblan, A. S., Al-Alfi, M. A., & Khan, M. Z. (2014). Mechanism linking diabetes mellitus and obesity. Diabetes, metabolic syndrome and obesity : targets and therapy, 7, 587–591. https://doi.org/10.2147/DMSO.S67400

[13] Tfayli, H., & Arslanian, S. (2009). Pathophysiology of type 2 diabetes mellitus in youth: the evolving chameleon. Arquivos brasileiros de endocrinologia e metabologia, 53(2), 165–174. https://doi.org/10.1590/s0004-27302009000200008

[14] World Health Organization (2011) 'Global status report on noncommunicable diseases 2010: Description of the global burden of NCDs, their risk factors and determinants', Noncommunicable diseases and mental health, Accessed Online Jan 13 2021: https://www.who.int/nmh/publications/ncd_report2010/en/

[15] Bommer et al (2018). Global Economic Burden of Diabetes in Adults: Projections From 2015 to 2030. Diabetes care, 41(5), 963–970. https://doi.org/10.2337/dc17-1962

[16] Wild et al (2004). "Global prevalence of diabetes: estimates for the year 2000 and projections for 2030". Diabetes Care. 27 (5): 1047–1053.

[17] World Health Organization (2009) 'GLOBAL HEALTH RISKS: Mortality and burden of disease attributable to selected major risks', WHO Library Cataloguing-in-Publication Data, Accessed Online Jan 13 2021: https://www.who.int/healthinfo/global_burden_disease/GlobalHealthRisks_report_full.pdf

[18] Roglic, G., Unwin, N., Bennett, P. H., Mathers, C., Tuomilehto, J., Nag, S., … King, H. (2005). The Burden of Mortality Attributable to Diabetes: Realistic estimates for the year 2000. Diabetes Care, 28(9), 2130–2135. doi:10.2337/diacare.28.9.2130

[19] Bitzur R. (2011). Diabetes and cardiovascular disease: when it comes to lipids, statins are all you need. Diabetes care, 34 Suppl 2(Suppl 2), S380–S382. https://doi.org/10.2337/dc11-s256

[20] Shah, A. D., Langenberg, C., Rapsomaniki, E., Denaxas, S., Pujades-Rodriguez, M., Gale, C. P., … Hemingway, H. (2015). Type 2 diabetes and incidence of cardiovascular diseases: a cohort study in 1·9 million people. The Lancet Diabetes & Endocrinology, 3(2), 105–113. doi:10.1016/s2213-8587(14)70219-0

[21] Ho, J. E., Paultre, F., & Mosca, L. (2003). Is Diabetes Mellitus a Cardiovascular Disease Risk Equivalent for Fatal Stroke in Women? Stroke, 34(12), 2812–2816. doi:10.1161/01.str.0000102901.41780.5c

[22] Morrish, N. J., Wang, S.-L., Stevens, L. K., Fuller, J. H., & Keen, H. (2001). Mortality and causes of death in the WHO multinational study of vascular disease in diabetes. Diabetologia, 44(S2), S14–S21. doi:10.1007/pl00002934

[23] NIDDK (2017) 'Diabetic Kidney Disease', Preventing Diabetes Problems, Accessed Online Jan 13 2021: https://www.niddk.nih.gov/health-information/diabetes/overview/preventing-problems/diabetic-kidney-disease

[24] Pasquier F. (2010). Diabetes and cognitive impairment: how to evaluate the cognitive status?. Diabetes & metabolism, 36 Suppl 3, S100–S105. https://doi.org/10.1016/S1262-3636(10)70475-4

[25] Boulton A. J. (1998). Lowering the risk of neuropathy, foot ulcers and amputations. Diabetic medicine : a journal of the British Diabetic Association, 15 Suppl 4, S57–S59. https://doi.org/10.1002/(sici)1096-9136(1998120)15:4+3.3.co;2-4

[26] Dwyer, M. S., Melton, L. J., 3rd, Ballard, D. J., Palumbo, P. J., Trautmann, J. C., & Chu, C. P. (1985). Incidence of diabetic retinopathy and blindness: a population-based study in Rochester, Minnesota. Diabetes care, 8(4), 316–322. https://doi.org/10.2337/diacare.8.4.316

[27] Kraft (2020) 'Detection of Diabetes Mellitus In Situ (Occult Diabetes)', Meridian Valley Labs, Accessed Online Jan 18 2021: http://meridianvalleylab.com/wp-content/uploads/2012/08/GITT-Article-Re-type1.pdf

[28] DiNicolantonio, J. J., Bhutani, J., OKeefe, J. H., & Crofts, C. (2017). Postprandial insulin assay as the earliest biomarker for diagnosing pre-diabetes, type 2 diabetes and increased cardiovascular risk. Open heart, 4(2), e000656. https://doi.org/10.1136/openhrt-2017-000656

[29] World Health Organization (2013) 'Diabetes', Fact Sheets, Accessed Online Jan 13 2021 https://web.archive.org/web/20130826174444/http://www.who.int/mediacentre/factsheets/fs312/en/

[30] American Diabetes Association (2010). Diagnosis and classification of diabetes mellitus. Diabetes care, 33 Suppl 1(Suppl 1), S62–S69. https://doi.org/10.2337/dc10-S062

[31] Vijan S. (2010). In the clinic. Type 2 diabetes. Annals of internal medicine, 152(5), ITC31–ITC316. https://doi.org/10.7326/0003-4819-152-5-201003020-01003

[32] International Expert Committee (2009). International Expert Committee report on the role of the A1C assay in the diagnosis of diabetes. Diabetes care, 32(7), 1327–1334. https://doi.org/10.2337/dc09-9033

[33] Nathan, D. M., & DCCT/EDIC Research Group (2014). The diabetes control and complications trial/epidemiology of diabetes interventions and complications study at 30 years: overview. Diabetes care, 37(1), 9–16. https://doi.org/10.2337/dc13-2112

[34] Nathan DM, Cleary PA, Backlund JY, Genuth SM, Lachin JM, Orchard TJ, Raskin P, Zinman B; Diabetes Control and Epidemiology of Diabetes Interventions and Complications (DCCT/EDIC) Study Research Group. Intensive diabetes treatment and cardiovascular disease in patients with type 1 diabetes. N Engl J Med. 2005 Dec 22;353(25):2643-53. doi: 10.1056/NEJMoa052187. PMID: 16371630; PMCID: PMC2637991.

[35] Intensive blood-glucose control with sulphonylureas or insulin compared with conventional treatment and risk of complications in patients with type 2 diabetes (UKPDS 33). UK Prospective Diabetes Study (UKPDS) Group. Lancet. 1998 Sep 12;352(9131):837-53. Erratum in: Lancet 1999 Aug 14;354(9178):602. PMID: 9742976.

[36] Adler et al (2000). Association of systolic blood pressure with macrovascular and microvascular complications of type 2 diabetes (UKPDS 36): prospective observational study. BMJ (Clinical research ed.), 321(7258), 412–419. https://doi.org/10.1136/bmj.321.7258.412

[37] Effect of intensive blood-glucose control with metformin on complications in overweight patients with type 2 diabetes (UKPDS 34). UK Prospective Diabetes Study (UKPDS) Group. (1998). Lancet (London, England), 352(9131), 854–865.

[38] Manson et al (1992). A prospective study of exercise and incidence of diabetes among US male physicians. JAMA, 268(1), 63–67.

[39] U.S. Department of Health and Human Services: Healthy People 2000: Summary Report, Washington, DC: U.S., Department of Health and Human Services; 1992:6-8, 55, 91-92.

[40] Tuomilehto et al (2001). Prevention of type 2 diabetes mellitus by changes in lifestyle among subjects with impaired glucose tolerance. The New England journal of medicine, 344(18), 1343–1350.

[41] Pan et al (1997). Effects of Diet and Exercise in Preventing NIDDM in People With Impaired Glucose Tolerance: The Da Qing IGT and Diabetes Study. Diabetes Care, 20(4), 537–544.

[42] Manson et al (1991). Physical activity and incidence of non-insulin-dependent diabetes mellitus in women. Lancet (London, England), 338(8770), 774–778.

[43] Zajac J, Shrestha A, Patel P, Poretsky L (2009). "The Main Events in the History of Diabetes Mellitus". In Poretsky L (ed.). Principles of diabetes mellitus (2nd ed.). New York: Springer. pp. 3–16. ISBN 978-0-387-09840-1. OCLC 663097550

[44] Ancient Egyptian Medicine, Ebers Papyrus, Accessed Online February 9th 2023: https://crystalinks.com/egyptmedicine.html

[45] Papaspyros (1964) 'The History of Diabetes', In: Verlag ed. The History of Diabetes Mellitus, Stuttgart: Thieme; 1964:4.

[46] Papaspyros NS. The history of diabetes. In: Verlag GT, ed. The History of Diabetes Mellitus. Stuttgart: Thieme; 1964:4–5.

[47] Mandal (2019) 'History of Diabetes', News Medical Life Sciences, Accessed Online Jan 17 2021: https://www.news-medical.net/health/History-of-Diabetes.aspx

[48] Medvei VC. The 16th century and the Renaissance. In: Medvei VC, ed. The History of Clinical Endocrinology: A Comprehensive Account of Endocrinology from Earliest Times to the Present Day. New York: Parthenon Publishing; 1993:55–56.

[49] Medvei VC. The 18th century and the beginning of the 19th century. In: Medvei VC, ed. The History of Clinical Endocrinology: A Comprehensive Account of Endocrinology from Earliest Times to the Present Day. New York: Parthenon Publishing; 1993:97.

[50] Medvei (1993) 'The Greco - Roman Period', In: Medvei 'The History of Clinical Endocrinology: A Comprehensive Account of Endycronology from Earliest Times to the Present Day,' New York: Parthenon Publishing, 1993:34, 37.

[51] Sanders LJ. From Thebes to Toronto and the 21st century: an incredible journey. Diabetes Spect. 2002;15:56–60.

[52] Medvei VC. The Greco – Roman period. In: Medvei VC, ed. The History of Clinical Endocrinology: A Comprehensive Account of Endocrinology from Earliest Times to the Present Day. New York: Parthenon Publishing; 1993:34, 37.

[53] Medvei (1993) 'The Greco - Roman Period', In: Medvei 'The History of Clinical Endocrinology: A Comprehensive Account of Endycronology from Earliest Times to the Present Day,' New York: Parthenon Publishing, 1993:34, 37.

[54] Sanders (2002) 'From Thebes to Toronto and the 21st Century: an Incredible Journey', Diabetes Spect. 2002;15:56-60.

[55] Papaspyros NS. The history of diabetes. In: Verlag GT, ed. The History of Diabetes Mellitus. Stuttgart: Thieme; 1964:4.

[56] Gardner, David G.; Shoback, Dolores, eds. (2011). "Chapter 17: Pancreatic hormones & diabetes mellitus". Greenspan's basic & clinical endocrinology (9th ed.). New York: McGraw-Hill Medical. ISBN 978-0-07-162243-1. OCLC 613429053

[57] Chiang, J. L., Kirkman, M. S., Laffel, L. M., Peters, A. L., & Type 1 Diabetes Sourcebook Authors (2014). Type 1 diabetes through the life span: a position statement of the American Diabetes Association. Diabetes care, 37(7), 2034–2054. https://doi.org/10.2337/dc14-1140

[58] WHO (2022) 'Diabetes' Fact Sheets, Accessed Online February 9th 2023: https://www.who.int/en/news-room/fact-sheets/detail/diabetes

[59] NIDDK (2016) 'What is Diabetes?', Diabetes Overview, Accessed Online February 9th 2023: https://www.niddk.nih.gov/health-information/diabetes/overview/symptoms-causes?dkrd=hispt0015

[60] Nguyen et al (2020). Type 3 Diabetes and Its Role Implications in Alzheimer's Disease. International journal of molecular sciences, 21(9), 3165. https://doi.org/10.3390/ijms21093165

[61] de la Monte, S. M., & Wands, J. R. (2008). Alzheimer's disease is type 3 diabetes-evidence reviewed. Journal of diabetes science and technology, 2(6), 1101–1113. https://doi.org/10.1177/193229680800200619

[62] D'Arrigo (2022) 'Alzheimer's and Diabetes: What's the Link?', WebMD, Accessed Online February 2nd 2023: https://www.webmd.com/alzheimers/alzheimers-diabetes-link

[63] Zhao et al (2017). Apolipoprotein E4 Impairs Neuronal Insulin Signaling by Trapping Insulin Receptor in the Endosomes. Neuron, 96(1), 115-129.e5. https://doi.org/10.1016/j.neuron.2017.09.003

[64] Medvei (1993) 'The 18th Century and the Beginning of the 19th Century ', In: Medvei The History of Clinical Endocrinology: A Comprehensive Account of Endocrinology from Earliest Times to the Present Day', New York: Parthenon Publishing, 1993:97.

[65] Jörgens, V., & Grüsser, M. (2013). Happy Birthday, Claude Bernard. Diabetes, 62(7), 2181–2182. https://doi.org/10.2337/db13-0700

[66] Medvei, V. C. (1993). Story of insulin. The History of Clinical Endocrinology: A Comprehensive Account of Endocrinology from Earliest Times to the Present Day. New York: Parthenon Publishing, 249-251.

[67] Anderson (1965) 'John Rollo's Patient', Journal of the History of Medicine and Allied Sciences, Volume XX, Issue 2, April 1965, Pages 163–164.

[68] Karamitsos D. T. (2011). The story of insulin discovery. Diabetes research and clinical practice, 93 Suppl 1, S2–S8. https://doi.org/10.1016/S0168-8227(11)70007-9

[69] Rogers, K. (2013). "Nicolas C. Paulescu". Encyclopædia Britannica. Encyclopædia Britannica Inc.

[70] Medvei (1993) 'Present Trends and Outlook for the Future - Part III', In: Medvei (1993) 'The History of Endocrinology: A Comprehensive Account of Endocrinology from Earliest Times to the Present Day.' New York: Parthenon Publishing, 1993: 380-383.

[71] Medvei (1993) 'Chronological Tables', In: Medvei (1993) 'The History of Endocrinology: A Comprehensive Account of Endocrinology from Earliest Times to the Present Day.' New York: Parthenon Publishing, 1993:495.

[72] Tof I (1994). "Recombinant DNA technology in the synthesis of human insulin". Little Tree Publishing. Retrieved 2009-11-03.

[73] FDA (2022) '100 Years of Insulin', Accessed Online February 10th 2023: https://www.fda.gov/about-fda/fda-history-exhibits/100-years-insulin#:~:text=signed%20an%20agreement%20with%20Genentech,that%20derived%20from%20this%20technology.

[74] Zajac et al (2010) 'The Main Events in the History of Diabetes Mellitus', In: Poretsky 'Principles of Diabetes Mellitus', Springer, New York, USA.

[75] WHO (2016) 'Global Report on Diabetes', World Health Organization 2016, Accessed Online February 11th 2023: https://apps.who.int/iris/bitstream/handle/10665/204871/9789241565257_eng.pdf

[76] Elflein (2021) 'Diabetics worldwide 2021, 2030, and 2045', Statista, Accessed Online February 11th 2023: https://www.statista.com/statistics/271442/number-of-diabetics-worldwide/

[77] Mozaffarian, D., Hao, T., Rimm, E. B., Willett, W. C., & Hu, F. B. (2011). Changes in Diet and Lifestyle and Long-Term Weight Gain in Women and Men. New England Journal of Medicine, 364(25), 2392–2404. https://doi.org/10.1056/nejmoa1014296

[78] Schwartz, M. W., Seeley, R. J., Zeltser, L. M., Drewnowski, A., Ravussin, E., Redman, L. M., & Leibel, R. L. (2017). Obesity Pathogenesis: An Endocrine Society Scientific Statement. Endocrine Reviews, 38(4), 267–296. https://doi.org/10.1210/er.2017-00111

[79] Centers for Disease Control and Prevention (CDC) (2004). Trends in intake of energy and macronutrients--United States, 1971-2000. MMWR. Morbidity and mortality weekly report, 53(4), 80–82.

[80] Rosenheck, R. (2008). Fast food consumption and increased caloric intake: a systematic review of a trajectory towards weight gain and obesity risk. Obesity Reviews, 9(6), 535–547. https://doi.org/10.1111/j.1467-789x.2008.00477.x

[81] Nielsen, S. J., Siega-Riz, A. M., & Popkin, B. M. (2002). Trends in energy intake in U.S. between 1977 and 1996: similar shifts seen across age groups. Obesity research, 10(5), 370–378. https://doi.org/10.1038/oby.2002.51

[82] FAO (2002) 'World agriculture: towards 2015/2030', Rome, Italy: Food and Agriculture Organization of the United Nations, 2002.

[83] Drewnowski, A., & Specter, S. (2004). Poverty and obesity: the role of energy density and energy costs. The American Journal of Clinical Nutrition, 79(1), 6–16. https://doi.org/10.1093/ajcn/79.1.6

[84] Hiza, HAB and Bente L (2007) 'Nutrient Content of the U.S. Food Supply, 1909-2004, A Summary Report', Center for Nutrition Policy and Promotion, Home Economics Research Report No. 57.

[85] Striegel-Moore, R. H., Thompson, D., Affenito, S. G., Franko, D. L., Obarzanek, E., Barton, B. A., Schreiber, G. B., Daniels, S. R., Schmidt, M., & Crawford, P. B. (2006). Correlates of beverage intake in adolescent girls: the National Heart, Lung, and Blood Institute Growth and Health Study. The Journal of pediatrics, 148(2), 183–187. https://doi.org/10.1016/j.jpeds.2005.11.025

[86] Rajeshwari, R., Yang, S.-J., Nicklas, T. A., & Berenson, G. S. (2005). Secular trends in children's sweetened-beverage consumption (1973 to 1994): The Bogalusa Heart Study. Journal of the American Dietetic Association, 105(2), 208–214. https://doi.org/10.1016/j.jada.2004.11.026

[87] Malik, V. S., Schulze, M. B., & Hu, F. B. (2006). Intake of sugar-sweetened beverages and weight gain: a systematic review. The American journal of clinical nutrition, 84(2), 274–288. https://doi.org/10.1093/ajcn/84.1.274

[88] Olsen, N. J., & Heitmann, B. L. (2009). Intake of calorically sweetened beverages and obesity. Obesity reviews : an official journal of the International Association for the Study of Obesity, 10(1), 68–75. https://doi.org/10.1111/j.1467-789X.2008.00523.x

[89] Centers for Disease Control and Prevention (CDC) (2003). Prevalence of physical activity, including lifestyle activities among adults--United States, 2000-2001. MMWR. Morbidity and mortality weekly report, 52(32), 764–769.

[90] McDonald N. C. (2007). Active transportation to school: trends among U.S. schoolchildren, 1969-2001. American journal of preventive medicine, 32(6), 509–516. https://doi.org/10.1016/j.amepre.2007.02.022

[91] DiNicolantonio, J. J., & Lucan, S. C. (2014). The wrong white crystals: not salt but sugar as aetiological in hypertension and cardiometabolic disease. Open heart, 1(1), e000167. https://doi.org/10.1136/openhrt-2014-000167

[92] DiNicolantonio, J. J., Lucan, S. C., & O'Keefe, J. H. (2016). The Evidence for Saturated Fat and for Sugar Related to Coronary Heart Disease. Progress in cardiovascular diseases, 58(5), 464–472. https://doi.org/10.1016/j.pcad.2015.11.006

[93] DiNicolantonio, J. J., Mehta, V., Onkaramurthy, N., & O'Keefe, J. H. (2018). Fructose-induced inflammation and increased cortisol: A new mechanism for how sugar induces visceral adiposity. Progress in cardiovascular diseases, 61(1), 3–9. https://doi.org/10.1016/j.pcad.2017.12.001

[94] DiNicolantonio, J. J., & OKeefe, J. H. (2017). Added sugars drive coronary heart disease via insulin resistance and hyperinsulinaemia: a new paradigm. Open heart, 4(2), e000729. https://doi.org/10.1136/openhrt-2017-000729

[95] DiNicolantonio, J. J., Subramonian, A. M., & O'Keefe, J. H. (2017). Added fructose as a principal driver of non-alcoholic fatty liver disease: a public health crisis. Open heart, 4(2), e000631. https://doi.org/10.1136/openhrt-2017-000631

[96] DiNicolantonio, J. J., & Berger, A. (2016). Added sugars drive nutrient and energy deficit in obesity: a new paradigm. Open heart, 3(2), e000469. https://doi.org/10.1136/openhrt-2016-000469

[97] DiNicolantonio, J. J., & O'Keefe, J. H. (2016). Hypertension Due to Toxic White Crystals in the Diet: Should We Blame Salt or Sugar?. Progress in cardiovascular diseases, 59(3), 219–225. https://doi.org/10.1016/j.pcad.2016.07.004

[98] DiNicolantonio, J. J., & Lucan, S. C. (2015). Is fructose malabsorption a cause of irritable bowel syndrome?. Medical hypotheses, 85(3), 295–297. https://doi.org/10.1016/j.mehy.2015.05.019

[99] DiNicolantonio, J. J., Mehta, V., Zaman, S. B., & O'Keefe, J. H. (2018). Not Salt But Sugar As Aetiological In Osteoporosis: A Review. Missouri medicine, 115(3), 247–252.

[100] DiNicolantonio J. J. (2016). Increase in the intake of refined carbohydrates and sugar may have led to the health decline of the Greenland Eskimos. Open heart, 3(2), e000444. https://doi.org/10.1136/openhrt-2016-000444

[101] DiNicolantonio, J. J., & O'Keefe, J. (2017). Markedly increased intake of refined carbohydrates and sugar is associated with the rise of coronary heart disease and diabetes among the Alaskan Inuit. Open heart, 4(2), e000673. https://doi.org/10.1136/openhrt-2017-000673

[102] Marriott, B. P., Olsho, L., Hadden, L., & Connor, P. (2010). Intake of Added Sugars and Selected Nutrients in the United States, National Health and Nutrition Examination Survey (NHANES) 2003—2006. Critical Reviews in Food Science and Nutrition, 50(3), 228–258. https://doi.org/10.1080/10408391003626223

[103] DiNicolantonio, J. J., & Lucan, S. C. (2014). The wrong white crystals: not salt but sugar as aetiological in hypertension and cardiometabolic disease. Open Heart, 1(1), e000167. https://doi.org/10.1136/openhrt-2014-000167

[104] Johnson et al (2007) 'Potential role of sugar (fructose) in the epidemic of hypertension, obesity and the metabolic syndrome, diabetes, kidney disease, and cardiovascular disease', The American Journal of Clinical Nutrition, Volume 86, Issue 4, October 2007, Pages 899–906, https://doi.org/10.1093/ajcn/86.4.899

[105] Strom (2012) 'U.S. Cuts Estimate of Sugar Intake', NY Times, 27th October 2012, Accessed Online March 3rd 2022: https://www.nytimes.com/2012/10/27/business/us-cuts-estimate-of-sugar-intake-of-typical-american.html

[106] Cordain, L., Eades, M. R., & Eades, M. D. (2003). Hyperinsulinemic diseases of civilization: more than just Syndrome X. Comparative biochemistry and physiology. Part A, Molecular & integrative physiology, 136(1), 95–112. https://doi.org/10.1016/s1095-6433(03)00011-4

[107] Yudkin (2012) 'Pure, white and deadly', Penguin Books

[108] Yudkin (2012) 'Pure, white and deadly', Penguin Books

[109] Johnson et al (2007), 'Potential role of sugar (fructose) in the epidemic of hypertension, obesity and the metabolic syndrome, diabetes, kidney disease, and cardiovascular disease', The American Journal of Clinical Nutrition, Volume 86, Issue 4, October 2007, Pages 899–906, https://doi.org/10.1093/ajcn/86.4.899

[110] Johnson et al (2007), 'Potential role of sugar (fructose) in the epidemic of hypertension, obesity and the metabolic syndrome, diabetes, kidney disease, and cardiovascular disease', The American Journal of Clinical Nutrition, Volume 86, Issue 4, October 2007, Pages 899–906, https://doi.org/10.1093/ajcn/86.4.899

[111] Cordain, L., Eades, M. R., & Eades, M. D. (2003). Hyperinsulinemic diseases of civilization: more than just Syndrome X. Comparative biochemistry and physiology. Part A, Molecular & integrative physiology, 136(1), 95–112. https://doi.org/10.1016/s1095-6433(03)00011-4

[112] Gross, L. S., Li, L., Ford, E. S., & Liu, S. (2004). Increased consumption of refined carbohydrates and the epidemic of type 2 diabetes in the United States: an ecologic assessment. The American journal of clinical nutrition, 79(5), 774–779. https://doi.org/10.1093/ajcn/79.5.774

[113] Tordoff, M. G., & Alleva, A. M. (1990). Effect of drinking soda sweetened with aspartame or high-fructose corn syrup on food intake and body weight. The American journal of clinical nutrition, 51(6), 963–969. https://doi.org/10.1093/ajcn/51.6.963

[114] Mattes, R. D. (1996). Dietary Compensation by Humans for Supplemental Energy Provided as Ethanol or Carbohydrate in Fluids. Physiology & Behavior, 59(1), 179–187. https://doi.org/10.1016/0031-9384(95)02007-1

[115] Raben, A., Vasilaras, T. H., Møller, A. C., & Astrup, A. (2002). Sucrose compared with artificial sweeteners: different effects on ad libitum food intake and body weight after 10 wk of supplementation in overweight subjects. The American journal of clinical nutrition, 76(4), 721–729. https://doi.org/10.1093/ajcn/76.4.721

[116] DiMeglio, D., & Mattes, R. (2000). Liquid versus solid carbohydrate: effects on food intake and body weight. International Journal of Obesity, 24(6), 794–800. https://doi.org/10.1038/sj.ijo.0801229

[117] Lucan, S. C., & DiNicolantonio, J. J. (2015). How calorie-focused thinking about obesity and related diseases may mislead and harm public health. An alternative. Public health nutrition, 18(4), 571–581. https://doi.org/10.1017/S1368980014002559

[118] DiNicolantonio, J. J., O'Keefe, J. H., & Lucan, S. C. (2015). Added fructose: a principal driver of type 2 diabetes mellitus and its consequences. Mayo Clinic proceedings, 90(3), 372–381. https://doi.org/10.1016/j.mayocp.2014.12.019

[119] Bray and Popkin (2014) 'Dietary Sugar and Body Weight: Have We Reached a Crisis in the Epidemic of Obesity and Diabetes?: Health Be Damned! Pour on the Sugar', Diabetes Care 2014;37(4):950–956

[120] Putnam and Allshouse (1999), 'Food Consumption, Prices and Expenditures, 1970–1997'. Washington, DC: Economic Research Service, US Dept of Agriculture.

[121] Duffey, K. J., & Popkin, B. M. (2007). Shifts in patterns and consumption of beverages between 1965 and 2002. Obesity (Silver Spring, Md.), 15(11), 2739–2747. https://doi.org/10.1038/oby.2007.326

[122] Reiser, S., Handler, H. B., Gardner, L. B., Hallfrisch, J. G., Michaelis, O. E., 4th, & Prather, E. S. (1979). Isocaloric exchange of dietary starch and sucrose in humans. II. Effect on fasting blood insulin, glucose, and glucagon and on insulin and glucose response to a sucrose load. The American journal of clinical nutrition, 32(11), 2206–2216. https://doi.org/10.1093/ajcn/32.11.2206

[123] Beck-Nielsen et al (1980) 'Impaired cellular insulin binding and insulin sensitivity induced by high-fructose feeding in normal subjects', The American Journal of Clinical Nutrition, Volume 33, Issue 2, February 1980, Pages 273–278, https://doi.org/10.1093/ajcn/33.2.273

[124] Stanhope, K. L., Schwarz, J. M., Keim, N. L., Griffen, S. C., Bremer, A. A., Graham, J. L., Hatcher, B., Cox, C. L., Dyachenko, A., Zhang, W., McGahan, J. P., Seibert, A., Krauss, R. M., Chiu, S., Schaefer, E. J., Ai, M., Otokozawa, S., Nakajima, K., Nakano, T., Beysen, C., … Havel, P. J. (2009). Consuming fructose-sweetened, not glucose-sweetened, beverages increases visceral adiposity and lipids and decreases insulin sensitivity in overweight/obese humans. The Journal of clinical investigation, 119(5), 1322–1334. https://doi.org/10.1172/JCI37385

[125] Trust for America's Health (2018) 'The State of Obesity 2018: Better Policies for a Healthier America', Accessed Online March 14th 2022: https://www.tfah.org/report-details/the-state-of-obesity-2018/

[126] Bray and Popkin (2014) 'Dietary Sugar and Body Weight: Have We Reached a Crisis in the Epidemic of Obesity and Diabetes?: Health Be Damned! Pour on the Sugar', Diabetes Care 2014;37(4):950–956

[127] Storlien et al (1988) 'Effects of sucrose vs starch diets on in vivo insulin action, thermogenesis, and obesity in rats', The American Journal of Clinical Nutrition, Volume 47, Issue 3, March 1988, Pages 420–427, https://doi.org/10.1093/ajcn/47.3.420

[128] Hulman, S., & Falkner, B. (1994). The effect of excess dietary sucrose on growth, blood pressure, and metabolism in developing Sprague-Dawley rats. Pediatric research, 36(1 Pt 1), 95–101. https://doi.org/10.1203/00006450-199407001-00017

[129] Pagliassotti, M. J., Shahrokhi, K. A., & Moscarello, M. (1994). Involvement of liver and skeletal muscle in sucrose-induced insulin resistance: dose-response studies. American Journal of Physiology-Regulatory, Integrative and Comparative Physiology, 266(5), R1637–R1644. https://doi.org/10.1152/ajpregu.1994.266.5.r1637

[130] Pugazhenthi, S., Angel, J. F., & Khandelwal, R. L. (1993). Effects of high sucrose diet on insulin-like effects of vanadate in diabetic rats. Molecular and cellular biochemistry, 122(1), 77–84. https://doi.org/10.1007/BF00925740

[131] Gutman et al (1987) 'Long-term hypertriglyceridemia and glucose intolerance in rats fed chronically an isocaloric sucrose-rich diet.', Metabolism: Clinical and Experimental, 01 Nov 1987, 36(11):1013-1020

[132] Wright, D. W., Hansen, R. I., Mondon, C. E., & Reaven, G. M. (1983). Sucrose-induced insulin resistance in the rat: modulation by exercise and diet. The American Journal of Clinical Nutrition, 38(6), 879–883. https://doi.org/10.1093/ajcn/38.6.879

[133] Reiser, S., & Hallfrisch, J. (1977). Insulin sensitivity and adipose tissue weight of rats fed starch or sucrose diets ad libitum or in meals. The Journal of nutrition, 107(1), 147–155. https://doi.org/10.1093/jn/107.1.147

[134] Reiser, S., Handler, H. B., Gardner, L. B., Hallfrisch, J. G., Michaelis, O. E., 4th, & Prather, E. S. (1979). Isocaloric exchange of dietary starch and sucrose in humans. II. Effect on fasting blood insulin, glucose, and glucagon and on insulin and glucose response to a sucrose load. The American journal of clinical nutrition, 32(11), 2206–2216. https://doi.org/10.1093/ajcn/32.11.2206

[135] Reiser, S., Bohn, E., Hallfrisch, J., Michaelis, O. E., 4th, Keeney, M., & Prather, E. S. (1981). Serum insulin and glucose in hyperinsulinemic subjects fed three different levels of sucrose. The American journal of clinical nutrition, 34(11), 2348–2358. https://doi.org/10.1093/ajcn/34.11.2348

[136] Gross, L. S., Li, L., Ford, E. S., & Liu, S. (2004). Increased consumption of refined carbohydrates and the epidemic of type 2 diabetes in the United States: an ecologic assessment. The American journal of clinical nutrition, 79(5), 774–779. https://doi.org/10.1093/ajcn/79.5.774

[137] Leaf A and Weber PC (1988) 'Cardiovascular effects of n-3 fatty acids', AGRIS, Accessed: http://agris.fao.org/agris-search/search.do?recordID=US8845581.

[138] PM Kris-Etherton, Denise Shaffer Taylor, Shaomei Yu-Poth, Peter Huth, Kristin Moriarty, Valerie Fishell, Rebecca L Hargrove, Guixiang Zhao, Terry D Etherton; Polyunsaturated fatty acids in the food chain in the United States, The American Journal of Clinical Nutrition, Volume 71, Issue 1, 1 January 2000, Pages 179S–188S.

[139] Simopoulos, A. P., & DiNicolantonio, J. J. (2016). The importance of a balanced ω-6 to ω-3 ratio in the prevention and management of obesity. Open Heart, 3(2), e000385. https://doi.org/10.1136/openhrt-2015-000385

[140] Russo GL (2009) 'Dietary n-6 and n-3 polyunsaturated fatty acids: from biochemistry to clinical implications in cardiovascular prevention', Biochem Pharmacol. 2009 Mar 15;77(6):937-46.

[141] Blasbalg, T. L., Hibbeln, J. R., Ramsden, C. E., Majchrzak, S. F., & Rawlings, R. R. (2011). Changes in consumption of omega-3 and omega-6 fatty acids in the United States during the 20th century. The American Journal of Clinical Nutrition, 93(5), 950–962. https://doi.org/10.3945/ajcn.110.006643

[142] Hiza, HAB and Bente L (2007) 'Nutrient Content of the U.S. Food Supply, 1909-2004, A Summary Report', Center for Nutrition Policy and Promotion, Home Economics Research Report No. 57.

[143] Guyenet, S. J., & Carlson, S. E. (2015). Increase in adipose tissue linoleic acid of US adults in the last half century. Advances in nutrition (Bethesda, Md.), 6(6), 660–664. https://doi.org/10.3945/an.115.009944

[144] Best, K. P., Gold, M., Kennedy, D., Martin, J., & Makrides, M. (2016). Omega-3 long-chain PUFA intake during pregnancy and allergic disease outcomes in the offspring: a systematic review and meta-analysis of observational studies and randomized controlled trials. The American Journal of Clinical Nutrition, 103(1), 128–143. doi:10.3945/ajcn.115.111104

[145] Guyenet, S. J., & Carlson, S. E. (2015). Increase in Adipose Tissue Linoleic Acid of US Adults in the Last Half Century. Advances in Nutrition, 6(6), 660–664. doi:10.3945/an.115.009944

[146] Simopoulos, A. P., & DiNicolantonio, J. J. (2016). The importance of a balanced ω-6 to ω-3 ratio in the prevention and management of obesity. Open Heart, 3(2), e000385. https://doi.org/10.1136/openhrt-2015-000385

[147] Alvheim, A. R., Torstensen, B. E., Lin, Y. H., Lillefosse, H. H., Lock, E. J., Madsen, L., Frøyland, L., Hibbeln, J. R., & Malde, M. K. (2014). Dietary linoleic acid elevates the endocannabinoids 2-AG and anandamide and promotes weight gain in mice fed a low fat diet. Lipids, 49(1), 59–69. https://doi.org/10.1007/s11745-013-3842-y

[148] Flachs, P., Rossmeisl, M., Kuda, O., & Kopecky, J. (2013). Stimulation of mitochondrial oxidative capacity in white fat independent of UCP1: A key to lean phenotype. Biochimica et Biophysica Acta (BBA) - Molecular and Cell Biology of Lipids, 1831(5), 986–1003. doi:10.1016/j.bbalip.2013.02.003

[149] Flachs, P., Mohamed-Ali, V., Horakova, O., Rossmeisl, M., Hosseinzadeh-Attar, M. J., Hensler, M., … Kopecky, J. (2006). Polyunsaturated fatty acids of marine origin induce adiponectin in mice fed a high-fat diet. Diabetologia, 49(2), 394–397. doi:10.1007/s00125-005-0053-y

[150] Hensler, M., Bardova, K., Jilkova, Z. M., Wahli, W., Meztger, D., Chambon, P., Kopecky, J., & Flachs, P. (2011). The inhibition of fat cell proliferation by n-3 fatty acids in dietary obese mice. Lipids in health and disease, 10, 128. https://doi.org/10.1186/1476-511X-10-128

[151] Ruzickova, J., Rossmeisl, M., Prazak, T., Flachs, P., Sponarova, J., Veck, M., Tvrzicka, E., Bryhn, M., & Kopecky, J. (2004). Omega-3 PUFA of marine origin limit diet-induced obesity in mice by reducing cellularity of adipose tissue. Lipids, 39(12), 1177–1185. https://doi.org/10.1007/s11745-004-1345-9

[152] Hill JO, Peters JC, Lin D, et al. Lipid accumulation and body fat distribution is influenced by type of dietary fat fed to rats. Int J Obes Relat Metab Disord. 1993 Apr;17(4):223-36.

[153] Blasbalg, T. L., Hibbeln, J. R., Ramsden, C. E., Majchrzak, S. F., & Rawlings, R. R. (2011). Changes in consumption of omega-3 and omega-6 fatty acids in the United States during the 20th century. The American Journal of Clinical Nutrition, 93(5), 950–962. https://doi.org/10.3945/ajcn.110.006643

154 Hall, K. D., Ayuketah, A., Brychta, R., Cai, H., Cassimatis, T., Chen, K. Y., Chung, S. T., Costa, E., Courville, A., Darcey, V., Fletcher, L. A., Forde, C. G., Gharib, A. M., Guo, J., Howard, R., Joseph, P. V., McGehee, S., Ouwerkerk, R., Raisinger, K., Rozga, I., … Zhou, M. (2019). Ultra-Processed Diets Cause Excess Calorie Intake and Weight Gain: An Inpatient Randomized Controlled Trial of Ad Libitum Food Intake. Cell metabolism, 30(1), 67–77.e3. https://doi.org/10.1016/j.cmet.2019.05.008

155 Bojanowska, E., & Ciosek, J. (2016). Can We Selectively Reduce Appetite for Energy-Dense Foods? An Overview of Pharmacological Strategies for Modification of Food Preference Behavior. Current Neuropharmacology, 14(2), 118–142. https://doi.org/10.2174/1570159x14666151109103147

[156] NIH (2016) 'Symptoms & Causes of Diabetes', Accessed Online February 17th 2023: https://www.niddk.nih.gov/health-information/diabetes/overview/symptoms-causes?dkrd=hiscr0005#causes

[157] Daneman D. (2006). Type 1 diabetes. Lancet (London, England), 367(9513), 847–858. https://doi.org/10.1016/S0140-6736(06)68341-4

[158] World Health Organization. (1999). Definition, diagnosis and classification of diabetes mellitus and its complications : report of a WHO consultation. Part 1, Diagnosis and classification of diabetes mellitus. World Health Organization. https://apps.who.int/iris/handle/10665/66040

[159] Oezkur et al (2015) Chronic hyperglycemia is associated with acute kidney injury in patients undergoing CABG surgery – a cohort study. BMC Cardiovasc Disord 15, 41.

[160] Dobretsov et al (2007). Early diabetic neuropathy: triggers and mechanisms. World journal of gastroenterology, 13(2), 175–191.

[161] Mohamed et al (2013). Hyperglycemia as a risk factor for the development of retinopathy of prematurity. BMC pediatrics, 13, 78.

[162] Arif, A. A., & Rohrer, J. E. (2006). The relationship between obesity, hyperglycemia symptoms, and health-related quality of life among Hispanic and non-Hispanic white children and adolescents. BMC Family Practice, 7(1).

[163] Flynn et al (2020). Transient Intermittent Hyperglycemia Accelerates Atherosclerosis by Promoting Myelopoiesis. Circulation Research, 127(7), 877–892.

[164] Weiss, M., Steiner, D. F., & Philipson, L. H. (2014). Insulin Biosynthesis, Secretion, Structure, and Structure-Activity Relationships. In K. R. Feingold (Eds.) et. al., Endotext. MDText.com, Inc.

[165] Sonksen, P., & Sonksen, J. (2000). Insulin: understanding its action in health and disease. British journal of anaesthesia, 85(1), 69–79. https://doi.org/10.1093/bja/85.1.69

[166] Stryer L (1995). Biochemistry (Fourth ed.). New York: W.H. Freeman and Company. pp. 773–74. ISBN 0-7167-2009-4.

[167] Koeslag et al (2003). A reappraisal of the blood glucose homeostat which comprehensively explains the type 2 diabetes mellitus-syndrome X complex. The Journal of physiology, 549(Pt 2), 333–346.

[168] Koeslag et al (2003). A reappraisal of the blood glucose homeostat which comprehensively explains the type 2 diabetes mellitus-syndrome X complex. The Journal of physiology, 549(Pt 2), 333–346.

[169] NIH (2018) 'Insulin Resistance & Prediabetes', NIDDK, Accessed Online March 29th 2022: https://www.niddk.nih.gov/health-information/diabetes/overview/what-is-diabetes/prediabetes-insulin-resistance

[170] Roden, M., Price, T. B., Perseghin, G., Petersen, K. F., Rothman, D. L., Cline, G. W., & Shulman, G. I. (1996). Mechanism of free fatty acid-induced insulin resistance in humans. The Journal of clinical investigation, 97(12), 2859–2865. https://doi.org/10.1172/JCI118742

[171] Koyama, K., Chen, G., Lee, Y., & Unger, R. H. (1997). Tissue triglycerides, insulin resistance, and insulin production: implications for hyperinsulinemia of obesity. The American journal of physiology, 273(4), E708–E713. https://doi.org/10.1152/ajpendo.1997.273.4.E708

[172] Schinner, S., Scherbaum, W. A., Bornstein, S. R., & Barthel, A. (2005). Molecular mechanisms of insulin resistance. Diabetic medicine : a journal of the British Diabetic Association, 22(6), 674–682. https://doi.org/10.1111/j.1464-5491.2005.01566.x

[173] Isganaitis, E., & Lustig, R. H. (2005). Fast food, central nervous system insulin resistance, and obesity. Arteriosclerosis, thrombosis, and vascular biology, 25(12), 2451–2462. https://doi.org/10.1161/01.ATV.0000186208.06964.91

[174] Wang G. (2014). Raison d'être of insulin resistance: the adjustable threshold hypothesis. Journal of the Royal Society, Interface, 11(101), 20140892. https://doi.org/10.1098/rsif.2014.0892

[175] Taylor, R. (2012). Insulin Resistance and Type 2 Diabetes. Diabetes, 61(4), 778–779. https://doi.org/10.2337/db12-0073

[176] Michael H et al (2008) 'Insulin Resistance and Hyperinsulinemia', Diabetes Care Feb 2008, 31 (Supplement 2) S262-S268.

[177] Modan, M., Halkin, H., Almog, S., Lusky, A., Eshkol, A., Shefi, M., Shitrit, A., … Fuchs, Z. (1985). Hyperinsulinemia. A link between hypertension obesity and glucose intolerance. The Journal of clinical investigation, 75(3), 809-17.

[178] Nguyen et al (2020). Type 3 Diabetes and Its Role Implications in Alzheimer's Disease. International journal of molecular sciences, 21(9), 3165. https://doi.org/10.3390/ijms21093165

[179] de la Monte, S. M., & Wands, J. R. (2008). Alzheimer's disease is type 3 diabetes-evidence reviewed. Journal of diabetes science and technology, 2(6), 1101–1113. https://doi.org/10.1177/193229680800200619

[180] Reno CM, Tanoli T, Bree A, Daphna-Iken D, Cui C, Maloney SE, Wozniak DF, Fisher SJ. Antecedent glycemic control reduces severe hypoglycemia-induced neuronal damage in diabetic rats. Am J Physiol Endocrinol Metab 304: E1331–E1337, 2013. doi:10.1152/ajpendo.00084.2013.

[181] Duarte AI, Santos MS, Seica R, de Oliveira CR. Insulin affects syn- aptosomal GABA and glutamate transport under oxidative stress conditions. Brain Res 977: 23–30, 2003. doi:10.1016/s0006-8993 (03)02679-9.

[182] Devaskar SU, Giddings SJ, Rajakumar PA, Carnaghi LR, Menon RK, Zahm DS. Insulin gene expression and insulin synthesis in mammalian neuronal cells. J Biol Chem 269: 8445–8454, 1994. doi:10.1016/S0021-9258(17)37214-9.

[183] Devaskar SU, Singh BS, Carnaghi LR, Rajakumar PA, Giddings SJ. Insulin II gene expression in rat central nervous system. Regul Pept 48: 55–63, 1993. doi:10.1016/0167-0115(93)90335-6.

[184] Lee J, Kim K, Cho JH, Bae JY, O'Leary TP, Johnson JD, Bae YC, Kim E-K. Insulin synthesized in the paraventricular nucleus of the hypothalamus regulates pituitary growth hormone production. JCI Insight 5: e135412, 2020. doi:10.1172/jci.insight.135412.

[185] Rojas, J. M., & Schwartz, M. W. (2014). Control of hepatic glucose metabolism by islet and brain. Diabetes, Obesity and Metabolism, 16(S1), 33-40.

[186] Hallschmid, M., Higgs, S., Thienel, M., Ott, V. & Lehnert, H. Postprandial administration of intranasal insulin intensifies satiety and reduces intake of palatable snacks in women. Diabetes 61, 782–789 (2012).

[187] Kullmann, S., Valenta, V., Wagner, R., Tschritter, O., Machann, J., Häring, H. U., … & Heni, M. (2020). Brain insulin sensitivity is linked to adiposity and body fat distribution. Nature communications, 11(1), 1-6.

[188] Jauch-Chara, K. et al. Intranasal Insulin suppresses food intake via enhancement of brain energy levels in humans. Diabetes 61, 2261–2268 (2012).

[189] Krug, R., Mohwinkel, L., Drotleff, B., Born, J. & Hallschmid, M. Insulin and estrogen independently and differentially reduce macronutrient intake in healthy men. J. Clin. Endocrinol. Metab. 103, 1393–1401 (2018).

[190] Hallschmid, M., Higgs, S., Thienel, M., Ott, V. & Lehnert, H. Postprandial administration of intranasal insulin intensifies satiety and reduces intake of palatable snacks in women. Diabetes 61, 782–789 (2012).

[191] Loh, K., Zhang, L., Brandon, A., Wang, Q., Begg, D., Qi, Y., Fu, M., Kulkarni, R., Teo, J., Baldock, P., Brüning, J. C., Cooney, G., Neely, G., & Herzog, H. (2017). Insulin controls food intake and energy balance via NPY neurons. Molecular Metabolism, 6(6), 574–584. https://doi.org/10.1016/j.molmet.2017.03.01

[192] Dodd GT, Tiganis T. Insulin action in the brain: roles in energy and glucose homeostasis. J Neuroendocrinol 29: e12513, 2017. doi:10.1111/jne.12513.

[193] Guthoff M, Grichisch Y, Canova C, Tschritter O, Veit R, Hallschmid M, Haring HU, Preissl H, Hennige AM, Fritsche A. Insulin modulates food-related activity in the central nervous system. J Clin Endocrinol Metab 95: 748–755, 2010. doi:10.1210/jc.2009-1677.

[194] Loh K, Zhang L, Brandon A, Wang Q, Begg D, Qi Y, Fu M, Kulkarni R, Teo J, Baldock P, Bruning JC, Cooney G, Neely GG, Herzog H. Insulin controls food intake and energy balance via NPY neurons. Mol Metab 6: 574–584, 2017. doi:10.1016/j.molmet.2017.03.013.

[195] Varela L, Horvath TL. Leptin and insulin pathways in POMC and AgRP neurons that modulate energy balance and glucose homeostasis. EMBO Rep 13: 1079–1086, 2012. doi:10.1038/embor.2012.174.

[196] Schneider, E., Spetter, M. S., Martin, E., Sapey, E., Yip, K. P., Manolopoulos, K. N., … & Higgs, S. (2022). The effect of intranasal insulin on appetite and mood in women with and without obesity: an experimental medicine study. International Journal of Obesity, 1-9.

[197] Kullmann, S., Valenta, V., Wagner, R., Tschritter, O., Machann, J., Häring, H. U., … & Heni, M. (2020). Brain insulin sensitivity is linked to adiposity and body fat distribution. Nature communications, 11(1), 1-6.

[198] Obici S, Zhang BB, Karkanias G, Rossetti L. Hypothalamic insulin signaling is required for inhibition of glucose production. Nat Med 8: 1376–1382, 2002. doi:10.1038/nm1202-798.

[199] Ramnanan CJ, Kraft G, Smith MS, Farmer B, Neal D, Williams PE, Lautz M, Farmer T, Donahue EP, Cherrington AD, Edgerton DS. Interaction between the central and peripheral effects of insulin in controlling hepatic glucose metabolism in the conscious dog. Diabetes 62: 74–84, 2013. doi:10.2337/db12-0148.

[200] Lewis GF, Carpentier AC, Pereira S, Hahn M, Giacca A. Direct and indirect control of hepatic glucose production by insulin. Cell Metab 33: 709–720, 2021. doi:10.1016/j.cmet.2021.03.007.

[201] Obici S, Zhang BB, Karkanias G, Rossetti L. Hypothalamic insulin signaling is required for inhibition of glucose production. Nat Med 2002; 8: 1376-82.

[202] Niijima A. Blood glucose levels modulate efferent activity in the vagal supply to the rat liver. J Physiol 1985; 364: 105-12.

[203] Schneider, E., Spetter, M. S., Martin, E., Sapey, E., Yip, K. P., Manolopoulos, K. N., … & Higgs, S. (2022). The effect of intranasal insulin on appetite and mood in women with and without obesity: an experimental medicine study. International Journal of Obesity, 1-9.

[204] Benedict C, Kern W, Schultes B, Born J, Hallschmid M. Differential sensitivity of men and women to anorexigenic and memory-improving effects of intranasal insulin. J Clin Endocrinol Metab 93: 1339 –1344, 2008.

[205] Hallschmid M, Benedict C, Schultes B, Fehm HL, Born J, Kern W. Intranasal insulin reduces body fat in men but not in women. Diabetes. 2004 Nov;53(11):3024-9. doi: 10.2337/diabetes.53.11.3024. PMID: 15504987.

[206] Sliwowska, J. H., Fergani, C., Gawałek, M., Skowronska, B., Fichna, P., & Lehman, M. N. (2014). Insulin: its role in the central control of reproduction. *Physiology & behavior, 133*, 197-206.

[207] Bruning JC, Gautam D, Burks DJ, Gillette J, Schubert M, Orban PC, Klein R, Krone W, Muller-Wieland D, Kahn CR. Role of brain in- sulin receptor in control of body weight and reproduction. Science 289: 2122–2125, 2000. doi:10.1126/science.289.5487.2122.

[208] Pitteloud et al (2008). Inhibition of Luteinizing Hormone Secretion by Testosterone in Men Requires Aromatization for Its Pituitary But Not Its Hypothalamic Effects: Evidence from the Tandem Study of Normal and Gonadotropin-Releasing Hormone-Deficient Men. The Journal of Clinical Endocrinology & Metabolism, 93(3), 784–791.

[209] Park et al (2007). Characteristics of the urinary luteinizing hormone surge in young ovulatory women. Fertility and sterility, 88(3), 684–690.

[210] 40. Soto M, Cai W, Konishi M, Kahn CR. Insulin signaling in the hippo- campus and amygdala regulates metabolism and neurobehavior. Proc Natl Acad Sci USA 116: 6379–6384, 2019. doi:10.1073/ pnas.1817391116.

[211] Chatterjee S, Mudher A. Alzheimer's disease and type 2 diabetes: a critical assessment of the shared pathological traits. Front Neurosci 12: 383, 2018. doi:10.3389/fnins.2018.00383.

[212] Han W, Li C. Linking type 2 diabetes and Alzheimer's disease. Proc Natl Acad Sci USA 107: 6557–6558, 2010. doi:10.1073/ pnas.1002555107.

[213] Talbot, K. (2014). Brain insulin resistance in Alzheimer's disease and its potential treatment with GLP-1 analogs. *Neurodegenerative disease management, 4*(1), 31-40.

[214] Talbot K, Wang H-Y, Kazi H, et al. Demonstrated brain insulin resistance in Alzheimer's disease patients is associated with IGF-1 resistance, IRS-1 dysregulation, and cognitive decline. *J Clin Invest.* 2012;122(4):1316–1338.

[215] Rorato et al (2017). LPS-Induced Low-Grade Inflammation Increases Hypothalamic JNK Expression and Causes Central Insulin Resistance Irrespective of Body Weight Changes. International journal of molecular sciences, 18(7), 1431.

[216] Boutagy et al (2016). Metabolic endotoxemia with obesity: Is it real and is it relevant?. Biochimie, 124, 11–20.

[217] Boroni Moreira, A. P. (2012). LA INFLUENCIA DE LA ENDOTOXEMIA EN LOS MECANISMOS MOLECULARES DE RESISTENCIA A LA INSULINA [JB]. NUTRICION HOSPITALARIA, 2, 382–390.

[218] Mohammad, S., & Thiemermann, C. (2021). Role of Metabolic Endotoxemia in Systemic Inflammation and Potential Interventions. Frontiers in Immunology, 11.

[219] Rizza, R.A., Mandarino, L.J., Genest, J. et al. Diabetologia (1985) 28: 70.

[220] Del Prato S et al (1994) 'Effect of sustained physiologic hyperinsulinaemia and hyperglycaemia on insulin secretion and insulin sensitivity in man', Diabetologia. 1994 Oct;37(10):1025-35.

[221] Tan, E., & Scott, E. M. (2014). Circadian rhythms, insulin action, and glucose homeostasis. Current opinion in clinical nutrition and metabolic care, 17(4), 343–348. https://doi.org/10.1097/MCO.0000000000000061

[222] Willi, C., Bodenmann, P., Ghali, W. A., Faris, P. D., & Cornuz, J. (2007). Active smoking and the risk of type 2 diabetes: a systematic review and meta-analysis. JAMA, 298(22), 2654–2664. https://doi.org/10.1001/jama.298.22.2654

[223] Attvall S et al (1993) 'Smoking induces insulin resistance--a potential link with the insulin resistance syndrome', J Intern Med. 1993 Apr;233(4):327-32.

[224] Koppes, L. L. J., Dekker, J. M., Hendriks, H. F. J., Bouter, L. M., & Heine, R. J. (2005). Moderate Alcohol Consumption Lowers the Risk of Type 2 Diabetes: A meta-analysis of prospective observational studies. Diabetes Care, 28(3), 719–725. doi:10.2337/diacare.28.3.719

[225] Brien, S. E., Ronksley, P. E., Turner, B. J., Mukamal, K. J., & Ghali, W. A. (2011). Effect of alcohol consumption on biological markers associated with risk of coronary heart disease: systematic review and meta-analysis of interventional studies. BMJ, 342(feb22 1), d636–d636. doi:10.1136/bmj.d636

[226] Joosten, M. M., Beulens, J. W. J., Kersten, S., & Hendriks, H. F. J. (2008). Moderate alcohol consumption increases insulin sensitivity and ADIPOQ expression in postmenopausal women: a randomised, crossover trial. Diabetologia, 51(8), 1375–1381. doi:10.1007/s00125-008-1031-y

[227] Ken C Chiu, Audrey Chu, Vay Liang W Go, Mohammed F Saad; Hypovitaminosis D is associated with insulin resistance and β cell dysfunction, The American Journal of Clinical Nutrition, Volume 79, Issue 5, 1 May 2004, Pages 820–825.

[228] DiNicolantonio JJ and O'Keefe JH. Sodium restriction and insulin resistance: A review of 23 clinical trials. Journal of Insulin Resistance. 2023 (accepted).

[229] Rosique-Esteban, N., Guasch-Ferré, M., Hernández-Alonso, P., & Salas-Salvadó, J. (2018). Dietary Magnesium and Cardiovascular Disease: A Review with Emphasis in Epidemiological Studies. Nutrients, 10(2), 168. doi:10.3390/nu10020168

[230] De Baaij, J. H. F., Hoenderop, J. G. J., & Bindels, R. J. M. (2015). Magnesium in Man: Implications for Health and Disease. Physiological Reviews, 95(1), 1–46. doi:10.1152/physrev.00012.2014

[231] El-Aal, A. A., El-Ghffar, E. A. A., Ghali, A. A., Zughbur, M. R., & Sirdah, M. M. (2018). The effect of vitamin C and/or E supplementations on type 2 diabetic adult males under metformin treatment: A single-blinded randomized controlled clinical trial. Diabetes & Metabolic Syndrome: Clinical Research & Reviews, 12(4), 483–489. doi:10.1016/j.dsx.2018.03.013

[232] Feng, W., Ding, Y., Zhang, W., Chen, Y., Li, Q., Wang, W., … Wu, X. (2018). Chromium malate alleviates high-glucose and insulin resistance in L6 skeletal muscle cells by regulating glucose uptake and insulin sensitivity signaling pathways. BioMetals, 31(5), 891–908. doi:10.1007/s10534-018-0132-4

[233] DiNicolantonio JJ and O'Keefe JH. Sodium restriction and insulin resistance: A review of 23 clinical trials. Journal of Insulin Resistance. 2023

[234] Page et al (2011). Thiamine deficiency in diabetes mellitus and the impact of thiamine replacement on glucose metabolism and vascular disease. International journal of clinical practice, 65(6), 684–690.

[235] Shahzad Alam, S. (2012). Effect of High Dose Thiamine Therapy on Risk Factors in Type 2 Diabetics. Journal of Diabetes & Metabolism, 03(10).

[236] Thornalley P. J. (2005). The potential role of thiamine (vitamin B1) in diabetic complications. Current diabetes reviews, 1(3), 287–298.

[237] VORHAUS, M. G. (1935). STUDIES ON CRYSTALLINE VITAMIN B1. Journal of the American Medical Association, 105(20), 1580.

[238] Williams, R.D., Mason, H.L., Wilder, R.M., & Smith, B.F. (1940). OBSERVATIONS ON INDUCED THIAMINE (VITAMIN B1) DEFICIENCY IN MAN. JAMA Internal Medicine, 66, 785-799.

[239] Chiu, K. C., Chu, A., Go, V. L., & Saad, M. F. (2004). Hypovitaminosis D is associated with insulin resistance and beta cell dysfunction. The American journal of clinical nutrition, 79(5), 820–825. https://doi.org/10.1093/ajcn/79.5.820

[240] Ivy J. L. (1997). Role of exercise training in the prevention and treatment of insulin resistance and non-insulin-dependent diabetes mellitus. Sports medicine (Auckland, N.Z.), 24(5), 321–336. https://doi.org/10.2165/00007256-199724050-00004

[241] Reutrakul, S., & Van Cauter, E. (2018). Sleep influences on obesity, insulin resistance, and risk of type 2 diabetes. Metabolism: clinical and experimental, 84, 56–66. https://doi.org/10.1016/j.metabol.2018.02.010

[242] Mesarwi, O., Polak, J., Jun, J., & Polotsky, V. Y. (2013). Sleep disorders and the development of insulin resistance and obesity. Endocrinology and metabolism clinics of North America, 42(3), 617–634. https://doi.org/10.1016/j.ecl.2013.05.001

[243] Stenvers, D. J., Scheer, F., Schrauwen, P., la Fleur, S. E., & Kalsbeek, A. (2019). Circadian clocks and insulin resistance. Nature reviews. Endocrinology, 15(2), 75–89. https://doi.org/10.1038/s41574-018-0122-1

[244] Isganaitis, E., & Lustig, R. H. (2005). Fast food, central nervous system insulin resistance, and obesity. Arteriosclerosis, thrombosis, and vascular biology, 25(12), 2451–2462. https://doi.org/10.1161/01.ATV.0000186208.06964.91

[245] A scientific review: the role of chromium in insulin resistance. (2004). The Diabetes educator, Suppl, 2–14.

[246] Guerrero-Romero, F., & Rodríguez-Morán, M. (2005). Complementary therapies for diabetes: the case for chromium, magnesium, and antioxidants. Archives of medical research, 36(3), 250–257. https://doi.org/10.1016/j.arcmed.2005.01.004

247 Rosique-Esteban, N., Guasch-Ferré, M., Hernández-Alonso, P., & Salas-Salvadó, J. (2018). Dietary Magnesium and Cardiovascular Disease: A Review with Emphasis in Epidemiological Studies. Nutrients, 10(2), 168. doi:10.3390/nu10020168

248 De Baaij, J. H. F., Hoenderop, J. G. J., & Bindels, R. J. M. (2015). Magnesium in Man: Implications for Health and Disease. Physiological Reviews, 95(1), 1–46. doi:10.1152/physrev.00012.2014

[249] Stone, M., Martyn, L., & Weaver, C. (2016). Potassium Intake, Bioavailability, Hypertension, and Glucose Control. Nutrients, 8(7), 444. doi:10.3390/nu8070444

[250] Wang, J., Persuitte, G., Olendzki, B. C., Wedick, N. M., Zhang, Z., Merriam, P. A., Fang, H., Carmody, J., Olendzki, G. F., & Ma, Y. (2013). Dietary magnesium intake improves insulin resistance among non-diabetic individuals with metabolic syndrome participating in a dietary trial. Nutrients, 5(10), 3910–3919. https://doi.org/10.3390/nu5103910

[251] Humphries, S. (1999). Low dietary magnesium is associated with insulin resistance in a sample of young, nondiabetic black Americans. American Journal of Hypertension, 12(8), 747–756. doi:10.1016/s0895-7061(99)00041-2

[252] Huerta, M. G., Roemmich, J. N., Kington, M. L., Bovbjerg, V. E., Weltman, A. L., Holmes, V. F., … Nadler, J. L. (2005). Magnesium Deficiency Is Associated With Insulin Resistance in Obese Children. Diabetes Care, 28(5), 1175–1181. doi:10.2337/diacare.28.5.1175

[253] Rodríguez-Morán, M., Simental Mendía, L. E., Zambrano Galván, G., & Guerrero-Romero, F. (2011). The role of magnesium in type 2 diabetes: a brief based-clinical review. Magnesium research, 24(4), 156–162. https://doi.org/10.1684/mrh.2011.0299

[254] Fantry L. E. (2003). Protease inhibitor-associated diabetes mellitus: a potential cause of morbidity and mortality. Journal of acquired immune deficiency syndromes (1999), 32(3), 243–244. https://doi.org/10.1097/00126334-200303010-00001

[255] Burghardt, K. J., Seyoum, B., Mallisho, A., Burghardt, P. R., Kowluru, R. A., & Yi, Z. (2018). Atypical antipsychotics, insulin resistance and weight; a meta-analysis of healthy volunteer studies. Progress in neuro-psychopharmacology & biological psychiatry, 83, 55–63. https://doi.org/10.1016/j.pnpbp.2018.01.004

[256] Balkau, B., Mhamdi, L., Oppert, J. M., Nolan, J., Golay, A., Porcellati, F., Laakso, M., Ferrannini, E., EGIR-RISC Study Group (2008). Physical activity and insulin sensitivity: the RISC study. Diabetes, 57(10), 2613-8.

[257] Lund, S., Holman, G. D., Schmitz, O., & Pedersen, O. (1995). Contraction stimulates translocation of glucose transporter GLUT4 in skeletal muscle through a mechanism distinct from that of insulin. Proceedings of the National Academy of Sciences of the United States of America, 92(13), 5817-21.

[258] Kyu, H. H., Bachman, V. F., Alexander, L. T., Mumford, J. E., Afshin, A., Estep, K., Veerman, J. L., Delwiche, K., Iannarone, M. L., Moyer, M. L., Cercy, K., Vos, T., Murray, C. J., & Forouzanfar, M. H. (2016). Physical activity and risk of breast cancer, colon cancer, diabetes, ischemic heart disease, and ischemic stroke events: systematic review and dose-response meta-analysis for the Global Burden of Disease Study 2013. BMJ (Clinical research ed.), 354, i3857. https://doi.org/10.1136/bmj.i3857

[259] Ishiguro, H., Kodama, S., Horikawa, C., Fujihara, K., Hirose, A. S., Hirasawa, R., Yachi, Y., Ohara, N., Shimano, H., Hanyu, O., & Sone, H. (2016). In Search of the Ideal Resistance Training Program to Improve Glycemic Control and its Indication for Patients with Type 2 Diabetes Mellitus: A Systematic Review and Meta-Analysis. Sports medicine (Auckland, N.Z.), 46(1), 67–77. https://doi.org/10.1007/s40279-015-0379-7

[260] Jessen, N., & Goodyear, L. J. (2005). Contraction signaling to glucose transport in skeletal muscle. Journal of Applied Physiology, 99(1), 330–337.

[261] Richter, E. A., & Hargreaves, M. (2013). Exercise, GLUT4, and Skeletal Muscle Glucose Uptake. Physiological Reviews, 93(3), 993–1017.

[262] Stöckli, J., Fazakerley, D. J., & James, D. E. (2011). GLUT4 exocytosis. Journal of Cell Science, 124(24), 4147–4159. https://doi.org/10.1242/jcs.097063

[263] Leto, D., Saltiel, A. Regulation of glucose transport by insulin: traffic control of GLUT4. Nat Rev Mol Cell Biol 13, 383–396 (2012). https://doi.org/10.1038/nrm3351

[264] Shiloah E et al (2003) 'Effect of Acute Psychotic Stress in Nondiabetic Subjects on β-Cell Function and Insulin Sensitivity', Diabetes Care 2003 May; 26(5): 1462-1467.

[265] Piroli GG et al (2007) 'Corticosterone Impairs Insulin-Stimulated Translocation of GLUT4 in the Rat Hippocampus', Neuroendocrinology 2007;85:71–80.

[266] Paul-Labrador M. et al (2006) 'Effects of a randomized controlled trial of transcendental meditation on components of the metabolic syndrome in subjects with coronary heart disease', Arch Intern Med. 2006 Jun 12;166(11):1218-24.

[267] Delarue and Magnan (2007) 'Free fatty acids and insulin resistance', Curr Opin Clin Nutr Metab Care. 2007 Mar;10(2):142-8.

[268] Shuldiner and McLenithan (2004) 'Genes and pathophysiology of type 2 diabetes: more than just the Randle cycle all over again', J Clin Invest. 2004 Nov;114(10):1414-7.

[269] Hue, L., & Taegtmeyer, H. (2009). The Randle cycle revisited: a new head for an old hat. American journal of physiology. Endocrinology and metabolism, 297 3, E578-91 .

[270] Bevilacqua et al (1990) 'Operation of Randle's cycle in patients with NIDDM', Diabetes. 1990 Mar;39(3):383-9.

[271] Randle et al (1963) 'THE GLUCOSE FATTY-ACID CYCLE ITS ROLE IN INSULIN SENSITIVITY AND THE METABOLIC DISTURBANCES OF DIABETES MELLITUS', The Lancet, ORIGINAL ARTICLES| VOLUME 281, ISSUE 7285, P785-789, APRIL 13, 1963.

[272] Randle et al (1963) 'The glucose fatty-acid cycle. Its role in insulin sensitivity and the metabolic disturbances of diabetes mellitus', Lancet. 1963 Apr 13;1(7285):785-9.

[273] Storlien LH et al (1991) 'Influence of Dietary Fat Composition on Development of Insulin Resistance in Rats: Relationship to Muscle Triglyceride and ω-3 Fatty Acids in Muscle Phospholipid', Diabetes 1991 Feb; 40(2): 280-289.

278

[274] Lucidi, P., Rossetti, P., Porcellati, F., Pampanelli, S., Candeloro, P., Andreoli, A. M., Perriello, G., Bolli, G. B., & Fanelli, C. G. (2010). Mechanisms of insulin resistance after insulin-induced hypoglycemia in humans: the role of lipolysis. Diabetes, 59(6), 1349–1357. https://doi.org/10.2337/db09-0745

[275] Abbate, S. L., & Brunzell, J. D. (1990). Pathophysiology of hyperlipidemia in diabetes mellitus. Journal of cardiovascular pharmacology, 16 Suppl 9, S1–S7.

[276] Mandaliya, D. K., & Seshadri, S. (2019). Short Chain Fatty Acids, pancreatic dysfunction and type 2 diabetes. Pancreatology, 19(4), 617–622. https://doi.org/10.1016/j.pan.2019.04.013

[277] Oh et al (2018). Fatty Acid-Induced Lipotoxity in Pancreatic Beta-Cells During Development of Type 2 Diabetes. Frontiers in Endocrinology, 9. https://doi.org/10.3389/fendo.2018.00384

[278] Shulman (2014) 'Ectopic Fat in Insulin Resistance, Dyslipidemia, and Cardiometabolic Disease', N Engl J Med 2014; 371:1131-1141.

[279] Omar-Hmeadi, M., Lund, P.-E., Gandasi, N. R., Tengholm, A., & Barg, S. (2020). Paracrine control of α-cell glucagon exocytosis is compromised in human type-2 diabetes. Nature Communications, 11(1). https://doi.org/10.1038/s41467-020-15717-8

[280] Isganaitis E and Lustig R.H. (2005) 'Fast Food, Central Nervous System Insulin Resistance, and Obesity', Arteriosclerosis, Thrombosis, and Vascular Biology. 2005;25:2451–2462.

[281] Clément L et al (2002) 'Dietary trans-10,cis-12 conjugated linoleic acid induces hyperinsulinemia and fatty liver in the mouse', J Lipid Res. 2002 Sep;43(9):1400-9.

[282] DiNicolantonio, J. J., O'Keefe, J. H., & Lucan, S. C. (2015). Added fructose: a principal driver of type 2 diabetes mellitus and its consequences. Mayo Clinic proceedings, 90(3), 372–381. https://doi.org/10.1016/j.mayocp.2014.12.019

[283] DiNicolantonio, J. J., Subramonian, A. M., & O'Keefe, J. H. (2017). Added fructose as a principal driver of non-alcoholic fatty liver disease: a public health crisis. Open heart, 4(2), e000631. https://doi.org/10.1136/openhrt-2017-000631

[284] DiNicolantonio, J. J., Mehta, V., Onkaramurthy, N., & O'Keefe, J. H. (2018). Fructose-induced inflammation and increased cortisol: A new mechanism for how sugar induces visceral adiposity. Progress in Cardiovascular Diseases, 61(1), 3–9. https://doi.org/10.1016/j.pcad.2017.12.001

[285] Goodpaster, B., & Kelley, D. E. (2008). Metabolic inflexibility and insulin resistance in skeletal muscle. Physical Activity and Type, 2, 59-66.

[286] Goodpaster, B. H., & Sparks, L. M. (2017). Metabolic Flexibility in Health and Disease. Cell Metabolism, 25(5), 1027–1036.

[287] Muoio D. M. (2014). Metabolic inflexibility: when mitochondrial indecision leads to metabolic gridlock. Cell, 159(6), 1253–1262.

[288] Lee, H. K. (2019). Fatty acid overload to compromised oxidative phosphorylation activates inflammation in type 2 diabetes: Hidden beasts and how to find them. Journal of Diabetes Investigation, 11(2), 290–293. Portico.

[289] Forrester et al (2018). Reactive Oxygen Species in Metabolic and Inflammatory Signaling. Circulation Research, 122(6), 877–902.

[290] Storlien, L., Oakes, N. D., & Kelley, D. E. (2004). Metabolic flexibility. Proceedings of the Nutrition Society, 63(2), 363–368. https://doi.org/10.1079/pns2004349

[291] Muoio (2014) 'Metabolic Inflexibility: When Mitochondrial Indecision Leads to Metabolic Gridlock', Cell, VOLUME 159, ISSUE 6, P1253-1262, DECEMBER 04, 2014.

[292] Bergouignan et al (2013). Effect of contrasted levels of habitual physical activity on metabolic flexibility. Journal of Applied Physiology, 114(3), 371–379.

[293] Palmer et al (2022) 'Metabolic Flexibility and Its Impact on Health Outcomes', Mayo Clinic Proceedings, VOLUME 97, ISSUE 4, P761-776.

[294] Baumeier et al (2015). Caloric restriction and intermittent fasting alter hepatic lipid droplet proteome and diacylglycerol species and prevent diabetes in NZO mice. Biochimica et Biophysica Acta (BBA) - Molecular and Cell Biology of Lipids, 1851(5), 566–576.

[295] de Cabo, R., & Mattson, M. P. (2019). Effects of Intermittent Fasting on Health, Aging, and Disease. New England Journal of Medicine, 381(26), 2541–2551.

[296] Anton et al (2018). Flipping the Metabolic Switch: Understanding and Applying the Health Benefits of Fasting. Obesity (Silver Spring, Md.), 26(2), 254–268.

[297] Gambelunghe et al (2001). Physical exercise intensity can be related to plasma glutathione levels. Journal of physiology and biochemistry, 57(2), 9–14.

[298] Elokda et al (2007). Effects of exercise training on the glutathione antioxidant system. European journal of cardiovascular prevention and rehabilitation : official journal of the European Society of Cardiology, Working Groups on Epidemiology & Prevention and Cardiac Rehabilitation and Exercise Physiology, 14(5), 630–637.

[299] Goodwin et al (1998) 'Regulation of energy metabolism of the heart during acute increase in heart work', J Biol Chem. 1998 Nov 6;273(45):29530-9.

[300] Mulligan et al (2007). Upregulation of AMPK during cold exposure occurs via distinct mechanisms in brown and white adipose tissue of the mouse. The Journal of physiology, 580(Pt. 2), 677–684.

[301] Wijngaarden et al (2013). Effects of prolonged fasting on AMPK signaling, gene expression, and mitochondrial respiratory chain content in skeletal muscle from lean and obese individuals. American journal of physiology. Endocrinology and metabolism, 304(9), E1012–E1021.

[302] Viollet, B. (2017). The Energy Sensor AMPK: Adaptations to Exercise, Nutritional and Hormonal Signals. Hormones, Metabolism and the Benefits of Exercise, 13–24.

[303] Li et al (2019). Skeletal Muscle Lipid Droplets and the Athlete's Paradox. Cells, 8(3), 249.

[304] van Loon et al (2004). Intramyocellular lipid content in type 2 diabetes patients compared with overweight sedentary men and highly trained endurance athletes. American Journal of Physiology-Endocrinology and Metabolism, 287(3), E558–E565.

[305] Daemen et al (2018) 'Distinct lipid droplet characteristics and distribution unmask the apparent contradiction of the athlete's paradox', Molecular Metabolism, Volume 17, November 2018, Pages 71-81.

[306] Wang, G (2014) 'Raison d'être of insulin resistance: the adjustable threshold hypothesis', Journal of the Royal Society, Vol 11(101).

[307] Kinzig, K. P., Honors, M. A., & Hargrave, S. L. (2010). Insulin sensitivity and glucose tolerance are altered by maintenance on a ketogenic diet. Endocrinology, 151(7), 3105–3114. https://doi.org/10.1210/en.2010-0175

[308] Kinzig, K. P., Honors, M. A., & Hargrave, S. L. (2010). Insulin sensitivity and glucose tolerance are altered by maintenance on a ketogenic diet. Endocrinology, 151(7), 3105–3114. https://doi.org/10.1210/en.2010-0175

[309] Webster, C. C., van Boom, K. M., Armino, N., Larmuth, K., Noakes, T. D., Smith, J. A., & Kohn, T. A. (2020). Reduced Glucose Tolerance and Skeletal Muscle GLUT4 and IRS1 Content in Cyclists Habituated to a Long-Term Low-Carbohydrate, High-Fat Diet. International Journal of Sport Nutrition and Exercise Metabolism, 30(3), 210–217. https://doi.org/10.1123/ijsnem.2019-0359

[310] Berry, M. N., Phillips, J. W., Henly, D. C., & Clark, D. G. (1993). Effects of fatty acid oxidation on glucose utilization by isolated hepatocytes. FEBS letters, 319(1-2), 26–30. https://doi.org/10.1016/0014-5793(93)80030-x

[311] Roy Moxham (7 February 2002). The Great Hedge of India: The Search for the Living Barrier that Divided a People. Basic Books. ISBN 978-0-7867-0976-2.

279

[312] Rolph, George (1873). Something about sugar: its history, growth, manufacture and distribution. San Francisco: J.J. Newbegin.

[313] Rolph, George (1873). Something about sugar: its history, growth, manufacture and distribution. San Francisco: J.J. Newbegin.

[314] Adas, Michael (January 2001). Agricultural and Pastoral Societies in Ancient and Classical History. Temple University Press. ISBN 1-56639-832-0. p. 311.

[315] Sen, Tansen. (2003). Buddhism, Diplomacy, and Trade: The Realignment of Sino-Indian Relations, 600–1400. Manoa: Asian Interactions and Comparisons, a joint publication of the University of Hawaii Press and the Association for Asian Studies. ISBN 0-8248-2593-4. pp. 38–40.

[316] Kieschnick, John (2003). The Impact of Buddhism on Chinese Material Culture Princeton University Press. ISBN 0-691-09676-7.

[317] Sen, Tansen. (2003). Buddhism, Diplomacy, and Trade: The Realignment of Sino-Indian Relations, 600–1400. Manoa: Asian Interactions and Comparisons, a joint publication of the University of Hawaii Press and the Association for Asian Studies. ISBN 0-8248-2593-4. pp. 38–40.

[318] Strong, Roy (2002), Feast: A History of Grand Eating, Jonathan Cape, ISBN 0224061380

[319] Jean-Pierre (1990) 'Jean Meyer. Histoire du Sucre', Annales de Démographie Historique, Année 1990, pp. 507-509.

[320] Ponting, Clive (2000) [2000]. World history: a new perspective. London: Chatto & Windus. p. 481.

[321] Barber, Malcolm (2004). The two cities: medieval Europe, 1050–1320 (2nd ed.). Routledge. p. 14.

[322] Manning, Patrick (2006). "Slavery & Slave Trade in West Africa 1450-1930". Themes in West Africa's history. Akyeampong, Emmanuel Kwaku. Athens: Ohio University. pp. 102–103. ISBN 978-0-8214-4566-2.

[323] Antonio Benítez Rojo (1996). The Repeating: The Caribbean and the Postmodern Perspective. James E. Maraniss (translation). Duke University Press. p. 93. ISBN 0-8223-1865-2.

[324] Abreu y Galindo, J. de (1977). A. Cioranescu (ed.). Historia de la conquista de las siete islas de Canarias. Tenerife: Goya ediciones.

[325] Marggraf (1747) "Experiences chimiques faites dans le dessein de tirer un veritable sucre de diverses plantes, qui croissent dans nos contrées" [Chemical experiments made with the intention of extracting real sugar from diverse plants that grow in our lands], Histoire de l'académie royale des sciences et belles-lettres de Berlin, pages 79–90.

[326] Hill, G.; Langer, R. H. M. (1991). Agricultural plants. Cambridge, UK: Cambridge University Press. pp. 197–199. ISBN 978-0-521-40563-8.

[327] Zucker-Museum im Haus Amrumer Straße(2004) 'Festveranstaltung zum 100jährigen Bestehen des Berliner Institut für Zuckerindustrie', Accessed Online April 10th 2022: https://web.archive.org/web/20070824035034/http://www2.tu-berlin.de/~zuckerinstitut/museum.html

[328] Otter, Chris (2020). Diet for a large planet. USA: University of Chicago Press. p. 73. ISBN 978-0-226-69710-9.

[329] The Sugar Association Inc (2015) 'Refining and Processing Sugar', Consumer Fact Sheet, Accessed Online April 10th 2022: https://web.archive.org/web/20150221031555/http://westernsugar.com/pdf/Refining%20and%20Processing%20Sugar.pdf

[330] DiNicolantonio JJ, Lucan SC. Sugar season. It's everywhere and addictive. The New York Times. 12 Dec 2014.

[331] Snow HL. Refined sugar: its use and misuse. The Improvement Era Magazine 1948;51.

[332] Moose (1944) 'SUGAR A "DILUTING" AGENT', JAMA. 1944;125(10):738-739. doi:10.1001/jama.1944.02850280054021

[333] Br Med J (1933) 'RELATION OF EXCESSIVE CARBOHYDRATE INGESTION TO CATARRHS AND OTHER DISEASES', 1:738, doi: https://doi.org/10.1136/bmj.1.3773.738

[334] Ludwig, D. S. (2002). The Glycemic Index. JAMA, 287(18), 2414. https://doi.org/10.1001/jama.287.18.2414

[335] Feinman, R. D., & Volek, J. S. (2008). Carbohydrate restriction as the default treatment for type 2 diabetes and metabolic syndrome. Scandinavian Cardiovascular Journal, 42(4), 256–263. https://doi.org/10.1080/14017430802014838

[336] Volek, J. S., & Feinman, R. D. (2005). Carbohydrate restriction improves the features of Metabolic Syndrome. Metabolic Syndrome may be defined by the response to carbohydrate restriction. Nutrition & metabolism, 2, 31. https://doi.org/10.1186/1743-7075-2-31

[337] Feinman, R. D., Pogozelski, W. K., Astrup, A., Bernstein, R. K., Fine, E. J., Westman, E. C., Accurso, A., Frassetto, L., Gower, B. A., McFarlane, S. I., Nielsen, J. V., Krarup, T., Saslow, L., Roth, K. S., Vernon, M. C., Volek, J. S., Wilshire, G. B., Dahlqvist, A., Sundberg, R., … Worm, N. (2015). Dietary carbohydrate restriction as the first approach in diabetes management: Critical review and evidence base. Nutrition, 31(1), 1–13. https://doi.org/10.1016/j.nut.2014.06.011

[338] Holesh JE, Aslam S, Martin A. Physiology, Carbohydrates. [Updated 2022 Jul 25]. In: StatPearls [Internet]. Treasure Island (FL): StatPearls Publishing; 2022 Jan-. Available from: https://www.ncbi.nlm.nih.gov/books/NBK459280/

[339] Teller, George L. (January 1918). "Sugars Other Than Cane or Beet". The American Food Journal: 23–24.

[340] FDA (2018) 'High Fructose Corn Syrup Questions and Answers', Accessed Online February 19th 2022: https://www.fda.gov/food/food-additives-petitions/high-fructose-corn-syrup-questions-and-answers

[341] Gromova et al (2021). Mechanisms of Glucose Absorption in the Small Intestine in Health and Metabolic Diseases and Their Role in Appetite Regulation. Nutrients, 13(7), 2474.

[342] Han et al (2016). Regulation of glucose metabolism from a liver-centric perspective. Experimental & molecular medicine, 48(3), e218.

[343] Alvim et al (2015). General aspects of muscle glucose uptake. Anais da Academia Brasileira de Ciencias, 87(1), 351–368.

[344] Ferraris, R. P., Choe, J. Y., & Patel, C. R. (2018). Intestinal Absorption of Fructose. Annual review of nutrition, 38, 41–67.

[345] Evans et al (2017). Fructose replacement of glucose or sucrose in food or beverages lowers postprandial glucose and insulin without raising triglycerides: a systematic review and meta-analysis. The American Journal of Clinical Nutrition, 106(2), 506–518.

[346] Jensen et al (2018). Fructose and sugar: A major mediator of non-alcoholic fatty liver disease. Journal of hepatology, 68(5), 1063–1075.

[347] Merino et al (2019). Intestinal Fructose and Glucose Metabolism in Health and Disease. Nutrients, 12(1), 94.

[348] Chiavaroli et al (2015). Effect of Fructose on Established Lipid Targets: A Systematic Review and Meta-Analysis of Controlled Feeding Trials. Journal of the American Heart Association, 4(9), e001700.

[349] Southgate D. A. (1995). Digestion and metabolism of sugars. The American journal of clinical nutrition, 62(1 Suppl), 203S–211S.

[350] ScienceDirect (2012) 'Sucrase' Quantitative Human Physiology, Accessed Online February 19th: https://www.sciencedirect.com/topics/biochemistry-genetics-and-molecular-biology/sucrase

[351] Hieronimus et al (2020). Synergistic effects of fructose and glucose on lipoprotein risk factors for cardiovascular disease in young adults. Metabolism, 112, 154356.

[352] Perez-Pozo, S. E., Schold, J., Nakagawa, T., Sánchez-Lozada, L. G., Johnson, R. J., & Lillo, J. L. (2009). Excessive fructose intake induces the features of metabolic syndrome in healthy adult men: role of uric acid in the hypertensive response. International Journal of Obesity, 34(3), 454–461. https://doi.org/10.1038/ijo.2009.259

[353] Reiser, S., Handler, H. B., Gardner, L. B., Hallfrisch, J. G., Michaelis, O. E., 4th, & Prather, E. S. (1979). Isocaloric exchange of dietary starch and sucrose in humans. II. Effect on fasting blood insulin, glucose, and glucagon and on insulin and glucose response to a sucrose load. The American journal of clinical nutrition, 32(11), 2206–2216. https://doi.org/10.1093/ajcn/32.11.2206

[354] Reiser, S., Michaelis, O. E., 4th, Cataland, S., & O'Dorisio, T. M. (1980). Effect of isocaloric exchange of dietary starch and sucrose in humans on the gastric inhibitory polypeptide response to a sucrose load. The American journal of clinical nutrition, 33(9), 1907–1911. https://doi.org/10.1093/ajcn/33.9.1907

[355] Hallfrisch, J., Ellwood, K. C., Michaelis, O. E., Reiser, S., O'Dorisio, T. M., & Prather, E. S. (1983). Effects of Dietary Fructose on Plasma Glucose and Hormone Responses in Normal and Hyperinsulinemic Men. The Journal of Nutrition, 113(9), 1819–1826. https://doi.org/10.1093/jn/113.9.1819

[356] Te Morenga et al (2014) 'Dietary sugars and cardiometabolic risk: systematic review and meta-analyses of randomized controlled trials of the effects on blood pressure and lipids', The American Journal of Clinical Nutrition, Volume 100, Issue 1, July 2014, Pages 65–79, https://doi.org/10.3945/ajcn.113.081521

[357] McCarty, M. F., & DiNicolantonio, J. J. (2014). The cardiometabolic benefits of glycine: Is glycine an 'antidote' to dietary fructose? Open Heart, 1(1), e000103. https://doi.org/10.1136/openhrt-2014-000103

[358] Basu, S., Yoffe, P., Hills, N., & Lustig, R. H. (2013). The Relationship of Sugar to Population-Level Diabetes Prevalence: An Econometric Analysis of Repeated Cross-Sectional Data. PLoS ONE, 8(2), e57873. https://doi.org/10.1371/journal.pone.0057873

[359] Bray, G. A., Nielsen, S. J., & Popkin, B. M. (2004). Consumption of high-fructose corn syrup in beverages may play a role in the epidemic of obesity. The American journal of clinical nutrition, 79(4), 537–543. https://doi.org/10.1093/ajcn/79.4.537

[360] YUDKIN, J. Sugar and Disease. Nature 239, 197–199 (1972). https://doi.org/10.1038/239197a0

[361] Shapiro, A., Mu, W., Roncal, C., Cheng, K.-Y., Johnson, R. J., & Scarpace, P. J. (2008). Fructose-induced leptin resistance exacerbates weight gain in response to subsequent high-fat feeding. American Journal of Physiology-Regulatory, Integrative and Comparative Physiology, 295(5), R1370–R1375. https://doi.org/10.1152/ajpregu.00195.2008

[362] DiNicolantonio, J. J., O'Keefe, J. H., & Lucan, S. C. (2014). An Unsavory Truth: Sugar, More than Salt, Predisposes to Hypertension and Chronic Disease. The American Journal of Cardiology, 114(7), 1126–1128. https://doi.org/10.1016/j.amjcard.2014.07.002

[363] Bray, G. A., & Popkin, B. M. (2014). Dietary Sugar and Body Weight: Have We Reached a Crisis in the Epidemic of Obesity and Diabetes? Diabetes Care, 37(4), 950–956. https://doi.org/10.2337/dc13-2085

[364] Brahm, A., & Hegele, R. A. (2013). Hypertriglyceridemia. Nutrients, 5(3), 981–1001.

[365] Kell et al (2014). Added sugars in the diet are positively associated with diastolic blood pressure and triglycerides in children. The American journal of clinical nutrition, 100(1), 46–52.

[366] Ma et al (2020). Triglyceride is independently correlated with insulin resistance and islet beta cell function: a study in population with different glucose and lipid metabolism states. Lipids in Health and Disease, 19(1).

[367] Van de Wiel, A. (2012). The Effect of Alcohol on Postprandial and Fasting Triglycerides. International Journal of Vascular Medicine, 2012, 1–4. https://doi.org/10.1155/2012/862504

[368] Taylor et al (2015). Exploring causal associations of alcohol with cardiovascular and metabolic risk factors in a Chinese population using Mendelian randomization analysis. Scientific Reports, 5(1).

[369] Mann, S., Beedie, C., & Jimenez, A. (2014). Differential effects of aerobic exercise, resistance training and combined exercise modalities on cholesterol and the lipid profile: review, synthesis and recommendations. Sports medicine (Auckland, N.Z.), 44(2), 211–221.

[370] Wang, Y., Shen, L., & Xu, D. (2019). Aerobic exercise reduces triglycerides by targeting apolipoprotein C3 in patients with coronary heart disease. Clinical cardiology, 42(1), 56–61.

[371] Yang, T. J., Wu, C. L., & Chiu, C. H. (2018). High-Intensity Intermittent Exercise Increases Fat Oxidation Rate and Reduces Postprandial Triglyceride Concentrations. Nutrients, 10(4), 492.

[372] Hannon et al (2018). Dietary Fiber Is Independently Related to Blood Triglycerides Among Adults with Overweight and Obesity. Current developments in nutrition, 3(2), nzy094.

[373] Whisner et al (2019). Effects of Low-Fat and High-Fat Meals, with and without Dietary Fiber, on Postprandial Endothelial Function, Triglyceridemia, and Glycemia in Adolescents. Nutrients, 11(11), 2626.

[374] Dibaba D. T. (2019). Effect of vitamin D supplementation on serum lipid profiles: a systematic review and meta-analysis. Nutrition reviews, 77(12), 890–902.

[375] Heden et al (2013). Meal frequency differentially alters postprandial triacylglycerol and insulin concentrations in obese women. Obesity (Silver Spring, Md.), 21(1), 123–129.

[376] Haslam et al (2020). Beverage Consumption and Longitudinal Changes in Lipoprotein Concentrations and Incident Dyslipidemia in US Adults: The Framingham Heart Study. Journal of the American Heart Association, 9(5).

[377] Zheng et al (2018). Association Between Triglyceride Level and Glycemic Control Among Insulin-Treated Patients With Type 2 Diabetes. The Journal of Clinical Endocrinology & Metabolism, 104(4), 1211–1220.

[378] Stanhope, K. L., & Havel, P. J. (2008). Fructose consumption: potential mechanisms for its effects to increase visceral adiposity and induce dyslipidemia and insulin resistance. Current opinion in lipidology, 19(1), 16–24.

[379] Dong et al (2020). The effects of low-carbohydrate diets on cardiovascular risk factors: A meta-analysis. PloS one, 15(1), e0225348.

[380] Gjuladin-Hellon et al (2018). Effects of carbohydrate-restricted diets on low-density lipoprotein cholesterol levels in overweight and obese adults: a systematic review and meta-analysis. Nutrition Reviews, 77(3), 161–180.

[381] Chawla et al (2020). The Effect of Low-Fat and Low-Carbohydrate Diets on Weight Loss and Lipid Levels: A Systematic Review and Meta-Analysis. Nutrients, 12(12), 3774.

[382] De Biase et al (2007). Vegetarian diet and cholesterol and triglycerides levels. Arquivos brasileiros de cardiologia, 88(1), 35–39.

[383] Ferdowsian, H. R., & Barnard, N. D. (2009). Effects of plant-based diets on plasma lipids. The American journal of cardiology, 104(7), 947–956.

[384] Jenkins et al (2001). Effect of a very-high-fiber vegetable, fruit, and nut diet on serum lipids and colonic function. Metabolism: clinical and experimental, 50(4), 494–503.

[385] Jenkins et al (1987). Low-glycemic index diet in hyperlipidemia: use of traditional starchy foods. The American Journal of Clinical Nutrition, 46(1), 66–71.

[386] Brouwer et al (2016) 'Effect of trans-fatty acid intake on blood lipids and lipoproteins: a systematic review and meta-regression analysis', World Health Organization, Accessed Online February 20th 2023: https://apps.who.int/iris/bitstream/handle/10665/246109/9789241510608-eng.pdf;jsessionid=516DEA1E80EC6901361A231E7207B493?sequence=1

[387] Raatz et al (2016). Twice weekly intake of farmed Atlantic salmon (Salmo salar) positively influences lipoprotein concentration and particle size in overweight men and women. Nutrition research (New York, N.Y.), 36(9), 899–906.

[388] Ghobadi et al (2019). Comparison of blood lipid-lowering effects of olive oil and other plant oils: A systematic review and meta-analysis of 27 randomized placebo-controlled clinical trials. Critical reviews in food science and nutrition, 59(13), 2110–2124.

[389] Lopez-Alvarenga et al (2010). Polyunsaturated fatty acids effect on serum triglycerides concentration in the presence of metabolic syndrome components. The Alaska-Siberia Project. Metabolism: clinical and experimental, 59(1), 86–92.

[390] Liu et al (2017). A healthy approach to dietary fats: understanding the science and taking action to reduce consumer confusion. Nutrition journal, 16(1), 53.

[391] Moose RM. Sugar a "diluting agent". JAMA 1944;125:738–9.

[392] Glushakova, O., Kosugi, T., Roncal, C., Mu, W., Heinig, M., Cirillo, P., Sánchez-Lozada, L. G., Johnson, R. J., & Nakagawa, T. (2008). Fructose Induces the Inflammatory Molecule ICAM-1 in Endothelial Cells. Journal of the American Society of Nephrology, 19(9), 1712–1720. https://doi.org/10.1681/asn.2007121304

[393] Nair, S., P Chacko, V., Arnold, C., & Diehl, A. M. (2003). Hepatic ATP reserve and efficiency of replenishing: comparison between obese and nonobese normal individuals. The American journal of gastroenterology, 98(2), 466–470. https://doi.org/10.1111/j.1572-0241.2003.07221.x

[394] Bode, J.C., Zelder, O., Rumpelt, H.J. and Wittkampy, U. (1973), Depletion of Liver Adenosine Phosphates and Metabolic Effects of Intravenous Infusion of Fructose or Sorbitol in Man and in the Rat,. European Journal of Clinical Investigation, 3: 436-441. https://doi.org/10.1111/j.1365-2362.1973.tb02211.x

[395] Bray, G. A. (2013). Energy and Fructose From Beverages Sweetened With Sugar or High-Fructose Corn Syrup Pose a Health Risk for Some People. Advances in Nutrition, 4(2), 220–225. https://doi.org/10.3945/an.112.002816

[396] Ahrens R. A. (1974). Sucrose, hypertension, and heart disease an historical perspective. The American journal of clinical nutrition, 27(4), 403–422. https://doi.org/10.1093/ajcn/27.4.403

[397] MacDonald and Thomas (1956) 'Studies on the genesis of experimental diffuse hepatic fibrosis.', Clinical Science, 01 Aug 1956, 15(3):373-387.

[398] Durand, A. M., Fisher, M., & Adams, M. (1968). The influence of type of dietary carbohydrate. Effect on histological findings in two strains of rats. Archives of pathology, 85(3), 318–324.

[399] DALDERUP, L. M., & VISSER, W. (1969). Influence of Extra Sucrose in the Daily Food on the Life-span of Wistar Albino Rats. Nature, 222(5198), 1050–1052. https://doi.org/10.1038/2221050a0

[400] Abdelmalek, M. F., Lazo, M., Horska, A., Bonekamp, S., Lipkin, E. W., Balasubramanyam, A., Bantle, J. P., Johnson, R. J., Diehl, A. M., Clark, J. M., & Fatty Liver Subgroup of Look AHEAD Research Group (2012). Higher dietary fructose is associated with impaired hepatic adenosine triphosphate homeostasis in obese individuals with type 2 diabetes. Hepatology (Baltimore, Md.), 56(3), 952–960. https://doi.org/10.1002/hep.25741

[401] Cannon, J. R., Harvison, P. J., & Rush, G. F. (1991). The effects of fructose on adenosine triphosphate depletion following mitochondrial dysfunction and lethal cell injury in isolated rat hepatocytes. Toxicology and applied pharmacology, 108(3), 407–416. https://doi.org/10.1016/0041-008x(91)90087-u

[402] Latta et al (1999) 'Metabolic Depletion of Atp by Fructose Inversely Controls Cd95- and Tumor Necrosis Factor Receptor 1–Mediated Hepatic Apoptosis', J Exp Med (2000) 191 (11): 1975–1986.

[403] Page, K. A., Chan, O., Arora, J., Belfort-DeAguiar, R., Dzuira, J., Roehmholdt, B., Cline, G. W., Naik, S., Sinha, R., Constable, R. T., & Sherwin, R. S. (2013). Effects of Fructose vs Glucose on Regional Cerebral Blood Flow in Brain Regions Involved With Appetite and Reward Pathways. JAMA, 309(1), 63. https://doi.org/10.1001/jama.2012.116975

[404] Welsh, J. A., Sharma, A. J., Grellinger, L., & Vos, M. B. (2011). Consumption of added sugars is decreasing in the United States. American Journal of Clinical Nutrition, 94(3), 726–734. https://doi.org/10.3945/ajcn.111.018366

[405] Cordain et al (2003) 'Hyperinsulinemic diseases of civilization: more than just Syndrome X', Comparative Biochemistry and Physiology Part A: Molecular & Integrative Physiology, Volume 136, Issue 1, September 2003, Pages 95-112.

[406] Malnik E. World Health Organisation advises halving sugar intake. The Telegraph. March 2014.

[407] Shanik et al (2008). Insulin resistance and hyperinsulinemia: is hyperinsulinemia the cart or the horse?. Diabetes care, 31 Suppl 2, S262–S268.

[408] Jenkins et al (1981) 'Glycemic index of foods: a physiological basis for carbohydrate exchange', The American Journal of Clinical Nutrition, Volume 34, Issue 3, March 1981, Pages 362–366.

[409] Glycemic Index Research (2018) 'Glycemic Index Defined', Accessed Online Feb 20th 2023: https://web.archive.org/web/20180927161417/http://www.glycemic.com/GlycemicIndex-LoadDefined.htm

[410] Diabetes Canada (2023) 'What is the Glycemic Index?', Accessed Online February 22nd 2023: https://www.diabetes.ca/en-CA/managing-my-diabetes/tools---resources/glycemic-index-education-portal

[411] Zeevi et al (2015). Personalized Nutrition by Prediction of Glycemic Responses. Cell, 163(5), 1079–1094.

[412] Glycemic Index Research (2018) 'Glycemic Index Defined', Accessed Online Feb 20th 2023: https://web.archive.org/web/20180927161417/http://www.glycemic.com/GlycemicIndex-LoadDefined.htm

[413] Holt et al (1997). An insulin index of foods: the insulin demand generated by 1000-kJ portions of common foods. The American journal of clinical nutrition, 66(5), 1264–1276.

[414] Holt et al (1997). An insulin index of foods: the insulin demand generated by 1000-kJ portions of common foods. The American journal of clinical nutrition, 66(5), 1264–1276.

[415] Blades, Mabel (2021). The glycemic load counter : a pocket guide to GL and GI values for over 800 foods. Berkeley, CA. ISBN 978-1-64604-249-4.

[416] Atkinson et al (2008). International tables of glycemic index and glycemic load values: 2008. Diabetes care, 31(12), 2281–2283.

[417] Gavin et al (1974). Insulin-dependent regulation of insulin receptor concentrations: a direct demonstration in cell culture. Proceedings of the National Academy of Sciences of the United States of America, 71(1), 84–88.

[418] Paz et al (1997). A molecular basis for insulin resistance. Elevated serine/threonine phosphorylation of IRS-1 and IRS-2 inhibits their binding to the juxtamembrane region of the insulin receptor and impairs their ability to undergo insulin-induced tyrosine phosphorylation. The Journal of biological chemistry, 272(47), 29911–29918.

[419] De Meyts et al (1973). Insulin interactions with its receptors: experimental evidence for negative cooperativity. Biochemical and biophysical research communications, 55 1, 154-61 .

[420] Rizza et al (1985). Production of insulin resistance by hyperinsulinaemia in man. Diabetologia, 28(2), 70–75.

[421] Koopmans et al (1996). Pulsatile intravenous insulin replacement in streptozotocin-diabetic rats is more efficient than continuous delivery: effects on glycaemic control, insulin-mediated glucose metabolism and lipolysis. Diabetologia, 39(4), 391–400.

[422] Bratusch-Marrain et al (1986). Efficacy of pulsatile versus continuous insulin administration on hepatic glucose production and glucose utilization in type I diabetic humans. Diabetes, 35(8), 922–926.

[423] Paolisso et al (1988). Pulsatile insulin delivery is more efficient than continuous infusion in modulating islet cell function in normal subjects and patients with type 1 diabetes. The Journal of clinical endocrinology and metabolism, 66(6), 1220–1226.

[424] Matthews et al (1983). Pulsatile insulin has greater hypoglycemic effect than continuous delivery. Diabetes, 32(7), 617–621.

[425] Goodner et al (1988). Rapid reduction and return of surface insulin receptors after exposure to brief pulses of insulin in perifused rat hepatocytes. Diabetes, 37(10), 1316–1323.

[426] Edwards, C. H., Grundy, M. M., Grassby, T., Vasilopoulou, D., Frost, G. S., Butterworth, P. J., Berry, S. E., Sanderson, J., & Ellis, P. R. (2015). Manipulation of starch bioaccessibility in wheat endosperm to regulate starch digestion, postprandial glycemia, insulinemia, and gut hormone responses: a randomized controlled trial in healthy ileostomy participants. The American Journal of Clinical Nutrition, 102(4), 791–800. https://doi.org/10.3945/ajcn.114.106203

[427] Putnam et al (2001) 'U. S. Per Capita Food Supply Trends: More Calories, Refined Carbohydrates, and Fats', Food Review/ National Food Review, Vol 25, Issue 3, Page 2-15.

[428] CDC (2017) 'Long-Term Trends in Diabetes', Accessed Online Feb 20th 2023: https://www.cdc.gov/diabetes/statistics/slides/long_term_trends.pdf

[429] Diabetes Research Institute (2020) 'Diabetes Statistics', Accessed Online Feb 20th 2023: https://diabetesresearch.org/diabetes-statistics/

[430] Storlien et al (1988) 'Effects of sucrose vs starch diets on in vivo insulin action, thermogenesis, and obesity in rats', The American Journal of Clinical Nutrition, Volume 47, Issue 3, March 1988, Pages 420–427, https://doi.org/10.1093/ajcn/47.3.420

[431] Hulman, S., & Falkner, B. (1994). The effect of excess dietary sucrose on growth, blood pressure, and metabolism in developing Sprague-Dawley rats. Pediatric research, 36(1 Pt 1), 95–101. https://doi.org/10.1203/00006450-199407001-00017

[432] Pagliassotti, M. J., Shahrokhi, K. A., & Moscarello, M. (1994). Involvement of liver and skeletal muscle in sucrose-induced insulin resistance: dose-response studies. American Journal of Physiology-Regulatory, Integrative and Comparative Physiology, 266(5), R1637–R1644. https://doi.org/10.1152/ajpregu.1994.266.5.r1637

[433] Pugazhenthi, S., Angel, J. F., & Khandelwal, R. L. (1993). Effects of high sucrose diet on insulin-like effects of vanadate in diabetic rats. Molecular and cellular biochemistry, 122(1), 77–84. https://doi.org/10.1007/BF00925740

[434] Gutman et al (1987) 'Long-term hypertriglyceridemia and glucose intolerance in rats fed chronically an isocaloric sucrose-rich diet.', Metabolism: Clinical and Experimental, 01 Nov 1987, 36(11):1013-1020

[435] Wright, D. W., Hansen, R. I., Mondon, C. E., & Reaven, G. M. (1983). Sucrose-induced insulin resistance in the rat: modulation by exercise and diet. The American Journal of Clinical Nutrition, 38(6), 879–883. https://doi.org/10.1093/ajcn/38.6.879

[436] Reiser, S., & Hallfrisch, J. (1977). Insulin sensitivity and adipose tissue weight of rats fed starch or sucrose diets ad libitum or in meals. The Journal of nutrition, 107(1), 147–155. https://doi.org/10.1093/jn/107.1.147

[437] Reiser, S., Handler, H. B., Gardner, L. B., Hallfrisch, J. G., Michaelis, O. E., 4th, & Prather, E. S. (1979). Isocaloric exchange of dietary starch and sucrose in humans. II. Effect on fasting blood insulin, glucose, and glucagon and on insulin and glucose response to a sucrose load. The American journal of clinical nutrition, 32(11), 2206–2216. https://doi.org/10.1093/ajcn/32.11.2206

[438] Beck-Nielsen et al (1980) 'Impaired cellular insulin binding and insulin sensitivity induced by high-fructose feeding in normal subjects', The American Journal of Clinical Nutrition, Volume 33, Issue 2, February 1980, Pages 273–278, https://doi.org/10.1093/ajcn/33.2.273

[439] Stanhope, K. L., Schwarz, J. M., Keim, N. L., Griffen, S. C., Bremer, A. A., Graham, J. L., Hatcher, B., Cox, C. L., Dyachenko, A., Zhang, W., McGahan, J. P., Seibert, A., Krauss, R. M., Chiu, S., Schaefer, E. J., Ai, M., Otokozawa, S., Nakajima, K., Nakano, T., Beysen, C., … Havel, P. J. (2009). Consuming fructose-sweetened, not glucose-sweetened, beverages increases visceral adiposity and lipids and decreases insulin sensitivity in overweight/obese humans. The Journal of clinical investigation, 119(5), 1322–1334. https://doi.org/10.1172/JCI37385

[440] Reiser, S., Handler, H. B., Gardner, L. B., Hallfrisch, J. G., Michaelis, O. E., 4th, & Prather, E. S. (1979). Isocaloric exchange of dietary starch and sucrose in humans. II. Effect on fasting blood insulin, glucose, and glucagon and on insulin and glucose response to a sucrose load. The American journal of clinical nutrition, 32(11), 2206–2216. https://doi.org/10.1093/ajcn/32.11.2206

[441] Reiser, S., Bohn, E., Hallfrisch, J., Michaelis, O. E., 4th, Keeney, M., & Prather, E. S. (1981). Serum insulin and glucose in hyperinsulinemic subjects fed three different levels of sucrose. The American journal of clinical nutrition, 34(11), 2348–2358. https://doi.org/10.1093/ajcn/34.11.2348

[442] DiNicolantonio et al (2015). Added fructose: a principal driver of type 2 diabetes mellitus and its consequences. Mayo Clinic proceedings, 90(3), 372–381.

[443] Buziau et al (2022). Fructose Intake From Fruit Juice and Sugar-Sweetened Beverages Is Associated With Higher Intrahepatic Lipid Content: The Maastricht Study. Diabetes care, 45(5), 1116–1123.

[444] Pereira et al (2017). Fructose Consumption in the Development of Obesity and the Effects of Different Protocols of Physical Exercise on the Hepatic Metabolism. Nutrients, 9(4), 405.

[445] Softic et al (2020). Fructose and hepatic insulin resistance. Critical reviews in clinical laboratory sciences, 57(5), 308–322.

[446] Merino et al (2019). Intestinal Fructose and Glucose Metabolism in Health and Disease. Nutrients, 12(1), 94.

[447] Sánchez-Lozada, L. G., Le, M., Segal, M., & Johnson, R. J. (2008). How safe is fructose for persons with or without diabetes?. The American journal of clinical nutrition, 88(5), 1189–1190. https://doi.org/10.3945/ajcn.2008.26812

[448] Segal, M. S., Gollub, E., & Johnson, R. J. (2007). Is the fructose index more relevant with regards to cardiovascular disease than the glycemic index?. European journal of nutrition, 46(7), 406–417. https://doi.org/10.1007/s00394-007-0680-9

[449] Bes-Rastrollo, M., Schulze, M. B., Ruiz-Canela, M., & Martinez-Gonzalez, M. A. (2013). Financial conflicts of interest and reporting bias regarding the association between sugar-sweetened beverages and weight gain: a systematic review of systematic reviews. PLoS medicine, 10(12), e1001578. https://doi.org/10.1371/journal.pmed.1001578

[450] Raben, A., Vasilaras, T. H., Møller, A. C., & Astrup, A. (2002). Sucrose compared with artificial sweeteners: different effects on ad libitum food intake and body weight after 10 wk of supplementation in overweight subjects. The American journal of clinical nutrition, 76(4), 721–729. https://doi.org/10.1093/ajcn/76.4.721

[451] Tordoff, M. G., & Alleva, A. M. (1990). Effect of drinking soda sweetened with aspartame or high-fructose corn syrup on food intake and body weight. The American journal of clinical nutrition, 51(6), 963–969. https://doi.org/10.1093/ajcn/51.6.963

[452] Ludwig, D. S., Peterson, K. E., & Gortmaker, S. L. (2001). Relation between consumption of sugar-sweetened drinks and childhood obesity: a prospective, observational analysis. The Lancet, 357(9255), 505–508. https://doi.org/10.1016/s0140-6736(00)04041-1

[453] Bes-Rastrollo, M., Schulze, M. B., Ruiz-Canela, M., & Martinez-Gonzalez, M. A. (2013). Financial conflicts of interest and reporting bias regarding the association between sugar-sweetened beverages and weight gain: a systematic review of systematic reviews. PLoS medicine, 10(12), e1001578. https://doi.org/10.1371/journal.pmed.1001578

[454] Stanhope et al (2009). Consuming fructose-sweetened, not glucose-sweetened, beverages increases visceral adiposity and lipids and decreases insulin sensitivity in overweight/obese humans. The Journal of clinical investigation, 119(5), 1322–1334.

[455] Price et al (August 2006). "Weight, shape, and mortality risk in older persons: elevated waist-hip ratio, not high body mass index, is associated with a greater risk of death". Am. J. Clin. Nutr. 84 (2): 449–60.

[456] Thomas, E. L., Parkinson, J. R., Frost, G. S., Goldstone, A. P., Doré, C. J., McCarthy, J. P., Collins, A. L., Fitzpatrick, J. A., Durighel, G., Taylor-Robinson, S. D., & Bell, J. D. (2012). The missing risk: MRI and MRS phenotyping of abdominal adiposity and ectopic fat. Obesity (Silver Spring, Md.), 20(1), 76–87. https://doi.org/10.1038/oby.2011.142

[457] Thomas, E. L., Frost, G., Taylor-Robinson, S. D., & Bell, J. D. (2012). Excess body fat in obese and normal-weight subjects. Nutrition research reviews, 25(1), 150–161. https://doi.org/10.1017/S0954422412000054

[458] Thomas, E. L., Parkinson, J. R., Frost, G. S., Goldstone, A. P., Doré, C. J., McCarthy, J. P., Collins, A. L., Fitzpatrick, J. A., Durighel, G., Taylor-Robinson, S. D., & Bell, J. D. (2012). The missing risk: MRI and MRS phenotyping of abdominal adiposity and ectopic fat. Obesity (Silver Spring, Md.), 20(1), 76–87. https://doi.org/10.1038/oby.2011.142

[459] Conus, F., Rabasa-Lhoret, R., & Péronnet, F. (2007). Characteristics of metabolically obese normal-weight (MONW) subjects. Applied physiology, nutrition, and metabolism = Physiologie appliquee, nutrition et metabolisme, 32(1), 4–12. https://doi.org/10.1139/h06-092

[460] Ruderman, N. B., Schneider, S. H., & Berchtold, P. (1981). The "metabolically-obese," normal-weight individual. The American journal of clinical nutrition, 34(8), 1617–1621. https://doi.org/10.1093/ajcn/34.8.1617

[461] Dimitriadis, G., Mitrou, P., Lambadiari, V., Maratou, E., & Raptis, S. A. (2011). Insulin effects in muscle and adipose tissue. Diabetes research and clinical practice, 93 Suppl 1, S52–S59. https://doi.org/10.1016/S0168-8227(11)70014-6

[462] Ohlson, L. O., Larsson, B., Svärdsudd, K., Welin, L., Eriksson, H., Wilhelmsen, L., Björntorp, P., & Tibblin, G. (1985). The influence of body fat distribution on the incidence of diabetes mellitus. 13.5 years of follow-up of the participants in the study of men born in 1913. Diabetes, 34(10), 1055–1058. https://doi.org/10.2337/diab.34.10.1055

[463] Donahue, R. P., Abbott, R. D., Bloom, E., Reed, D. M., & Yano, K. (1987). Central obesity and coronary heart disease in men. Lancet (London, England), 1(8537), 821–824. https://doi.org/10.1016/s0140-6736(87)91605-9

[464] Ducimetiere and Cambien (1986) 'The pattern of subcutaneous fat distribution in middle-aged men and the risk of coronary heart disease: the Paris Prospective Study.', International Journal of Obesity, 01 Jan 1986, 10(3):229-240.

[465] Lapidus, L., Bengtsson, C., Larsson, B., Pennert, K., Rybo, E., & Sjöström, L. (1984). Distribution of adipose tissue and risk of cardiovascular disease and death: a 12 year follow up of participants in the population study of women in Gothenburg, Sweden. British medical journal (Clinical research ed.), 289(6454), 1257–1261. https://doi.org/10.1136/bmj.289.6454.1257

[466] Larsson et al (1984) 'Abdominal adipose tissue distribution, obesity, and risk of cardiovascular disease and death: 13 year follow up of participants in the study of men born in 1913.', Br Med J (Clin Res Ed) 1984; 288 doi: https://doi.org/10.1136/bmj.288.6428.1401

[467] Pou, K. M., Massaro, J. M., Hoffmann, U., Vasan, R. S., Maurovich-Horvat, P., Larson, M. G., Keaney, J. F., Jr, Meigs, J. B., Lipinska, I., Kathiresan, S., Murabito, J. M., O'Donnell, C. J., Benjamin, E. J., & Fox, C. S. (2007). Visceral and subcutaneous adipose tissue volumes are cross-sectionally related to markers of inflammation and oxidative stress: the Framingham Heart Study. Circulation, 116(11), 1234–1241. https://doi.org/10.1161/CIRCULATIONAHA.107.710509

[468] Pischon, T., Boeing, H., Hoffmann, K., Bergmann, M., Schulze, M. B., Overvad, K., van der Schouw, Y. T., Spencer, E., Moons, K. G., Tjønneland, A., Halkjaer, J., Jensen, M. K., Stegger, J., Clavel-Chapelon, F., Boutron-Ruault, M. C., Chajes, V., Linseisen, J., Kaaks, R., Trichopoulou, A., Trichopoulos, D., ... Riboli, E. (2008). General and abdominal adiposity and risk of death in Europe. The New England journal of medicine, 359(20), 2105–2120. https://doi.org/10.1056/NEJMoa0801891

[469] Kern, P. A., Ranganathan, S., Li, C., Wood, L., & Ranganathan, G. (2001). Adipose tissue tumor necrosis factor and interleukin-6 expression in human obesity and insulin resistance. American journal of physiology. Endocrinology and metabolism, 280(5), E745–E751. https://doi.org/10.1152/ajpendo.2001.280.5.E745

[470] Mokdad, A. H., Ford, E. S., Bowman, B. A., Dietz, W. H., Vinicor, F., Bales, V. S., & Marks, J. S. (2003). Prevalence of obesity, diabetes, and obesity-related health risk factors, 2001. JAMA, 289(1), 76–79. https://doi.org/10.1001/jama.289.1.76

[471] Marette A. (2003). Molecular mechanisms of inflammation in obesity-linked insulin resistance. International journal of obesity and related metabolic disorders : journal of the International Association for the Study of Obesity, 27 Suppl 3, S46–S48. https://doi.org/10.1038/sj.ijo.0802500

[472] Montague, C. T., & O'Rahilly, S. (2000). The perils of portliness: causes and consequences of visceral adiposity. Diabetes, 49(6), 883–888. https://doi.org/10.2337/diabetes.49.6.883

[473] Maresky, H. S., Sharfman, Z., Ziv-Baran, T., Gomori, J. M., Copel, L., & Tal, S. (2015). Anthropometric Assessment of Neck Adipose Tissue and Airway Volume Using Multidetector Computed Tomography: An Imaging Approach and Association With Overall Mortality. Medicine, 94(45), e1991. https://doi.org/10.1097/MD.0000000000001991

[474] Batra, A., & Siegmund, B. (2012). The role of visceral fat. Digestive diseases (Basel, Switzerland), 30(1), 70–74. https://doi.org/10.1159/000335722

[475] Ibrahim M. M. (2010). Subcutaneous and visceral adipose tissue: structural and functional differences. Obesity reviews : an official journal of the International Association for the Study of Obesity, 11(1), 11–18. https://doi.org/10.1111/j.1467-789X.2009.00623.x

[476] Kuo, L. E., Czarnecka, M., Kitlinska, J. B., Tilan, J. U., Kvetnanský, R., & Zukowska, Z. (2008). Chronic stress, combined with a high-fat/high-sugar diet, shifts sympathetic signaling toward neuropeptide Y and leads to obesity and the metabolic syndrome. Annals of the New York Academy of Sciences, 1148, 232–237. https://doi.org/10.1196/annals.1410.035

[477] Björntorp P. (1996). The regulation of adipose tissue distribution in humans. International journal of obesity and related metabolic disorders : journal of the International Association for the Study of Obesity, 20(4), 291–302.

[478] Mårin, P., Darin, N., Amemiya, T., Andersson, B., Jern, S., & Björntorp, P. (1992). Cortisol secretion in relation to body fat distribution in obese premenopausal women. Metabolism: clinical and experimental, 41(8), 882–886. https://doi.org/10.1016/0026-0495(92)90171-6

[479] Price et al (August 2006). "Weight, shape, and mortality risk in older persons: elevated waist-hip ratio, not high body mass index, is associated with a greater risk of death". Am. J. Clin. Nutr. 84 (2): 449–60.

[480] Tchernof, A., & Després, P. (2013). Pathophysiology of human visceral obesity: an update. Physiological reviews, 93(1), 359–404. https://doi.org/10.1152/physrev.00033.2011

[481] Chielle, E. O., Feltez, A., & Rossi, E. M. (2017). Influence of obesity on the serum concentration of retinol-binding protein 4 (RBP4) in young adults. Jornal Brasileiro de Patologia e Medicina Laboratorial. https://doi.org/10.5935/1676-2444.20170012

[482] Chang, X., Yan, H., Bian, H., Xia, M., Zhang, L., Gao, J., & Gao, X. (2015). Serum retinol binding protein 4 is associated with visceral fat in human with nonalcoholic fatty liver disease without known diabetes: a cross-sectional study. Lipids in health and disease, 14, 28. https://doi.org/10.1186/s12944-015-0033-2

[483] Patel, P., & Abate, N. (2013). Body fat distribution and insulin resistance. Nutrients, 5(6), 2019–2027. https://doi.org/10.3390/nu5062019

[484] Havel P. J. (2005). Dietary fructose: implications for dysregulation of energy homeostasis and lipid/carbohydrate metabolism. Nutrition reviews, 63(5), 133–157. https://doi.org/10.1301/nr.2005.may.133-157

[485] Lustig R. H. (2010). Fructose: metabolic, hedonic, and societal parallels with ethanol. Journal of the American Dietetic Association, 110(9), 1307–1321. https://doi.org/10.1016/j.jada.2010.06.008

[486] Stanhope, K. L., Schwarz, J. M., Keim, N. L., Griffen, S. C., Bremer, A. A., Graham, J. L., Hatcher, B., Cox, C. L., Dyachenko, A., Zhang, W., McGahan, J. P., Seibert, A., Krauss, R. M., Chiu, S., Schaefer, E. J., Ai, M., Otokozawa, S., Nakajima, K., Nakano, T., Beysen, C., ... Havel, P. J. (2009). Consuming fructose-sweetened, not glucose-sweetened, beverages increases visceral adiposity and lipids and decreases insulin sensitivity in overweight/obese humans. The Journal of clinical investigation, 119(5), 1322–1334. https://doi.org/10.1172/JCI37385

[487] Tchernof, A., & Després, J. P. (2013). Pathophysiology of human visceral obesity: an update. Physiological reviews, 93(1), 359–404. https://doi.org/10.1152/physrev.00033.2011

[488] Walker, B. R., & Andrew, R. (2006). Tissue production of cortisol by 11beta-hydroxysteroid dehydrogenase type 1 and metabolic disease. Annals of the New York Academy of Sciences, 1083, 165–184. https://doi.org/10.1196/annals.1367.012

[489] Thieringer, R., Le Grand, C. B., Carbin, L., Cai, T. Q., Wong, B., Wright, S. D., & Hermanowski-Vosatka, A. (2001). 11 Beta-hydroxysteroid dehydrogenase type 1 is induced in human monocytes upon differentiation to macrophages. Journal of immunology (Baltimore, Md. : 1950), 167(1), 30–35. https://doi.org/10.4049/jimmunol.167.1.30

[490] Beck-Nielsen, H., Pedersen, O., & Lindskov, H. O. (1980). Impaired cellular insulin binding and insulin sensitivity induced by high-fructose feeding in normal subjects. The American journal of clinical nutrition, 33(2), 273–278. https://doi.org/10.1093/ajcn/33.2.273

[491] Stanhope, K. L., Schwarz, J. M., Keim, N. L., Griffen, S. C., Bremer, A. A., Graham, J. L., Hatcher, B., Cox, C. L., Dyachenko, A., Zhang, W., McGahan, J. P., Seibert, A., Krauss, R. M., Chiu, S., Schaefer, E. J., Ai, M., Otokozawa, S., Nakajima, K., Nakano, T., Beysen, C., ... Havel, P. J. (2009). Consuming fructose-sweetened, not glucose-sweetened, beverages increases visceral adiposity and lipids and decreases insulin sensitivity in overweight/obese humans. The Journal of clinical investigation, 119(5), 1322–1334. https://doi.org/10.1172/JCI37385

[492] Glushakova, O., Kosugi, T., Roncal, C., Mu, W., Heinig, M., Cirillo, P., Sánchez-Lozada, L. G., Johnson, R. J., & Nakagawa, T. (2008). Fructose induces the inflammatory molecule ICAM-1 in endothelial cells. Journal of the American Society of Nephrology : JASN, 19(9), 1712–1720. https://doi.org/10.1681/ASN.2007121304

[493] Basciano, H., Federico, L., & Adeli, K. (2005). Fructose, insulin resistance, and metabolic dyslipidemia. Nutrition & metabolism, 2(1), 5. https://doi.org/10.1186/1743-7075-2-5

[494] DiNicolantonio, J. J., Mehta, V., Onkaramurthy, N., & O'Keefe, J. H. (2018). Fructose-induced inflammation and increased cortisol: A new mechanism for how sugar induces visceral adiposity. Progress in cardiovascular diseases, 61(1), 3–9. https://doi.org/10.1016/j.pcad.2017.12.001

[495] London, E., & Castonguay, T. W. (2011). High fructose diets increase 11β-hydroxysteroid dehydrogenase type 1 in liver and visceral adipose in rats within 24-h exposure. Obesity (Silver Spring, Md.), 19(5), 925–932. https://doi.org/10.1038/oby.2010.284

[496] Vasiljević, A., Bursać, B., Djordjevic, A., Milutinović, D. V., Nikolić, M., Matić, G., & Veličković, N. (2014). Hepatic inflammation induced by high-fructose diet is associated with altered 11βHSD1 expression in the liver of Wistar rats. European journal of nutrition, 53(6), 1393–1402. https://doi.org/10.1007/s00394-013-0641-4

[497] Snel, M., Jonker, J. T., Schoones, J., Lamb, H., de Roos, A., Pijl, H., Smit, J. W., Meinders, A. E., & Jazet, I. M. (2012). Ectopic fat and insulin resistance: pathophysiology and effect of diet and lifestyle interventions. International journal of endocrinology, 2012, 983814. https://doi.org/10.1155/2012/983814

[498] Dekker, M. J., Su, Q., Baker, C., Rutledge, A. C., & Adeli, K. (2010). Fructose: a highly lipogenic nutrient implicated in insulin resistance, hepatic steatosis, and the metabolic syndrome. American Journal of Physiology-Endocrinology and Metabolism, 299(5), E685–E694. https://doi.org/10.1152/ajpendo.00283.2010

[499] Rizkalla S. W. (2010). Health implications of fructose consumption: A review of recent data. Nutrition & metabolism, 7, 82. https://doi.org/10.1186/1743-7075-7-82

[500] Morino, K., Petersen, K. F., & Shulman, G. I. (2006). Molecular mechanisms of insulin resistance in humans and their potential links with mitochondrial dysfunction. Diabetes, 55 Suppl 2(Suppl 2), S9–S15. https://doi.org/10.2337/db06-S002

[501] White J. S. (2013). Challenging the fructose hypothesis: new perspectives on fructose consumption and metabolism. Advances in nutrition (Bethesda, Md.), 4(2), 246–256. https://doi.org/10.3945/an.112.003137

[502] Marriott, B. P., Cole, N., & Lee, E. (2009). National estimates of dietary fructose intake increased from 1977 to 2004 in the United States. The Journal of nutrition, 139(6), 1228S–1235S. https://doi.org/10.3945/jn.108.098277

[503] Bernadette P. Marriott, Lauren Olsho, Louise Hadden & Patty Connor (2010) Intake of Added Sugars and Selected Nutrients in the United States, National Health and Nutrition Examination Survey (NHANES) 2003—2006, Critical Reviews in Food Science and Nutrition, 50:3, 228-258, DOI: 10.1080/10408391003626223

[504] Walker, R. W., Dumke, K. A., & Goran, M. I. (2014). Fructose content in popular beverages made with and without high-fructose corn syrup. Nutrition, 30(7–8), 928–935. https://doi.org/10.1016/j.nut.2014.04.003

[505] Ventura, E. E., Davis, J. N., & Goran, M. I. (2011). Sugar Content of Popular Sweetened Beverages Based on Objective Laboratory Analysis: Focus on Fructose Content. Obesity, 19(4), 868–874. Portico. https://doi.org/10.1038/oby.2010.255

[506] Michael I. Goran, Stanley J. Ulijaszek & Emily E. Ventura (2013) High fructose corn syrup and diabetes prevalence: A global perspective, Global Public Health, 8:1, 55-64, DOI: 10.1080/17441692.2012.736257

[507] Nour, M., Lutze, S. A., Grech, A., & Allman-Farinelli, M. (2018). The Relationship between Vegetable Intake and Weight Outcomes: A Systematic Review of Cohort Studies. Nutrients, 10(11), 1626. https://doi.org/10.3390/nu10111626

[508] Ledoux, T. A., Hingle, M. D., & Baranowski, T. (2011). Relationship of fruit and vegetable intake with adiposity: a systematic review. Obesity reviews : an official journal of the International Association for the Study of Obesity, 12(5), e143–e150. https://doi.org/10.1111/j.1467-789X.2010.00786.x

[509] Basciano et al (2005). Fructose, insulin resistance, and metabolic dyslipidemia. Nutrition & metabolism, 2(1), 5.

[510] USDA (2021) 'Sugar & Sweeteners', Background, Accessed Online: Feb 21st 2023: https://www.ers.usda.gov/topics/crops/sugar-and-sweeteners/background/

[511] Hanover et al (1993). Manufacturing, composition, and applications of fructose. The American journal of clinical nutrition, 58(5 Suppl), 724S–732S.

[512] Goran et al (2013). High fructose corn syrup and diabetes prevalence: a global perspective. Global public health, 8(1), 55–64.

[513] Engber (2009) 'Dark Sugar: The decline and fall of high-fructose corn syrup', Accessed Online Feb 21 2023: https://slate.com/technology/2009/04/the-decline-and-fall-of-high-fructose-corn-syrup.html

[514] Bray, 2004 & U.S. Department of Agriculture, Economic Research Service, Sugar and Sweetener Yearbook series, Tables 50–52

[515] Everstine et al (2013). Economically motivated adulteration (EMA) of food: common characteristics of EMA incidents. Journal of food protection, 76(4), 723–735.

[516] White, J. S. (2008). Straight talk about high-fructose corn syrup: what it is and what it ain't. The American Journal of Clinical Nutrition, 88(6), 1716S-1721S.

[517] USDA (2021) 'Sugar & Sweeteners', Background, Accessed Online: Feb 21st 2023: https://www.ers.usda.gov/topics/crops/sugar-and-sweeteners/background/

[518] Daniels (1984) 'COKE, PEPSI TO USE MORE CORN SYRUP', The New York Times, Accessed Online Feb 21st 2023: https://www.nytimes.com/1984/11/07/business/coke-pepsi-to-use-more-corn-syrup.html

[519] USDA (2022) 'Difference in availability of refined sugars and corn sweeteners grew over the last 10 years', Accessed Online Feb 21st 2023: https://www.ers.usda.gov/data-products/chart-gallery/gallery/chart-detail/?chartId=58332

[520] Chung et al (2014). Fructose, high-fructose corn syrup, sucrose, and nonalcoholic fatty liver disease or indexes of liver health: a systematic review and meta-analysis. The American journal of clinical nutrition, 100(3), 833–849.

[521] Fattore, E., Botta, F., & Bosetti, C. (2021). Effect of fructose instead of glucose or sucrose on cardiometabolic markers: a systematic review and meta-analysis of isoenergetic intervention trials. Nutrition reviews, 79(2), 209–226.

[522] Stanhope et al (2009). Consuming fructose-sweetened, not glucose-sweetened, beverages increases visceral adiposity and lipids and decreases insulin sensitivity in overweight/obese humans. The Journal of clinical investigation, 119(5), 1322–1334.

[523] Reiser et al (1980). Effect of isocaloric exchange of dietary starch and sucrose in humans on the gastric inhibitory polypeptide response to a sucrose load. The American journal of clinical nutrition, 33(9), 1907–1911.

[524] Reiser et al (1979). Isocaloric exchange of dietary starch and sucrose in humans. II. Effect on fasting blood insulin, glucose, and glucagon and on insulin and glucose response to a sucrose load. The American journal of clinical nutrition, 32(11), 2206–2216.

[525] KARLAMANGLA (2016) 'Doctors' message to Asian Americans: Watch out for diabetes even if you're young and thin', LA Times, Accessed Online Feb 21st 2023: https://www.latimes.com/health/la-me-asian-americans-diabetes-20160419-story.html

[526] CDC (2022) 'Diabetes and Asian American People', Accessed Online Feb 21st 2023: https://www.cdc.gov/diabetes/library/spotlights/diabetes-asian-americans.html

[527] Menke et al (2015). Prevalence of and Trends in Diabetes Among Adults in the United States, 1988-2012. JAMA, 314(10), 1021.

[528] Yi et al (2015). Weighing in on the hidden Asian American obesity epidemic. Preventive medicine, 73, 6–9.

[529] Miller (2016) 'Asians and Obesity: Looks Can Be Deceiving', U.S. News, Accessed Online Feb 21st 2023: https://health.usnews.com/wellness/articles/2016-03-11/asians-and-obesity-looks-can-be-deceiving

[530] Wild et al (2004). "Global prevalence of diabetes: estimates for the year 2000 and projections for 2030". Diabetes Care. 27 (5): 1047–1053.

[531] Taylor, R., & Holman, R. R. (2015). Normal weight individuals who develop type 2 diabetes: the personal fat threshold. Clinical science (London, England : 1979), 128(7), 405–410. https://doi.org/10.1042/CS20140553

[532] Virtue, S., & Vidal-Puig, A. (2010). Adipose tissue expandability, lipotoxicity and the Metabolic Syndrome--an allostatic perspective. Biochimica et biophysica acta, 1801(3), 338–349. https://doi.org/10.1016/j.bbalip.2009.12.006

[533] Rochlani, Y., Pothineni, N. V., Kovelamudi, S., & Mehta, J. L. (2017). Metabolic syndrome: pathophysiology, management, and modulation by natural compounds. Therapeutic Advances in Cardiovascular Disease, 11(8), 215–225. doi:10.1177/1753944717711379

[534] Falkner, B., & Cossrow, N. D. (2014). Prevalence of metabolic syndrome and obesity-associated hypertension in the racial ethnic minorities of the United States. Current hypertension reports, 16(7), 449.

[535] Grundy, S. M., Hansen, B., Smith, S. C., Cleeman, J. I., & Kahn, R. A. (2004). Clinical Management of Metabolic Syndrome. Arteriosclerosis, Thrombosis, and Vascular Biology, 24(2). doi:10.1161/01.atv.0000112379.88385.67

[536] Mottillo, S., Filion, K. B., Genest, J., Joseph, L., Pilote, L., Poirier, P., ... Eisenberg, M. J. (2010). The Metabolic Syndrome and Cardiovascular Risk. Journal of the American College of Cardiology, 56(14), 1113–1132. doi:10.1016/j.jacc.2010.05.034

[537] Price et al (August 2006). "Weight, shape, and mortality risk in older persons: elevated waist-hip ratio, not high body mass index, is associated with a greater risk of death". Am. J. Clin. Nutr. 84 (2): 449–60.

[538] Edwardson et al (2012). Association of sedentary behaviour with metabolic syndrome: a meta-analysis. PloS one, 7(4), e34916.

[539] Sun et al (2014). Alcohol consumption and risk of metabolic syndrome: a meta-analysis of prospective studies. Clinical nutrition (Edinburgh, Scotland), 33(4), 596–602.

[540] He et al (2014). Association between leisure time physical activity and metabolic syndrome: a meta-analysis of prospective cohort studies. Endocrine, 46(2), 231–240.

[541] Bremer et al (2012). Toward a unifying hypothesis of metabolic syndrome. Pediatrics, 129(3), 557–570.

[542] Malik et al (2010). Sugar-sweetened beverages and risk of metabolic syndrome and type 2 diabetes: a meta-analysis. Diabetes care, 33(11), 2477–2483.

[543] Merlotti, C., Ceriani, V., Morabito, A., & Pontiroli, A. E. (2017). Subcutaneous fat loss is greater than visceral fat loss with diet and exercise, weight-loss promoting drugs and bariatric surgery: a critical review and meta-analysis. International journal of obesity (2005), 41(5), 672–682. https://doi.org/10.1038/ijo.2017.31

[544] Hu, F. B., & Malik, V. S. (2010). Sugar-sweetened beverages and risk of obesity and type 2 diabetes: epidemiologic evidence. Physiology & behavior, 100(1), 47–54. https://doi.org/10.1016/j.physbeh.2010.01.036

[545] Stanhope, K. L., Schwarz, J. M., Keim, N. L., Griffen, S. C., Bremer, A. A., Graham, J. L., Hatcher, B., Cox, C. L., Dyachenko, A., Zhang, W., McGahan, J. P., Seibert, A., Krauss, R. M., Chiu, S., Schaefer, E. J., Ai, M., Otokozawa, S., Nakajima, K., Nakano, T., Beysen, C., ... Havel, P. J. (2009). Consuming fructose-sweetened, not glucose-sweetened, beverages increases visceral adiposity and lipids and decreases insulin sensitivity in overweight/obese humans. The Journal of clinical investigation, 119(5), 1322–1334. https://doi.org/10.1172/JCI37385

[546] Ma, J., Sloan, M., Fox, C. S., Hoffmann, U., Smith, C. E., Saltzman, E., Rogers, G. T., Jacques, P. F., & McKeown, N. M. (2014). Sugar-sweetened beverage consumption is associated with abdominal fat partitioning in healthy adults. The Journal of nutrition, 144(8), 1283–1290. https://doi.org/10.3945/jn.113.188599

[547] Stanhope, K. L., Griffen, S. C., Bair, B. R., Swarbrick, M. M., Keim, N. L., & Havel, P. J. (2008). Twenty-four-hour endocrine and metabolic profiles following consumption of high-fructose corn syrup-, sucrose-, fructose-, and glucose-sweetened beverages with meals. The American journal of clinical nutrition, 87(5), 1194–1203. https://doi.org/10.1093/ajcn/87.5.1194

[548] Stanhope, K. L., & Havel, P. J. (2008). Endocrine and metabolic effects of consuming beverages sweetened with fructose, glucose, sucrose, or high-fructose corn syrup. The American journal of clinical nutrition, 88(6), 1733S–1737S. https://doi.org/10.3945/ajcn.2008.25825D

[549] Schwarz, J. M., Noworolski, S. M., Erkin-Cakmak, A., Korn, N. J., Wen, M. J., Tai, V. W., Jones, G. M., Palii, S. P., Velasco-Alin, M., Pan, K., Patterson, B. W., Gugliucci, A., Lustig, R. H., & Mulligan, K. (2017). Effects of Dietary Fructose Restriction on Liver Fat, De Novo Lipogenesis, and Insulin Kinetics in Children With Obesity. Gastroenterology, 153(3), 743–752. https://doi.org/10.1053/j.gastro.2017.05.043

[550] Jensen et al (2018). Fructose and sugar: A major mediator of non-alcoholic fatty liver disease. Journal of hepatology, 68(5), 1063–1075.

[551] Bendsen, N. T., Christensen, R., Bartels, E. M., Kok, F. J., Sierksma, A., Raben, A., & Astrup, A. (2013). Is beer consumption related to measures of abdominal and general obesity? A systematic review and meta-analysis. Nutrition reviews, 71(2), 67–87. https://doi.org/10.1111/j.1753-4887.2012.00548.x

[552] Dorn et al (2003) 'Alcohol Drinking Patterns Differentially Affect Central Adiposity as Measured by Abdominal Height in Women and Men', The Journal of Nutrition, Volume 133, Issue 8, August 2003, Pages 2655–2662, https://doi.org/10.1093/jn/133.8.2655

[553] Kim, K. H., Oh, S. W., Kwon, H., Park, J. H., Choi, H., & Cho, B. (2012). Alcohol consumption and its relation to visceral and subcutaneous adipose tissues in healthy male Koreans. Annals of nutrition & metabolism, 60(1), 52–61. https://doi.org/10.1159/000334710

[554] Cigolini, M., Targher, G., Bergamo Andreis, I. A., Tonoli, M., Filippi, F., Muggeo, M., & De Sandre, G. (1996). Moderate alcohol consumption and its relation to visceral fat and plasma androgens in healthy women. International journal of obesity and related metabolic disorders : journal of the International Association for the Study of Obesity, 20(3), 206–212.

[555] Dorn et al (2003) 'Alcohol Drinking Patterns Differentially Affect Central Adiposity as Measured by Abdominal Height in Women and Men', The Journal of Nutrition, Volume 133, Issue 8, August 2003, Pages 2655–2662.

[556] de Souze et al (2015) 'Intake of saturated and trans unsaturated fatty acids and risk of all cause mortality, cardiovascular disease, and type 2 diabetes: systematic review and meta-analysis of observational studies', BMJ 2015; 351 doi: https://doi.org/10.1136/bmj.h3978

[557] Mozaffarian, D., Aro, A., & Willett, W. C. (2009). Health effects of trans-fatty acids: experimental and observational evidence. European journal of clinical nutrition, 63 Suppl 2, S5–S21. https://doi.org/10.1038/sj.ejcn.1602973

[558] Kavanagh, K., Jones, K. L., Sawyer, J., Kelley, K., Carr, J. J., Wagner, J. D., & Rudel, L. L. (2007). Trans fat diet induces abdominal obesity and changes in insulin sensitivity in monkeys. Obesity (Silver Spring, Md.), 15(7), 1675–1684. https://doi.org/10.1038/oby.2007.200

[559] US FDA, Trans Fat, Accessed 2018: https://www.fda.gov/food/ucm292278.htm

[560] Verheggen, R. J., Maessen, M. F., Green, D. J., Hermus, A. R., Hopman, M. T., & Thijssen, D. H. (2016). A systematic review and meta-analysis on the effects of exercise training versus hypocaloric diet: distinct effects on body weight and visceral adipose tissue. Obesity reviews : an official journal of the International Association for the Study of Obesity, 17(8), 664–690. https://doi.org/10.1111/obr.12406

[561] Ohkawara, K., Tanaka, S., Miyachi, M., Ishikawa-Takata, K., & Tabata, I. (2007). A dose-response relation between aerobic exercise and visceral fat reduction: systematic review of clinical trials. International journal of obesity (2005), 31(12), 1786–1797. https://doi.org/10.1038/sj.ijo.0803683

[562] Ross, R., & Rissanen, J. (1994). Mobilization of visceral and subcutaneous adipose tissue in response to energy restriction and exercise. The American journal of clinical nutrition, 60(5), 695–703. https://doi.org/10.1093/ajcn/60.5.695

[563] Khalafi, M., Malandish, A., Rosenkranz, S. K., & Ravasi, A. A. (2021). Effect of resistance training with and without caloric restriction on visceral fat: A systemic review and meta-analysis. Obesity reviews : an official journal of the International Association for the Study of Obesity, 22(9), e13275. https://doi.org/10.1111/obr.13275

[564] Hejnová, J., Majercík, M., Polák, J., Richterová, B., Crampes, F., deGlisezinski, I., & Stich, V. (2004). Vliv silove-dynamického tréninku na inzulínovou senzitivitu u inzulínorezistentních mužů [Effect of dynamic strength training on insulin sensitivity in men with insulin resistance]. Casopis lekaru ceskych, 143(11), 762–765.

[565] Coker, R. H., Williams, R. H., Kortebein, P. M., Sullivan, D. H., & Evans, W. J. (2009). Influence of exercise intensity on abdominal fat and adiponectin in elderly adults. Metabolic syndrome and related disorders, 7(4), 363–368. https://doi.org/10.1089/met.2008.0060

[566] Irving, B. A., Davis, C. K., Brock, D. W., Weltman, J. Y., Swift, D., Barrett, E. J., Gaesser, G. A., & Weltman, A. (2008). Effect of exercise training intensity on abdominal visceral fat and body composition. Medicine and science in sports and exercise, 40(11), 1863–1872. https://doi.org/10.1249/MSS.0b013e3181801d40

[567] Vissers, D., Hens, W., Taeymans, J., Baeyens, J. P., Poortmans, J., & Van Gaal, L. (2013). The effect of exercise on visceral adipose tissue in overweight adults: a systematic review and meta-analysis. PloS one, 8(2), e56415. https://doi.org/10.1371/journal.pone.0056415

[568] Thomas, E. L., Brynes, A. E., McCarthy, J., Goldstone, A. P., Hajnal, J. V., Saeed, N., Frost, G., & Bell, J. D. (2000). Preferential loss of visceral fat following aerobic exercise, measured by magnetic resonance imaging. Lipids, 35(7), 769–776. https://doi.org/10.1007/s11745-000-0584-0

[569] Ismail, I., Keating, S. E., Baker, M. K., & Johnson, N. A. (2012). A systematic review and meta-analysis of the effect of aerobic vs. resistance exercise training on visceral fat. Obesity reviews : an official journal of the International Association for the Study of Obesity, 13(1), 68–91. https://doi.org/10.1111/j.1467-789X.2011.00931.x

[570] Patel, S. R., Malhotra, A., White, D. P., Gottlieb, D. J., & Hu, F. B. (2006). Association between reduced sleep and weight gain in women. American journal of epidemiology, 164(10), 947–954. https://doi.org/10.1093/aje/kwj280

[571] Hairston, K. G., Bryer-Ash, M., Norris, J. M., Haffner, S., Bowden, D. W., & Wagenknecht, L. E. (2010). Sleep duration and five-year abdominal fat accumulation in a minority cohort: the IRAS family study. Sleep, 33(3), 289–295. https://doi.org/10.1093/sleep/33.3.289

[572] Beccuti, G., & Pannain, S. (2011). Sleep and obesity. Current opinion in clinical nutrition and metabolic care, 14(4), 402–412. https://doi.org/10.1097/MCO.0b013e3283479109

[573] Theorell-Haglöw, J., Berne, C., Janson, C., Sahlin, C., & Lindberg, E. (2010). Associations between short sleep duration and central obesity in women. Sleep, 33(5), 593–598.

[574] Pillar and Shehadeh (2008) 'Abdominal Fat and Sleep Apnea: The chicken or the egg?', Diabetes Care 2008;31(Supplement_2):S303–S309.

[575] Toyama, Y., Tanizawa, K., Kubo, T., Chihara, Y., Harada, Y., Murase, K., Azuma, M., Hamada, S., Hitomi, T., Handa, T., Oga, T., Chiba, T., Mishima, M., & Chin, K. (2015). Impact of Obstructive Sleep Apnea on Liver Fat Accumulation According to Sex and Visceral Obesity. PLOS ONE, 10(6), e0129513. https://doi.org/10.1371/journal.pone.0129513

[576] Kim, N. H., Lee, S. K., Eun, C. R., Seo, J. A., Kim, S. G., Choi, K. M., Baik, S. H., Choi, D. S., Yun, C. H., Kim, N. H., & Shin, C. (2013). Short sleep duration combined with obstructive sleep apnea is associated with visceral obesity in Korean adults. Sleep, 36(5), 723–729. https://doi.org/10.5665/sleep.2636

[577] Chaput, J. P., Bouchard, C., & Tremblay, A. (2014). Change in sleep duration and visceral fat accumulation over 6 years in adults. Obesity (Silver Spring, Md.), 22(5), E9–E12. https://doi.org/10.1002/oby.20701

[578] Broussard JL, Ehrmann DA, Van Cauter E, Tasali E, Brady MJ. Impaired Insulin Signaling in Human Adipocytes After Experimental Sleep Restriction: A Randomized, Crossover Study. Ann Intern Med. 2012;157:549–557. doi: 10.7326/0003-4819-157-8-201210160-00005

[579] Jones (2013) 'In U.S., 40% Get Less Than Recommended Amount of Sleep', Gallup, WELL-BEING, DECEMBER 19, 2013, Accessed Online: https://news.gallup.com/poll/166553/less-recommended-amount-sleep.aspx

[580] Mattson, M. P., Longo, V. D., & Harvie, M. (2017). Impact of intermittent fasting on health and disease processes. Ageing Research Reviews, 39, 46–58. https://doi.org/10.1016/j.arr.2016.10.005

[581] Arnason, T. G., Bowen, M. W., & Mansell, K. D. (2017). Effects of intermittent fasting on health markers in those with type 2 diabetes: A pilot study. World journal of diabetes, 8(4), 154–164. https://doi.org/10.4239/wjd.v8.i4.154

[582] Barnosky, A. R., Hoddy, K. K., Unterman, T. G., & Varady, K. A. (2014). Intermittent fasting vs daily calorie restriction for type 2 diabetes prevention: a review of human findings. Translational Research, 164(4), 302–311. https://doi.org/10.1016/j.trsl.2014.05.013

[583] Volek, J., Sharman, M., Gómez, A., Judelson, D., Rubin, M., Watson, G., Sokmen, B., Silvestre, R., French, D., & Kraemer, W. (2004). Comparison of energy-restricted very low-carbohydrate and low-fat diets on weight loss and body composition in overweight men and women. Nutrition & metabolism, 1(1), 13. https://doi.org/10.1186/1743-7075-1-13

[584] Gower, B. A., & Goss, A. M. (2015). A lower-carbohydrate, higher-fat diet reduces abdominal and intermuscular fat and increases insulin sensitivity in adults at risk of type 2 diabetes. The Journal of nutrition, 145(1), 177S–83S. https://doi.org/10.3945/jn.114.195065

[585] Sasakabe, T., Haimoto, H., Umegaki, H., & Wakai, K. (2015). Association of decrease in carbohydrate intake with reduction in abdominal fat during 3-month moderate low-carbohydrate diet among non-obese Japanese patients with type 2 diabetes. Metabolism: clinical and experimental, 64(5), 618–625. https://doi.org/10.1016/j.metabol.2015.01.012

[586] Goss, A. M., Goree, L. L., Ellis, A. C., Chandler-Laney, P. C., Casazza, K., Lockhart, M. E., & Gower, B. A. (2013). Effects of diet macronutrient composition on body composition and fat distribution during weight maintenance and weight loss. Obesity (Silver Spring, Md.), 21(6), 1139–1142. https://doi.org/10.1002/oby.20191

587 Hall, K. D., Guyenet, S. J., & Leibel, R. L. (2018). The Carbohydrate-Insulin Model of Obesity Is Difficult to Reconcile With Current Evidence. JAMA internal medicine, 178(8), 1103–1105. https://doi.org/10.1001/jamainternmed.2018.2920

588 Gardner, C. D., Trepanowski, J. F., Del Gobbo, L. C., Hauser, M. E., Rigdon, J., Ioannidis, J. P. A., ... King, A. C. (2018). Effect of Low-Fat vs Low-Carbohydrate Diet on 12-Month Weight Loss in Overweight Adults and the Association With Genotype Pattern or Insulin Secretion. JAMA, 319(7), 667. doi:10.1001/jama.2018.0245

589 Schoeller, D. A., & Buchholz, A. C. (2005). Energetics of obesity and weight control: does diet composition matter?. Journal of the American Dietetic Association, 105(5 Suppl 1), S24–S28. https://doi.org/10.1016/j.jada.2005.02.025

590 Howell, S., & Kones, R. (2017). "Calories in, calories out" and macronutrient intake: the hope, hype, and science of calories. American journal of physiology. Endocrinology and metabolism, 313(5), E608–E612. https://doi.org/10.1152/ajpendo.00156.2017

591 Nordmann, A. J., Nordmann, A., Briel, M., Keller, U., Yancy, W. S., Jr, Brehm, B. J., & Bucher, H. C. (2006). Effects of low-carbohydrate vs low-fat diets on weight loss and cardiovascular risk factors: a meta-analysis of randomized controlled trials. Archives of internal medicine, 166(3), 285–293. https://doi.org/10.1001/archinte.166.3.285

592 Manninen A. H. (2004). Is a calorie really a calorie? Metabolic advantage of low-carbohydrate diets. Journal of the International Society of Sports Nutrition, 1(2), 21–26. https://doi.org/10.1186/1550-2783-1-2-21

593 Brehm, B. J., Spang, S. E., Lattin, B. L., Seeley, R. J., Daniels, S. R., & D'Alessio, D. A. (2005). The role of energy expenditure in the differential weight loss in obese women on low-fat and low-carbohydrate diets. The Journal of clinical endocrinology and metabolism, 90(3), 1475–1482. https://doi.org/10.1210/jc.2004-1540

594 Hendrickson, S., & Mattes, R. (2007). Financial incentive for diet recall accuracy does not affect reported energy intake or number of underreporters in a sample of overweight females. Journal of the American Dietetic Association, 107(1), 118–121. https://doi.org/10.1016/j.jada.2006.10.003

595 Champagne, C. M., Bray, G. A., Kurtz, A. A., Monteiro, J. B., Tucker, E., Volaufova, J., & Delany, J. P. (2002). Energy intake and energy expenditure: a controlled study comparing dietitians and non-dietitians. Journal of the American Dietetic Association, 102(10), 1428–1432. https://doi.org/10.1016/s0002-8223(02)90316-0

596 Schoeller, D. A., Thomas, D., Archer, E., Heymsfield, S. B., Blair, S. N., Goran, M. I., Hill, J. O., Atkinson, R. L., Corkey, B. E., Foreyt, J., Dhurandhar, N. V., Kral, J. G., Hall, K. D., Hansen, B. C., Heitmann, B. L., Ravussin, E., & Allison, D. B. (2013). Self-report-based estimates of energy intake offer an inadequate basis for scientific conclusions. The American journal of clinical nutrition, 97(6), 1413–1415. https://doi.org/10.3945/ajcn.113.062125

597 Layman, D. K., Boileau, R. A., Erickson, D. J., Painter, J. E., Shiue, H., Sather, C., & Christou, D. D. (2003). A reduced ratio of dietary carbohydrate to protein improves body composition and blood lipid profiles during weight loss in adult women. The Journal of nutrition, 133(2), 411–417. https://doi.org/10.1093/jn/133.2.411

[598] Hairston, K. G., Vitolins, M. Z., Norris, J. M., Anderson, A. M., Hanley, A. J., & Wagenknecht, L. E. (2012). Lifestyle factors and 5-year abdominal fat accumulation in a minority cohort: the IRAS Family Study. Obesity (Silver Spring, Md.), 20(2), 421–427. https://doi.org/10.1038/oby.2011.171

599 Wanders, A. J., van den Borne, J. J., de Graaf, C., Hulshof, T., Jonathan, M. C., Kristensen, M., Mars, M., Schols, H. A., & Feskens, E. J. (2011). Effects of dietary fibre on subjective appetite, energy intake and body weight: a systematic review of randomized controlled trials. Obesity reviews : an official journal of the International Association for the Study of Obesity, 12(9), 724–739. https://doi.org/10.1111/j.1467-789X.2011.00895.x

600 Clark, M. J., & Slavin, J. L. (2013). The effect of fiber on satiety and food intake: a systematic review. Journal of the American College of Nutrition, 32(3), 200–211. https://doi.org/10.1080/07315724.2013.791194

601 Burton-Freeman B. (2000). Dietary fiber and energy regulation. The Journal of nutrition, 130(2S Suppl), 272S–275S. https://doi.org/10.1093/jn/130.2.272S

[602] Morrison, D. J., & Preston, T. (2016). Formation of short chain fatty acids by the gut microbiota and their impact on human metabolism. Gut microbes, 7(3), 189–200. https://doi.org/10.1080/19490976.2015.1134082

[603] Byrne, C. S., Chambers, E. S., Morrison, D. J., & Frost, G. (2015). The role of short chain fatty acids in appetite regulation and energy homeostasis. International journal of obesity (2005), 39(9), 1331–1338. https://doi.org/10.1038/ijo.2015.84

[604] Tolhurst, G., Heffron, H., Lam, Y. S., Parker, H. E., Habib, A. M., Diakogiannaki, E., Cameron, J., Grosse, J., Reimann, F., & Gribble, F. M. (2012). Short-chain fatty acids stimulate glucagon-like peptide-1 secretion via the G-protein-coupled receptor FFAR2. Diabetes, 61(2), 364–371. https://doi.org/10.2337/db11-1019

605 Kristensen, M., Jensen, M. G., Aarestrup, J., Petersen, K. E., Søndergaard, L., Mikkelsen, M. S., & Astrup, A. (2012). Flaxseed dietary fibers lower cholesterol and increase fecal fat excretion, but magnitude of effect depend on food type. Nutrition & metabolism, 9, 8. https://doi.org/10.1186/1743-7075-9-8

606 Uebelhack, R., Busch, R., Alt, F., Beah, Z. M., & Chong, P. W. (2014). Effects of cactus fiber on the excretion of dietary fat in healthy subjects: a double blind, randomized, placebo-controlled, crossover clinical investigation. Current therapeutic research, clinical and experimental, 76, 39–44. https://doi.org/10.1016/j.curtheres.2014.02.001

[607] Ogawa, A., Kobayashi, T., Sakai, F., Kadooka, Y., & Kawasaki, Y. (2015). Lactobacillus gasseri SBT2055 suppresses fatty acid release through enlargement of fat emulsion size in vitro and promotes fecal fat excretion in healthy Japanese subjects. Lipids in health and disease, 14, 20. https://doi.org/10.1186/s12944-015-0019-0

[608] Kadooka, Y., Sato, M., Imaizumi, K., Ogawa, A., Ikuyama, K., Akai, Y., Okano, M., Kagoshima, M., & Tsuchida, T. (2010). Regulation of abdominal adiposity by probiotics (Lactobacillus gasseri SBT2055) in adults with obese tendencies in a randomized controlled trial. European journal of clinical nutrition, 64(6), 636–643. https://doi.org/10.1038/ejcn.2010.19

[609] Kadooka, Y., Sato, M., Ogawa, A., Miyoshi, M., Uenishi, H., Ogawa, H., Ikuyama, K., Kagoshima, M., & Tsuchida, T. (2013). Effect of Lactobacillus gasseri SBT2055 in fermented milk on abdominal adiposity in adults in a randomised controlled trial. The British journal of nutrition, 110(9), 1696–1703. https://doi.org/10.1017/S0007114513001037

[610] Pasiakos, S. M., Lieberman, H. R., & Fulgoni, V. L., 3rd (2015). Higher-protein diets are associated with higher HDL cholesterol and lower BMI and waist circumference in US adults. The Journal of nutrition, 145(3), 605–614. https://doi.org/10.3945/jn.114.205203

[611] Loenneke, J.P., Wilson, J.M., Manninen, A.H. et al. Quality protein intake is inversely related with abdominal fat. Nutr Metab (Lond) 9, 5 (2012). https://doi.org/10.1186/1743-7075-9-5

[612] Belko, A. Z., Barbieri, T. F., & Wong, E. C. (1986). Effect of energy and protein intake and exercise intensity on the thermic effect of food. The American journal of clinical nutrition, 43(6), 863–869. https://doi.org/10.1093/ajcn/43.6.863

[613] Fukagawa, N. K., Bandini, L. G., Lim, P. H., Roingeard, F., Lee, M. A., & Young, J. B. (1991). Protein-induced changes in energy expenditure in young and old individuals. The American journal of physiology, 260(3 Pt 1), E345–E352. https://doi.org/10.1152/ajpendo.1991.260.3.E345

[614] Shimabukuro et al (1998). Fatty acid-induced beta cell apoptosis: a link between obesity and diabetes. Proceedings of the National Academy of Sciences of the United States of America, 95(5), 2498–2502.

[615] Maedler et al (2001). Distinct effects of saturated and monounsaturated fatty acids on beta-cell turnover and function. Diabetes, 50(1), 69–76.

[616] Unger R. H. (1995). Lipotoxicity in the pathogenesis of obesity-dependent NIDDM. Genetic and clinical implications. Diabetes, 44(8), 863–870.

[617] McGarry JD: Dysregulation of fatty acid metabolism in the etiology of type 2 diabetes. Diabetes 51:7–18,2002

[618] Boden G. (1997). Role of fatty acids in the pathogenesis of insulin resistance and NIDDM. Diabetes, 46(1), 3–10.

[619] Grill*, V., & Björklund, A. (2000). Dysfunctional insulin secretion in type 2 diabetes: role of metabolic abnormalities. Cellular and Molecular Life Sciences, 57(3), 429–440.

[620] Lewis et al (2002) 'Disordered Fat Storage and Mobilization in the Pathogenesis of Insulin Resistance and Type 2 Diabetes', Endocrine Reviews, Volume 23, Issue 2, 1 April 2002, Pages 201–229.

[621] Paolisso et al (1995). A high concentration of fasting plasma non-esterified fatty acids is a risk factor for the development of NIDDM. Diabetologia, 38(10), 1213–1217.

[622] Charles et al (1997). The role of non-esterified fatty acids in the deterioration of glucose tolerance in Caucasian subjects: results of the Paris Prospective Study. Diabetologia, 40(9), 1101–1106.

[623] Busch et al (2002). Expression profiling of palmitate- and oleate-regulated genes provides novel insights into the effects of chronic lipid exposure on pancreatic beta-cell function. Diabetes, 51(4), 977–987.

[624] Segall et al (1999). Lipid rather than glucose metabolism is implicated in altered insulin secretion caused by oleate in INS-1 cells. The American journal of physiology, 277(3), E521–E528.

[625] Iizuka et al (2002). Metabolic consequence of long-term exposure of pancreatic beta cells to free fatty acid with special reference to glucose insensitivity. Biochimica et biophysica acta, 1586(1), 23–31.

[626] Liang et al (1997). Chronic effect of fatty acids on insulin release is not through the alteration of glucose metabolism in a pancreatic beta-cell line (beta HC9). Diabetologia, 40(9), 1018–1027.

[627] Liu et al (1998). Fatty acid-induced beta cell hypersensitivity to glucose. Increased phosphofructokinase activity and lowered glucose-6-phosphate content. Journal of Clinical Investigation, 101(9), 1870–1875.

[628] Bollheimer et al (1998). Chronic exposure to free fatty acid reduces pancreatic beta cell insulin content by increasing basal insulin secretion that is not compensated for by a corresponding increase in proinsulin biosynthesis translation. The Journal of clinical investigation, 101(5), 1094–1101.

[629] Oh et al (2018). Fatty Acid-Induced Lipotoxicity in Pancreatic Beta-Cells During Development of Type 2 Diabetes. Frontiers in Endocrinology, 9.

[630] Maedler et al (2001). Distinct effects of saturated and monounsaturated fatty acids on beta-cell turnover and function. Diabetes, 50(1), 69–76.

[631] Shimabukuro et al (1998). Fatty acid-induced beta cell apoptosis: a link between obesity and diabetes. Proceedings of the National Academy of Sciences of the United States of America, 95(5), 2498–2502.

[632] Zhou, Y. P., & Grill, V. E. (1994). Long-term exposure of rat pancreatic islets to fatty acids inhibits glucose-induced insulin secretion and biosynthesis through a glucose fatty acid cycle. Journal of Clinical Investigation, 93(2), 870–876.

[633] Liang et al (1997). Chronic effect of fatty acids on insulin release is not through the alteration of glucose metabolism in a pancreatic beta-cell line (beta HC9). Diabetologia, 40(9), 1018–1027.

[634] Eto et al (2002). Genetic manipulations of fatty acid metabolism in beta-cells are associated with dysregulated insulin secretion. Diabetes, 51 Suppl 3, S414–S420.

[635] Schmitz-Peiffer, C. (2000). Signalling aspects of insulin resistance in skeletal muscle: mechanisms induced by lipid oversupply. Cellular signalling, 12 9-10, 583–94 .

[636] Chan et al (2001). Increased uncoupling protein-2 levels in beta-cells are associated with impaired glucose-stimulated insulin secretion: mechanism of action. Diabetes, 50(6), 1302–1310.

[637] Tordjman et al (2002). PPARalpha suppresses insulin secretion and induces UCP2 in insulinoma cells. Journal of lipid research, 43(6), 936–943.

[638] Newsholme et al (2006). Life and death decisions of the pancreatic β-cell: the role of fatty acids. Clinical Science, 112(1), 27–42.

[639] Hagman DK, Hays LB, Parazzoli SD, Poitout V. Palmitate inhibits insulin gene expression by altering PDX-1 nuclear localization and reducing MafA expression in isolated rat islets of Langerhans. J Biol Chem. (2005) 280:32413–8.

[640] Acosta-Montaño et al (2018). Effects of Dietary Fatty Acids in Pancreatic Beta Cell Metabolism, Implications in Homeostasis. Nutrients, 10(4), 393.

[641] Keane et al (2010). Arachidonic acid actions on functional integrity and attenuation of the negative effects of palmitic acid in a clonal pancreatic β-cell line. Clinical Science, 120(5), 195–206.

[642] Baynes et al (2018). The role of polyunsaturated fatty acids (n-3 PUFAs) on the pancreatic β-cells and insulin action. Adipocyte, 1–7.

[643] Weir et al (2020). Associations between omega-6 polyunsaturated fatty acids, hyperinsulinemia and incident diabetes by race/ethnicity: The Multi-Ethnic Study of Atherosclerosis. Clinical Nutrition, 39(10), 3031–3041.

[644] Bowen et al (2016). Omega-3 Fatty Acids and Cardiovascular Disease: Are There Benefits?. Current treatment options in cardiovascular medicine, 18(11), 69.

[645] Kromhout et al (1985). The inverse relation between fish consumption and 20-year mortality from coronary heart disease. The New England journal of medicine, 312(19), 1205–1209. https://doi.org/10.1056/NEJM198505093121901

[646] Oomen et al (2000). Fish consumption and coronary heart disease mortality in Finland, Italy, and The Netherlands. American journal of epidemiology, 151(10), 999–1006. https://doi.org/10.1093/oxfordjournals.aje.a010144

[647] Keli, S. O., Feskens, E. J., & Kromhout, D. (1994). Fish consumption and risk of stroke. The Zutphen Study. Stroke, 25(2), 328–332. https://doi.org/10.1161/01.str.25.2.328

[648] De Lorgeril, M., Salen, P., Defaye, P., & Rabaeus, M. (2013). Recent findings on the health effects of omega-3 fatty acids and statins, and their interactions: do statins inhibit omega-3? BMC Medicine, 11(1). doi:10.1186/1741-7015-11-5

[649] Hooper et al (2006). Risks and benefits of omega 3 fats for mortality, cardiovascular disease, and cancer: systematic review. BMJ (Clinical research ed.), 332(7544), 752–760. https://doi.org/10.1136/bmj.38755.366331.2F

[650] Tavazzi et al (2008). Effect of n-3 polyunsaturated fatty acids in patients with chronic heart failure (the GISSI-HF trial): a randomised, double-blind, placebo-controlled trial. Lancet (London, England), 372(9645), 1223–1230.

[651] Dietary supplementation with n-3 polyunsaturated fatty acids and vitamin E after myocardial infarction: results of the GISSI-Prevenzione trial. Gruppo Italiano per lo Studio della Sopravvivenza nell'Infarto miocardico. (1999). Lancet (London, England), 354(9177), 447–455.

[652] Marchioli et al (2002). Early protection against sudden death by n-3 polyunsaturated fatty acids after myocardial infarction: time-course analysis of the results of the Gruppo Italiano per lo Studio della Sopravvivenza nell'Infarto Miocardico (GISSI)-Prevenzione. Circulation, 105(16), 1897–1903.

[653] Sierra, S., Lara-Villoslada, F., Comalada, M., Olivares, M., & Xaus, J. (2006). Dietary fish oil n−3 fatty acids increase regulatory cytokine production and exert anti-inflammatory effects in two murine models of inflammation. Lipids, 41(12), 1115–1125. doi:10.1007/s11745-006-5061-2

[654] Huang YJ et al (1997) 'Amelioration of insulin resistance and hypertension in a fructose-fed rat model with fish oil supplementation', Metabolism Clinical and Experimental, November 1997Volume 46, Issue 11, Pages 1252–1258.

[655] Hill JO, Peters JC, Lin D, et al. Lipid accumulation and body fat distribution is influenced by type of dietary fat fed to rats. Int J Obes Relat Metab Disord. 1993 Apr;17(4):223-36.

[656] Mazidi et al (2021). Omega-6 fatty acids and the Risk of Cardiovascular Disease: Insights from a Systematic Review and Meta-Analysis of Randomized Controlled Trials and a Mendelian Randomization Study. Archives of Medical Science.

[657] Hooper et al (2018). Omega-6 fats for the primary and secondary prevention of cardiovascular disease. Cochrane Database of Systematic Reviews, 2018(11).

[658] Ramsden et al (2013). Use of dietary linoleic acid for secondary prevention of coronary heart disease and death: evaluation of recovered data from the Sydney Diet Heart Study and updated meta-analysis. BMJ (Clinical research ed.), 346, e8707.

[659] Ramsden et al (2010). n-6 fatty acid-specific and mixed polyunsaturate dietary interventions have different effects on CHD risk: a meta-analysis of randomised controlled trials. The British journal of nutrition, 104(11), 1586–1600.

[660] Ramsden et al (2013). Use of dietary linoleic acid for secondary prevention of coronary heart disease and death: evaluation of recovered data from the Sydney Diet Heart Study and updated meta-analysis. BMJ (Clinical research ed.), 346, e8707.

[661] Marklund et al (2019). Biomarkers of Dietary Omega-6 Fatty Acids and Incident Cardiovascular Disease and Mortality. Circulation, 139(21), 2422–2436.

[662] Wu et al (2017) 'Omega-6 fatty acid biomarkers and incident type 2 diabetes: pooled analysis of individual-level data for 39 740 adults from 20 prospective cohort studies', The Lancet, VOLUME 5, ISSUE 12, P965-974.

[663] Weir et al (2020). Associations between omega-6 polyunsaturated fatty acids, hyperinsulinemia and incident diabetes by race/ethnicity: The Multi-Ethnic Study of Atherosclerosis. Clinical Nutrition, 39(10), 3031–3041.

[664] Hodgson et al (1993). Can linoleic acid contribute to coronary artery disease?. The American journal of clinical nutrition, 58(2), 228–234.

[665] Schwertner, H. A., & Mosser, E. L. (1993). Comparison of lipid fatty acids on a concentration basis vs weight percentage basis in patients with and without coronary artery disease or diabetes. Clinical chemistry, 39(4), 659–663.

[666] DiNicolantonio J. J. (2014). The cardiometabolic consequences of replacing saturated fats with carbohydrates or Ω-6 polyunsaturated fats: Do the dietary guidelines have it wrong?. Open heart, 1(1), e000032.

[667] Weintraub et al (1988). Dietary polyunsaturated fats of the W-6 and W-3 series reduce postprandial lipoprotein levels. Chronic and acute effects of fat saturation on postprandial lipoprotein metabolism. The Journal of clinical investigation, 82(6), 1884–1893.

[668] Gago-Dominguez, M., Jiang, X., & Castelao, J. E. (2007). Lipid peroxidation, oxidative stress genes and dietary factors in breast cancer protection: a hypothesis. Breast cancer research : BCR, 9(1), 201. https://doi.org/10.1186/bcr1628

[669] Kew, S., Banerjee, T., Minihane, A. M., Finnegan, Y. E., Williams, C. M., & Calder, P. C. (2003). Relation between the fatty acid composition of peripheral blood mononuclear cells and measures of immune cell function in healthy, free-living subjects aged 25–72 y. The American Journal of Clinical Nutrition, 77(5), 1278–1286. doi:10.1093/ajcn/77.5.1278

[670] Kanner J. (2007). Dietary advanced lipid oxidation endproducts are risk factors to human health. Molecular nutrition & food research, 51(9), 1094–1101. https://doi.org/10.1002/mnfr.200600303

[671] Colas et al (2010). Increased lipid peroxidation in LDL from type-2 diabetic patients. Lipids, 45(8), 723–731.

[672] Gorelik, S., Ligumsky, M., Kohen, R., & Kanner, J. (2008). The stomach as a "bioreactor": when red meat meets red wine. Journal of agricultural and food chemistry, 56(13), 5002–5007.

[673] Kanner, J., & Lapidot, T. (2001). The stomach as a bioreactor: dietary lipid peroxidation in the gastric fluid and the effects of plant-derived antioxidants. Free radical biology & medicine, 31(11), 1388–1395.

[674] Kanner J. (2007). Dietary advanced lipid oxidation endproducts are risk factors to human health. Molecular nutrition & food research, 51(9), 1094–1101. https://doi.org/10.1002/mnfr.200600303

[675] Aviram, M., & Eias, K. (1993). Dietary Olive Oil Reduces Low-Density Lipoprotein Uptake by Macrophages and Decreases the Susceptibility of the Lipoprotein to Undergo Lipid Peroxidation. Annals of Nutrition and Metabolism, 37(2), 75–84. doi:10.1159/000177753

[676] Norwegian Scientific Committee for Food Safety (2011) 'Description of the processes in the value chain and risk assessment of decomposition substances and oxidation products in fish oils', Opinion of Steering Committee of the Norwegian Scientific Committee for Food Safety, 08-504-4-final, Accessed Online: https://web.archive.org/web/20160909213119/http://english.vkm.no/dav/0fd42c8b08.pdf

[677] Consumerlab.com (2018) 'Fish Oil and Omega-3 and -7 Supplements Review (Including Krill, Algae, Calamari, and Sea Buckthorn)', Product Reviews, Accessed Online: https://www.consumerlab.com/reviews/fish_oil_supplements_review/omega3/

[678] Sanguanwong et al (2016) 'Oral Supplementation of Vitamin C Reduced Lipid Peroxidation and Insulin Resistance in Patients with Type 2 Diabetes Mellitus', International Journal of Toxicological and Pharmacological Research 8(3):114-119.

[679] Viitala et al. (2004). Lipids in Health and Disease, 3(1), 14.

[680] Loffredo, L., Perri, L., Di Castelnuovo, A., Iacoviello, L., De Gaetano, G., & Violi, F. (2015). Supplementation with vitamin E alone is associated with reduced myocardial infarction: A meta-analysis. Nutrition, Metabolism and Cardiovascular Diseases, 25(4), 354–363. doi:10.1016/j.numecd.2015.01.008

[681] Huang (2002) 'Effects of vitamin C and vitamin E on in vivo lipid peroxidation: results of a randomized controlled trial', The American Journal of Clinical Nutrition, Volume 76, Issue 3, September 2002, Pages 549–555, https://doi.org/10.1093/ajcn/76.3.549

[682] Kanter et al (1993). Effects of an antioxidant vitamin mixture on lipid peroxidation at rest and postexercise. Journal of applied physiology (Bethesda, Md. : 1985), 74(2), 965–969. https://doi.org/10.1152/jappl.1993.74.2.965

[683] Dillard et al (1978). Effects of exercise, vitamin E, and ozone on pulmonary function and lipid peroxidation. Journal of applied physiology: respiratory, environmental and exercise physiology, 45(6), 927–932.

[684] Kanter et al (1993). Effects of an antioxidant vitamin mixture on lipid peroxidation at rest and postexercise. Journal of applied physiology (Bethesda, Md. : 1985), 74(2), 965–969.

[685] Patlar et al (2017) 'Effect of Vitamin C Supplementation on Lipid Peroxidation and Lactate Levels in Individuals Performing Exhaustion Exercise', Annals of Applied Sport Science 5(2):21-27.

[686] Xiao N. N. (2015). Effects of Resveratrol Supplementation on Oxidative Damage and Lipid Peroxidation Induced by Strenuous Exercise in Rats. Biomolecules & therapeutics, 23(4), 374–378.

[687] Helalizadeh et al (2020). Effect of ginger supplement on lipid peroxidation induced by exercise- A meta-analysis study. Journal of Medicinal Plants, 19(74), 25–38.

[688] Mirzaei et al (2013) 'Effects of creatine monohydrate supplementation on oxidative DNA damage and lipid peroxidation induced by acute incremental exercise to exhaustion in wrestlers', Kinesiology 45(1):30-40.

[689] Beavers et al (2010). Effect of exercise training on chronic inflammation. Clinica chimica acta; international journal of clinical chemistry, 411(11-12), 785–793.

[690] Myers, J. (2003). Exercise and Cardiovascular Health. Circulation, 107(1). doi:10.1161/01.cir.0000048890.59383.8d

[691] Jaarin, K., & Kamisah, Y. (2012). Repeatedly Heated Vegetable Oils and Lipid Peroxidation. Lipid Peroxidation. doi:10.5772/46076

[692] Doll, S. and Conrad, M. (2017), Iron and ferroptosis: A still ill-defined liaison. IUBMB Life, 69: 423-434. doi:10.1002/iub.1616

[693] Lee HS, Cui L, Li Y, Choi JS, Choi J-H, Li Z, et al. (2016) Correction: Influence of Light Emitting Diode-Derived Blue Light Overexposure on Mouse Ocular Surface. PLoS ONE 11(11): e0167671. https://doi.org/10.1371/journal.pone.0167671

[694] Torti, S. V., & Torti, F. M. (2013). Iron and cancer: more ore to be mined. Nature reviews. Cancer, 13(5), 342–355. https://doi.org/10.1038/nrc3495

[695] Fleming, R. E., & Ponka, P. (2012). Iron overload in human disease. The New England journal of medicine, 366(4), 348–359. https://doi.org/10.1056/NEJMra1004967

[696] Chisté et al (2014) 'Carotenoids inhibit lipid peroxidation and hemoglobin oxidation, but not the depletion of glutathione induced by ROS in human erythrocytes', Life Sciences, Volume 99, Issues 1–2, 18 March 2014, Pages 52-60.

[697] Zhang et al (1991). Carotenoids enhance gap junctional communication and inhibit lipid peroxidation in C3H/10T1/2 cells: relationship to their cancer chemopreventive action. Carcinogenesis, 12(11), 2109–2114. https://doi.org/10.1093/carcin/12.11.2109

[698] McNulty et al (2007). Differential effects of carotenoids on lipid peroxidation due to membrane interactions: X-ray diffraction analysis. Biochimica et Biophysica Acta (BBA) - Biomembranes, 1768(1), 167–174. doi:10.1016/j.bbamem.2006.09.010

[699] Lu et al (2006). Preventive effects of Spirulina platensis on skeletal muscle damage under exercise-induced oxidative stress. European journal of applied physiology, 98(2), 220–226. https://doi.org/10.1007/s00421-006-0263-0

[700] Ould Amara-Leffad, L., Ramdane, H., Nekhoul, K., Ouznadji, A., & Koceir, E. A. (2018). Spirulina effect on modulation of toxins provided by food, impact on hepatic and renal functions. Archives of Physiology and Biochemistry, 125(2), 184–194. doi:10.1080/13813455.2018.1444059

[701] Jabbari et al (2005). Comparison between swallowing and chewing of garlic on levels of serum lipids, cyclosporine, creatinine and lipid peroxidation in Renal Transplant Recipients, Lipids in Health and Disease, 4(1), 11. doi:10.1186/1476-511x-4-11

[702] Reddy, A. C., & Lokesh, B. R. (1994). Effect of dietary turmeric (Curcuma longa) on iron-induced lipid peroxidation in the rat liver. Food and chemical toxicology : an international journal published for the British Industrial Biological Research Association, 32(3), 279–283. https://doi.org/10.1016/0278-6915(94)90201-1

[703] Ji Z. (2010). Targeting DNA damage and repair by curcumin. Breast cancer : basic and clinical research, 4, 1–3.

[704] Kanner, J., Selhub, J., Shpaizer, A., Rabkin, B., Shacham, I., & Tirosh, O. (2017). Redox homeostasis in stomach medium by foods: The Postprandial Oxidative Stress Index (POSI) for balancing nutrition and human health. Redox Biology, 12, 929–936. doi:10.1016/j.redox.2017.04.029

[705] Li, Z., Henning, S. M., Zhang, Y., Rahnama, N., Zerlin, A., Thames, G., … Heber, D. (2013). Decrease of postprandial endothelial dysfunction by spice mix added to high-fat hamburger meat in men with Type 2 diabetes mellitus. Diabetic Medicine, 30(5), 590–595. doi:10.1111/dme.12120

[706] Kanner, J. (2007). Dietary advanced lipid oxidation endproducts are risk factors to human health. Molecular Nutrition & Food Research, 51(9), 1094–1101. doi:10.1002/mnfr.200600303

[707] Skulas-Ray, A. C., Kris-Etherton, P. M., Teeter, D. L., Chen, C.-Y. O., Vanden Heuvel, J. P., & West, S. G. (2011). A High Antioxidant Spice Blend Attenuates Postprandial Insulin and Triglyceride Responses and Increases Some Plasma Measures of Antioxidant Activity in Healthy, Overweight Men. The Journal of Nutrition, 141(8), 1451–1457. doi:10.3945/jn.111.138966

[708] Li, Z., Henning, S. M., Zhang, Y., Zerlin, A., Li, L., Gao, K., … Heber, D. (2010). Antioxidant-rich spice added to hamburger meat during cooking results in reduced meat, plasma, and urine malondialdehyde concentrations. The American Journal of Clinical Nutrition, 91(5), 1180–1184. doi:10.3945/ajcn.2009.28526

[709] Zhang, H., Zhang, H., Troise, A. D., & Fogliano, V. (2019). Melanoidins from Coffee, Cocoa, and Bread Are Able to Scavenge α-Dicarbonyl Compounds under Simulated Physiological Conditions. Journal of Agricultural and Food Chemistry, 67(39), 10921–10929. doi:10.1021/acs.jafc.9b03744

[710] Sirota et al (2013) 'Coffee polyphenols protect human plasma from postprandial carbonyl modifications', Molecular Nutrition & Food Research 57(5).

[711] Urquiaga, I., Troncoso, D., Mackenna, M., Urzúa, C., Pérez, D., Dicenta, S., … Rigotti, A. (2018). The Consumption of Beef Burgers Prepared with Wine Grape Pomace Flour Improves Fasting Glucose, Plasma Antioxidant Levels, and Oxidative Damage Markers in Humans: A Controlled Trial. Nutrients, 10(10), 1388. doi:10.3390/nu10101388

[712] Basu, A., Newman, E. D., Bryant, A. L., Lyons, T. J., & Betts, N. M. (2013). Pomegranate Polyphenols Lower Lipid Peroxidation in Adults with Type 2 Diabetes but Have No Effects in Healthy Volunteers: A Pilot Study. Journal of Nutrition and Metabolism, 2013, 1–7. doi:10.1155/2013/708381

[713] Basu, A., Sanchez, K., Leyva, M. J., Wu, M., Betts, N. M., Aston, C. E., & Lyons, T. J. (2010). Green Tea Supplementation Affects Body Weight, Lipids, and Lipid Peroxidation in Obese Subjects with Metabolic Syndrome. Journal of the American College of Nutrition, 29(1), 31–40. doi:10.1080/07315724.2010.10719814

[714] Tagliazucchi, D. (2015). Melanoidins from Coffee and Lipid Peroxidation. Coffee in Health and Disease Prevention, 859–867. doi:10.1016/b978-0-12-409517-5.00095-4

[715] Devasagayam, T. P., Kamat, J. P., Mohan, H., & Kesavan, P. C. (1996). Caffeine as an antioxidant: inhibition of lipid peroxidation induced by reactive oxygen species. Biochimica et biophysica acta, 1282(1), 63–70. https://doi.org/10.1016/0005-2736(96)00040-5

[716] Zeb, A., & Rahman, S. U. (2017). Protective effects of dietary glycine and glutamic acid toward the toxic effects of oxidized mustard oil in rabbits. Food & Function, 8(1), 429–436. doi:10.1039/c6fo01329e

[717] Zhong, Z., Jones, S., & Thurman, R. G. (1996). Glycine minimizes reperfusion injury in a low-flow, reflow liver perfusion model in the rat. American Journal of Physiology-Gastrointestinal and Liver Physiology, 270(2), G332–G338. doi:10.1152/ajpgi.1996.270.2.g332

[718] Bloomer, R. J., Tschume, L. C., & Smith, W. A. (2009). Glycine Propionyl-L-carnitine Modulates Lipid Peroxidation and Nitric Oxide in Human Subjects. International Journal for Vitamin and Nutrition Research, 79(3), 131–141. doi:10.1024/0300-9831.79.3.131

[719] McCarty, M. F., Iloki-Assanga, S., Lujan, L. M. L., & DiNicolantonio, J. J. (2019). Activated glycine receptors may decrease endosomal NADPH oxidase activity by opposing ClC-3-mediated efflux of chloride from endosomes. Medical Hypotheses, 123, 125–129.

[720] Kumar et al (2021). Glycine and N-acetylcysteine (GlyNAC) supplementation in older adults improves glutathione deficiency, oxidative stress, mitochondrial dysfunction, inflammation, insulin resistance, endothelial dysfunction, genotoxicity, muscle strength, and cognition: Results of a pilot clinical trial. Clinical and translational medicine, 11(3), e372.

[721] McCarty et al (2019) 'Activated Glycine Receptors May Decrease Endosomal NADPH Oxidase Activity by Opposing ClC-3-Mediated Efflux of Chloride from Endosomes', Medical Hypotheses 123, DOI: 10.1016/j.mehy.2019.01.012

[722] DiNicolantonio, J. J., & O'Keefe, J. H. (2018). Importance of maintaining a low omega–6/omega–3 ratio for reducing inflammation. Open Heart, 5(2), e000946. doi:10.1136/openhrt-2018-000946

[723] PM Kris-Etherton, Denise Shaffer Taylor, Shaomei Yu-Poth, Peter Huth, Kristin Moriarty, Valerie Fishell, Rebecca L Hargrove, Guixiang Zhao, Terry D Etherton; Polyunsaturated fatty acids in the food chain in the United States, The American Journal of Clinical Nutrition, Volume 71, Issue 1, 1 January 2000, Pages 179S–188S.

[724] Leaf A and Weber PC (1988) 'Cardiovascular effects of n-3 fatty acids', AGRIS, Accessed: http://agris.fao.org/agris-search/search.do?recordID=US8845581.

[725] RAHEJA, B. S., SADIKOT, S. M., PHATAK, R. B., & RAO, M. B. (1993). Significance of the N-6/N-3 Ratio for Insulin Action in Diabetes. Annals of the New York Academy of Sciences, 683(1 Dietary Lipid), 258–271. doi:10.1111/j.1749-6632.1993.tb35715.x

[726] Simopoulos, A. P., & DiNicolantonio, J. J. (2016). The importance of a balanced ω-6 to ω-3 ratio in the prevention and management of obesity. Open Heart, 3(2), e000385. doi:10.1136/openhrt-2015-000385

[727] Russo GL (2009) 'Dietary n-6 and n-3 polyunsaturated fatty acids: from biochemistry to clinical implications in cardiovascular prevention', Biochem Pharmacol. 2009 Mar 15;77(6):937-46.

[728] Simopoulos (1999) 'Essential fatty acids in health and chronic disease 1,2', American Journal of Clinical Nutrition 70(3 Suppl):560S-569S

[729] Hiza, HAB and Bente L (2007) 'Nutrient Content of the U.S. Food Supply, 1909-2004, A Summary Report', Center for Nutrition Policy and Promotion, Home Economics Research Report No. 57.

[730] Lalia, A., & Lanza, I. (2016). Insulin-Sensitizing Effects of Omega-3 Fatty Acids: Lost in Translation? Nutrients, 8(6), 329.

[731] Brown (2019). Omega-3, omega-6, and total dietary polyunsaturated fat for prevention and treatment of type 2 diabetes mellitus: systematic review and meta-analysis of randomised controlled trials. BMJ (Clinical research ed.), 366, l4697.

[732] Song et al (2020) 'Effects of Omega-3 PUFA Supplementation on Insulin Resistance and Lipid Metabolism in Patients with T2DM: A Systematic Review and Meta-Analysis', Current Developments in Nutrition, Volume 4, Issue Supplement_2, June 2020, Page 77.

[733] Farsi et al (2014). Effects of supplementation with omega-3 on insulin sensitivity and non-esterified free fatty acid (NEFA) in type 2 diabetic patients. Arquivos brasileiros de endocrinologia e metabologia, 58(4), 335–340.

[734] Lardinois C. K. (1987). The role of omega 3 fatty acids on insulin secretion and insulin sensitivity. Medical hypotheses, 24(3), 243–248.

[735] Gao et al (2017). Fish oil supplementation and insulin sensitivity: a systematic review and meta-analysis. Lipids in health and disease, 16(1), 131.

[736] Lepretti et al (2018). Omega-3 Fatty Acids and Insulin Resistance: Focus on the Regulation of Mitochondria and Endoplasmic Reticulum Stress. Nutrients, 10(3), 350.

[737] Azadbakht et al (2011). Omega-3 fatty acids, insulin resistance and type 2 diabetes. Journal of research in medical sciences : the official journal of Isfahan University of Medical Sciences, 16(10), 1259–1260.

[738] Thota et al (2019). Curcumin and/or omega-3 polyunsaturated fatty acids supplementation reduces insulin resistance and blood lipids in individuals with high risk of type 2 diabetes: a randomised controlled trial. Lipids in Health and Disease, 18(1).

[739] Udupa et al (2013). A comparative study of effects of omega-3 Fatty acids, alpha lipoic Acid and vitamin e in type 2 diabetes mellitus. Annals of medical and health sciences research, 3(3), 442–446.

[740] Li et al (2021). Omega-3FAs Can Inhibit the Inflammation and Insulin Resistance of Adipose Tissue Caused by HHcy Induced Lipids Profile Changing in Mice. Frontiers in Physiology, 12.

[741] Albert et al (2014). Higher omega-3 index is associated with increased insulin sensitivity and more favourable metabolic profile in middle-aged overweight men. Scientific Reports, 4(1).

[742] VanWinden et al (2017). The Use of Omega-3 Fatty Acids to Improve Insulin Sensitivity in Pregnancy: A Pilot Study of Safety and Tolerability [6Q]. Obstetrics & Gynecology, 129(1), S174–S174.

[743] Oomen et al (2000). Fish consumption and coronary heart disease mortality in Finland, Italy, and The Netherlands. American journal of epidemiology, 151(10), 999–1006. https://doi.org/10.1093/oxfordjournals.aje.a010144

[744] Keli, S. O., Feskens, E. J., & Kromhout, D. (1994). Fish consumption and risk of stroke. The Zutphen Study. Stroke, 25(2), 328–332. https://doi.org/10.1161/01.str.25.2.328

[745] DiNicolantonio, J. J., & O'Keefe, J. H. (2018). Omega-6 vegetable oils as a driver of coronary heart disease: the oxidized linoleic acid hypothesis. Open Heart, 5(2), e000898. doi:10.1136/openhrt-2018-000898

[746] Guyenet, S. J., & Carlson, S. E. (2015). Increase in Adipose Tissue Linoleic Acid of US Adults in the Last Half Century. Advances in Nutrition, 6(6), 660–664. doi:10.3945/an.115.009944

[747] Li et al (2020). Dietary intake and biomarkers of linoleic acid and mortality: systematic review and meta-analysis of prospective cohort studies. The American journal of clinical nutrition, 112(1), 150–167.

[748] Warensjö, E., Sundström, J., Vessby, B., Cederholm, T., & Risérus, U. (2008). Markers of dietary fat quality and fatty acid desaturation as predictors of total and cardiovascular mortality: a population-based prospective study. The American Journal of Clinical Nutrition, 88(1), 203–209. doi:10.1093/ajcn/88.1.203

[749] De Goede, J., Verschuren, W. M. M., Boer, J. M. A., Verberne, L. D. M., Kromhout, D., & Geleijnse, J. M. (2013). N-6 and N-3 Fatty Acid Cholesteryl Esters in Relation to Fatal CHD in a Dutch Adult Population: A Nested Case-Control Study and Meta-Analysis. PLoS ONE, 8(5), e59408. doi:10.1371/journal.pone.0059408

[750] Fernandez-Real, J.-M., Broch, M., Vendrell, J., & Ricart, W. (2003). Insulin Resistance, Inflammation, and Serum Fatty Acid Composition. Diabetes Care, 26(5), 1362–1368. doi:10.2337/diacare.26.5.1362

[751] Miettinen, T. A., Naukkarinen, V., Huttunen, J. K., Mattila, S., & Kumlin, T. (1982). Fatty-acid composition of serum lipids predicts myocardial infarction. BMJ, 285(6347), 993–996. doi:10.1136/bmj.285.6347.993

[752] Wu, J. H. Y., Lemaitre, R. N., King, I. B., Song, X., Psaty, B. M., Siscovick, D. S., & Mozaffarian, D. (2014). Circulating Omega-6 Polyunsaturated Fatty Acids and Total and Cause-Specific Mortality. Circulation, 130(15), 1245–1253. doi:10.1161/circulationaha.114.011590

[753] PM Kris-Etherton, Denise Shaffer Taylor, Shaomei Yu-Poth, Peter Huth, Kristin Moriarty, Valerie Fishell, Rebecca L Hargrove, Guixiang Zhao, Terry D Etherton; Polyunsaturated fatty acids in the food chain in the United States, The American Journal of Clinical Nutrition, Volume 71, Issue 1, 1 January 2000, Pages 179S–188S.

[754] Kris-Etherton, P., Taylor, D. S., Yu-Poth, S., Huth, P., Moriarty, K., Fishell, V., … Etherton, T. D. (2000). Polyunsaturated fatty acids in the food chain in the United States. The American Journal of Clinical Nutrition, 71(1), 179S–188S. doi:10.1093/ajcn/71.1.179s

[755] Eaton, S. B., Eaton III, S. B., Sinclair, A. J., Cordain, L., & Mann, N. J. (1998). Dietary Intake of Long-Chain Polyunsaturated Fatty Acids during the Paleolithic. The Return of W3 Fatty Acids into the Food Supply, 12–23. doi:10.1159/000059672

[756] Singh, R. B., Demeester, F., & Wilczynska, A. (2010). The tsim tsoum approaches for prevention of cardiovascular disease. Cardiology research and practice, 2010, 824938. https://doi.org/10.4061/2010/824938

[757] Kuipers, R. S., Luxwolda, M. F., Janneke Dijck-Brouwer, D. A., Eaton, S. B., Crawford, M. A., Cordain, L., & Muskiet, F. A. J. (2010). Estimated macronutrient and fatty acid intakes from an East African Paleolithic diet. British Journal of Nutrition, 104(11), 1666–1687. doi:10.1017/s0007114510002679

[758] Rodriguez-Leyva, D., Bassett, C. M. C., McCullough, R., & Pierce, G. N. (2010). The cardiovascular effects of flaxseed and its omega-3 fatty acid, alpha-linolenic acid. Canadian Journal of Cardiology, 26(9), 489–496. doi:10.1016/s0828-282x(10)70455-4

[759] Sprecher H. Dietary w3 and w6 fatty acids: biological effects and nutritional essentiality. NATO Series A, Life Sciences. 1989 Jan:69-79.

[760] Cordain, L., Watkins, B., Florant, G., Kelher, M., Rogers, L., & Li, Y. (2002). Fatty acid analysis of wild ruminant tissues: evolutionary implications for reducing diet-related chronic disease. European Journal of Clinical Nutrition, 56(3), 181–191. doi:10.1038/sj.ejcn.1601307

[761] Cordain, L., Watkins, B., Florant, G. et al. Fatty acid analysis of wild ruminant tissues: evolutionary implications for reducing diet-related chronic disease. Eur J Clin Nutr 56, 181–191 (2002).

[762] Simopoulos, A. P., Leaf, A., & Salem, N., Jr (1999). Essentiality of and recommended dietary intakes for omega-6 and omega-3 fatty acids. Annals of nutrition & metabolism, 43(2), 127–130. https://doi.org/10.1159/000012777

[763] Harris, W. S., & von Schacky, C. (2004). The Omega-3 Index: a new risk factor for death from coronary heart disease? Preventive Medicine, 39(1), 212–220. doi:10.1016/j.ypmed.2004.02.030

[764] Acosta-Montaño, P., & García-González, V. (2018). Effects of Dietary Fatty Acids in Pancreatic Beta Cell Metabolism, Implications in Homeostasis. Nutrients, 10(4), 393.

[765] Oh et al (2018). Fatty Acid-Induced Lipotoxicity in Pancreatic Beta-Cells During Development of Type 2 Diabetes. Frontiers in Endocrinology, 9.

[766] Hagman DK, Hays LB, Parazzoli SD, Poitout V. Palmitate inhibits insulin gene expression by altering PDX-1 nuclear localization and reducing MafA expression in isolated rat islets of Langerhans. J Biol Chem. (2005) 280:32413–8.

[767] Volk et al (2014) 'Effects of Step-Wise Increases in Dietary Carbohydrate on Circulating Saturated Fatty Acids and Palmitoleic Acid in Adults with Metabolic Syndrome', PLoS ONE 9(11): e113605.

[768] Merrill et al (2020). Low-Carbohydrate and Very-Low-Carbohydrate Diets in Patients With Diabetes. Diabetes Spectrum, 33(2), 133–142.

[769] Bolla et al (2019). Low-Carb and Ketogenic Diets in Type 1 and Type 2 Diabetes. Nutrients, 11(5), 962.

[770] Unwin et al (2020). Insights from a general practice service evaluation supporting a lower carbohydrate diet in patients with type 2 diabetes mellitus and prediabetes: a secondary analysis of routine clinic data including HbA1c, weight and prescribing over 6 years. BMJ Nutrition, Prevention & Health, 3(2), 285–294.

[771] Goldenberg et al (2021). Efficacy and safety of low and very low carbohydrate diets for type 2 diabetes remission: systematic review and meta-analysis of published and unpublished randomized trial data. BMJ, m4743.

[772] McMacken, M., & Shah, S. (2017). A plant-based diet for the prevention and treatment of type 2 diabetes. Journal of geriatric cardiology : JGC, 14(5), 342–354.

[773] Olfert, M. D., & Wattick, R. A. (2018). Vegetarian Diets and the Risk of Diabetes. Current diabetes reports, 18(11), 101.

[774] Nielsen, S. J., Siega-Riz, A. M., & Popkin, B. M. (2002). Trends in energy intake in U.S. between 1977 and 1996: similar shifts seen across age groups. Obesity research, 10(5), 370–378. https://doi.org/10.1038/oby.2002.51

[775] FAO (2002) 'World agriculture: towards 2015/2030', Rome, Italy: Food and Agriculture Organization of the United Nations, 2002.

[776] Campbell, J. D. (2001). Lifestyle, minerals and health. Medical Hypotheses, 57(5), 521–531. doi:10.1054/mehy.2001.1351

[777] DiNicolantonio, J. J., O'Keefe, J. H., & Wilson, W. (2018). Subclinical magnesium deficiency: a principal driver of cardiovascular disease and a public health crisis. Open heart, 5(1), e000668.

[778] DiNicolantonio, J. J., Mangan, D., & O'Keefe, J. H. (2018). Copper deficiency may be a leading cause of ischaemic heart disease. Open Heart, 5(2), e000784. doi:10.1136/openhrt-2018-000784

[779] Ames, B. N., Atamna, H., & Killilea, D. W. (2005). Mineral and vitamin deficiencies can accelerate the mitochondrial decay of aging. Molecular Aspects of Medicine, 26(4-5), 363–378. doi:10.1016/j.mam.2005.07.007

[780] Römer-Lüthi, C. (2006). Mineralstoffe und Spurenelemente im Kohlenhydratstoffwechsel. Ihre potenzielle Bedeutung für die Prävention und Therapie von Krankheiten. Schweizerische Zeitschrift Für Ganzheitsmedizin / Swiss Journal of Integrative Medicine, 18(4), 207–212. doi:10.1159/000282053

[781] Markham, G. D., & Pajares, M. A. (2008). Structure-function relationships in methionine adenosyltransferases. Cellular and Molecular Life Sciences, 66(4), 636–648. doi:10.1007/s00018-008-8516-1

[782] Hamon et al (1978) 'Activation of Tryptophan Hydroxylase by Adenosine Triphosphate, Magnesium, and Calcium', Molecular Pharmacology January 1978, 14 (1) 99-110.

[783] Wasserbauer (2017) 'Does Dietary Melatonin Play a Role in Bone Mineralization?', Theses - ALL. 120.

[784] Billyard et al (2006) 'Dietary magnesium deficiency decreases plasma melatonin in rats.', Magnesium Research, 01 Sep 2006, 19(3):157-161.

[785] Rondanelli, M., Opizzi, A., Monteferrario, F., Antoniello, N., Manni, R., & Klersy, C. (2011). The Effect of Melatonin, Magnesium, and Zinc on Primary Insomnia in Long-Term Care Facility Residents in Italy: A Double-Blind, Placebo-Controlled Clinical Trial. Journal of the American Geriatrics Society, 59(1), 82–90. doi:10.1111/j.1532-5415.2010.03232.x

[786] Peuhkuri, K., Sihvola, N., & Korpela, R. (2012). Dietary factors and fluctuating levels of melatonin. Food & Nutrition Research, 56(1), 17252. doi:10.3402/fnr.v56i0.17252

[787] Sugden, D. (1989). Melatonin biosynthesis in the mammalian pineal gland. Experientia, 45(10), 922–932. doi:10.1007/bf01953049

[788] Majewski, M., Kozlowska, A., Thoene, M., Lepiarczyk, E., & Grzegorzewski, W. J. (2016). Overview of the role of vitamins and minerals on the kynurenine pathway in health and disease. Journal of physiology and pharmacology : an official journal of the Polish Physiological Society, 67(1), 3–19.

[789] Takaya, J., Higashino, H., & Kobayashi, Y. (2004). Intracellular magnesium and insulin resistance. Magnesium research, 17(2), 126–136.

[790] Wesselink, E., Koekkoek, W. A. C., Grefte, S., Witkamp, R. F., & van Zanten, A. R. H. (2019). Feeding mitochondria: Potential role of nutritional components to improve critical illness convalescence. Clinical Nutrition, 38(3), 982–995. doi:10.1016/j.clnu.2018.08.032

[791] Hruby, A., O'Donnell, C. J., Jacques, P. F., Meigs, J. B., Hoffmann, U., & McKeown, N. M. (2014). Magnesium Intake Is Inversely Associated With Coronary Artery Calcification. JACC: Cardiovascular Imaging, 7(1), 59–69. doi:10.1016/j.jcmg.2013.10.006

[792] Houston, M. (2011). The Role of Magnesium in Hypertension and Cardiovascular Disease. The Journal of Clinical Hypertension, 13(11), 843–847. doi:10.1111/j.1751-7176.2011.00538.x

[793] DiNicolantonio, J. J., Liu, J., & O'Keefe, J. H. (2018). Magnesium for the prevention and treatment of cardiovascular disease. Open Heart, 5(2), e000775. doi:10.1136/openhrt-2018-000775

[794] Yang, Q. (2011). Sodium and Potassium Intake and Mortality Among US Adults. Archives of Internal Medicine, 171(13), 1183. doi:10.1001/archinternmed.2011.257

[795] D'Elia, L., Barba, G., Cappuccio, F. P., & Strazzullo, P. (2011). Potassium Intake, Stroke, and Cardiovascular Disease. Journal of the American College of Cardiology, 57(10), 1210–1219. doi:10.1016/j.jacc.2010.09.070

[796] Piazza (2017) 'How too little potassium may contribute to cardiovascular disease', NIH National Institute of Health, NIH Research Matters, Accessed Online Nov 15 2020: https://www.nih.gov/news-events/nih-research-matters/how-too-little-potassium-may-contribute-cardiovascular-disease

[797] DiNicolantonio, J. J., & Berger, A. (2016). Added sugars drive nutrient and energy deficit in obesity: a new paradigm. Open Heart, 3(2), e000469. doi:10.1136/openhrt-2016-000469

[798] Sakamaki, Y., Goto, K., Watanabe, Y., Takata, T., Yamazaki, H., Imai, N., Ito, Y., & Narita, I. (2014). Nephrotic syndrome and end-stage kidney disease accompanied by bicytopenia due to copper deficiency. Internal medicine (Tokyo, Japan), 53(18), 2101–2106. https://doi.org/10.2169/internalmedicine.53.2338

[799] DiNicolantonio, J. J., Bhutani, J., & O'Keefe, J. H. (2016). Added sugars drive chronic kidney disease and its consequences: A comprehensive review. Journal of Insulin Resistance, 1(1). doi:10.4102/jir.v1i1.3

[800] DiNicolantonio, J. J., O'Keefe, J. H., & Wilson, W. (2018). Subclinical magnesium deficiency: a principal driver of cardiovascular disease and a public health crisis. Open Heart, 5(1), e000668. doi:10.1136/openhrt-2017-000668

[801] Kahn, B. B. (1998). Type 2 Diabetes: When Insulin Secretion Fails to Compensate for Insulin Resistance. Cell, 92(5), 593–596.

[802] De Felice et al (2022). Impaired insulin signalling and allostatic load in Alzheimer disease. Nature Reviews Neuroscience, 23(4), 215–230.

[803] Clark et al (2001) 'Decreased insulin secretion in type 2 diabetes: a problem of cellular mass or function?', Diabetes 2001;50(suppl_1):S169.

[804] Wolf, F. (2003). Cell physiology of magnesium. Molecular Aspects of Medicine, 24(1-3), 11–26. doi:10.1016/s0098-2997(02)00088-2

[805] Takaya et al (2004). Intracellular magnesium and insulin resistance. Magnesium research, 17(2), 126–136.

[806] Ha, B. G., Park, J.-E., Cho, H.-J., & Shon, Y. H. (2015). Stimulatory Effects of Balanced Deep Sea Water on Mitochondrial Biogenesis and Function. PLOS ONE, 10(6), e0129972. doi:10.1371/journal.pone.0129972

[807] Wang, J., Persuitte, G., Olendzki, B. C., Wedick, N. M., Zhang, Z., Merriam, P. A., Fang, H., Carmody, J., Olendzki, G. F., & Ma, Y. (2013). Dietary magnesium intake improves insulin resistance among non-diabetic individuals with metabolic syndrome participating in a dietary trial. Nutrients, 5(10), 3910–3919. https://doi.org/10.3390/nu5103910

[808] Humphries, S. (1999). Low dietary magnesium is associated with insulin resistance in a sample of young, nondiabetic black Americans. American Journal of Hypertension, 12(8), 747–756. doi:10.1016/s0895-7061(99)00041-2

[809] Huerta, M. G., Roemmich, J. N., Kington, M. L., Bovbjerg, V. E., Weltman, A. L., Holmes, V. F., … Nadler, J. L. (2005). Magnesium Deficiency Is Associated With Insulin Resistance in Obese Children. Diabetes Care, 28(5), 1175–1181. doi:10.2337/diacare.28.5.1175

[810] Weglicki and Phillips (1992) 'Pathobiology of magnesium deficiency: a cytokine/neurogenic inflammation hypothesis', American Journal of Physiology-Regulatory, Integrative and Comparative Physiology 1992 263:3, R734-R737

[811] Laurant et al (1999) 'Effect of Magnesium Deficiency on Blood Pressure and Mechanical Properties of Rat Carotid Artery', Hypertension. 1999;33:1105–1110.

[812] Shibutani, Y., Sakamoto, K., Katsuno, S., Yoshimoto, S., & Matsuura, T. (1988). Serum and erythrocyte magnesium levels in junior high school students: relation to blood pressure and a family history of hypertension. Magnesium, 7(4), 188–194.

[813] Rodríguez-Morán, M., Simental Mendía, L. E., Zambrano Galván, G., & Guerrero-Romero, F. (2011). The role of magnesium in type 2 diabetes: a brief based-clinical review. Magnesium research, 24(4), 156–162. https://doi.org/10.1684/mrh.2011.0299

[814] Takaya, J., Higashino, H., & Kobayashi, Y. (2004). Intracellular magnesium and insulin resistance. Magnesium research, 17(2), 126–136.

[815] el-Hindi HM, Amer HA. Effect of thiamine, magnesium, and sulfate salts on growth, thiamine levels, and serum lipid constituents in rats. J Nutr Sci Vitaminol 1989;35:505–10.

[816] Altura, B. T., Brust, M., Bloom, S., Barbour, R. L., Stempak, J. G., & Altura, B. M. (1990). Magnesium dietary intake modulates blood lipid levels and atherogenesis. Proceedings of the National Academy of Sciences of the United States of America, 87(5), 1840–1844. https://doi.org/10.1073/pnas.87.5.1840

[817] World Health Organization. Calcium and Magnesium in Drinking Water: Public health significance. Geneva: World Health Organization Press; 2009.

[818] Schulze et al (2007). Fiber and magnesium intake and incidence of type 2 diabetes: a prospective study and meta-analysis. Archives of internal medicine, 167(9), 956–965.

[819] Larsson, S. C., & Wolk, A. (2007). Magnesium intake and risk of type 2 diabetes: a meta-analysis. Journal of internal medicine, 262(2), 208–214.

[820] Larsson et al (2012). Dietary magnesium intake and risk of stroke: a meta-analysis of prospective studies. The American journal of clinical nutrition, 95(2), 362–366.

[821] Hruby et al (2014) 'Magnesium Intake Is Inversely Associated with Coronary Artery Calcification: The Framingham Heart Study', JACC: Cardiovascular Imaging, Volume 7, Issue 1, January 2014, Pages 59-69.

[822] Nielsen, F. H., Milne, D. B., Gallagher, S., Johnson, L., & Hoverson, B. (2007). Moderate magnesium deprivation results in calcium retention and altered potassium and phosphorus excretion by postmenopausal women. Magnesium research, 20(1), 19–31.

[823] Tipton IH, Stewart PL, Dickson J. Patterns of elemental excretion in long term balance studies. Health Phys 1969;16:455–62.

[824] DiNicolantonio JJ, O'Keefe JH, Wilson W. Correction: Subclinical magnesium deficiency: a principal driver of cardiovascular disease and a public health crisis. Open Heart 2018;5.

[825] Hunt, C. D., & Johnson, L. K. (2006). Magnesium requirements: new estimations for men and women by cross-sectional statistical analyses of metabolic magnesium balance data. The American journal of clinical nutrition, 84(4), 843–852. https://doi.org/10.1093/ajcn/84.4.843

[826] Uğurlu, V., Binay, Ç., Şimşek, E., & Bal, C. (2016). Cellular Trace Element Changes in Type 1 Diabetes Patients. Journal of Clinical Research in Pediatric Endocrinology, 8(2), 180–186. doi:10.4274/jcrpe.2449

[827] Schnack, C., Bauer, I., Pregant, P., Hopmeier, P., & Schernthaner, G. (1992). Hypomagnesaemia in Type 2 (non-insulin-dependent) diabetes mellitus is not corrected by improvement of long-term metabolic control. Diabetologia, 35(1), 77–79. doi:10.1007/bf00400855

[828] Djurhuus, M. S., Skøtt, P., Hother-Nielsen, O., Klitgaard, N. A. H., & Beck-Nielsen, H. (1995). Insulin Increases Renal Magnesium Excretion: A Possible Cause of Magnesium Depletion in Hyperinsulinaemic States. Diabetic Medicine, 12(8), 664–669. doi:10.1111/j.1464-5491.1995.tb00566.x

[829] Hwang, D. L., Yen, C. F., & Nadler, J. L. (1993). Insulin increases intracellular magnesium transport in human platelets. The Journal of Clinical Endocrinology & Metabolism, 76(3), 549–553. doi:10.1210/jcem.76.3.8445010

[830] de Lourdes Lima et al (2006) '[Magnesium deficiency and insulin resistance in patients with type 2 diabetes mellitus]', Arquivos Brasileiros de Endocrinologia & Metabologia 49(6):959-63.

[831] DiNicolantonio, J. J., O'Keefe, J. H., & Wilson, W. (2018). Subclinical magnesium deficiency: a principal driver of cardiovascular disease and a public health crisis. Open Heart, 5(1), e000668. doi:10.1136/openhrt-2017-000668

[832] NIH (2020) 'Magnesium: Fact Sheet for Health Professionals', Dietary Supplement Fact Sheets, Accessed Online Jan 26 2021: https://ods.od.nih.gov/factsheets/Magnesium-HealthProfessional/

[833] Bohn et al (2004). Fractional magnesium absorption is significantly lower in human subjects from a meal served with an oxalate-rich vegetable, spinach, as compared with a meal served with kale, a vegetable with a low oxalate content. The British journal of nutrition, 91(4), 601–606.

[834] Melse-Boonstra, A. (2020). Bioavailability of Micronutrients From Nutrient-Dense Whole Foods: Zooming in on Dairy, Vegetables, and Fruits. Frontiers in Nutrition, 7.

[835] Ekmekcioglu C. (2000). Intestinal bioavailability of minerals and trace elements from milk and beverages in humans. Die Nahrung, 44(6), 390–397. https://doi.org/10.1002/1521-3803(20001201)44:6<390::AID-FOOD390>3.0.CO;2-Y

[836] Spätling L, Classen HG, Külpmann WR, et al. [Diagnosing magnesium deficiency. Current recommendations of the Society for Magnesium Research]. Fortschr Med Orig 2000;118(Suppl 2):49–53.

[837] Elin, R. J. (2011). Re-evaluation of the concept of chronic, latent, magnesium deficiency. Magnesium Research, 24(4), 225–227. doi:10.1684/mrh.2011.0298

[838] Costello, R. B., Elin, R. J., Rosanoff, A., Wallace, T. C., Guerrero-Romero, F., Hruby, A., … Van Horn, L. V. (2016). Perspective: The Case for an Evidence-Based Reference Interval for Serum Magnesium: The Time Has Come. Advances in Nutrition: An International Review Journal, 7(6), 977–993. doi:10.3945/an.116.012765

[839] Gullestad, L., Midtvedt, K., Dolva, L. ø., Norseth, J., & Kjekshus, J. (1994). The magnesium loading test: Reference values in healthy subjects. Scandinavian Journal of Clinical and Laboratory Investigation, 54(1), 23–31. doi:10.3109/00365519409086506

[840] Gullestad, L., Dolva, L. ø, Waage, A., Falch, D., Fagerthun, H., & Kjekshus, J. (1992). Magnesium deficiency diagnosed by an intravenous loading test. Scandinavian Journal of Clinical and Laboratory Investigation, 52(4), 245–253. doi:10.3109/00365519209088355

[841] Caddell JL. Magnesium deficiency in man. Del Med J 1968;40:133–8.

[842] Gullestad, L., Nes, M., Rønneberg, R., Midtvedt, K., Falch, D., & Kjekshus, J. (1994). Magnesium status in healthy free-living elderly Norwegians. Journal of the American College of Nutrition, 13(1), 45–50. doi:10.1080/07315724.1994.10718370

[843] DiNicolantonio, J. J., O'Keefe, J. H., & Wilson, W. (2018). Subclinical magnesium deficiency: a principal driver of cardiovascular disease and a public health crisis. Open Heart, 5(1), e000668. doi:10.1136/openhrt-2017-000668

[844] Shils ME. Experimental human magnesium depletion. Medicine 1969;48:61–85.

[845] De Carvalho, M., Kiernan, M. C., & Swash, M. (2017). Fasciculation in amyotrophic lateral sclerosis: origin and pathophysiological relevance. Journal of Neurology, Neurosurgery & Psychiatry, 88(9), 773–779. doi:10.1136/jnnp-2017-315574

[846] Cieslewicz et al (2012) 'The role of magnesium in cardiac arrhythmias', Journal of Elementology 18(2/2013), DOI: 10.5601/jelem.2013.18.2.11

[847] Sun-Edelstein, C., & Mauskop, A. (2009). Role of magnesium in the pathogenesis and treatment of migraine. Expert review of neurotherapeutics, 9(3), 369–379. https://doi.org/10.1586/14737175.9.3.369

[848] Grobin W. A New Syndrome, Magnesium-Deficiency Tetany. Can Med Assoc J 1960;82:1034–5.

[849] Jooste, P. L., Wolfswinkel, J. M., Schoeman, J. J., & Strydom, N. B. (1979). Epileptic-type convulsions and magnesium deficiency. Aviation, space, and environmental medicine, 50(7), 734–735.

[850] Johnson, S. (2001). The multifaceted and widespread pathology of magnesium deficiency. Medical Hypotheses, 56(2), 163–170. doi:10.1054/mehy.2000.1133

[851] Alloui, A., Begon, S., Chassaing, C., Eschalier, A., Gueux, E., Rayssiguier, Y., & Dubray, C. (2003). Does Mg2+ deficiency induce a long-term sensitization of the central nociceptive pathways? European Journal of Pharmacology, 469(1-3), 65–69. doi:10.1016/s0014-2999(03)01719-9

[852] Durlach J, Pagès N, Bac P, et al. Headache due to photosensitive magnesium depletion. Magnes Res 2005;18:109–22.

[853] Cevette, M. J., Barrs, D. M., Patel, A., Conroy, K. P., Sydlowski, S., Noble, B. N., Nelson, G. A., & Stepanek, J. (2011). Phase 2 study examining magnesium-dependent tinnitus. The international tinnitus journal, 16(2), 168–173.

[854] Cevette, M. J., Vormann, J., & Franz, K. (2003). Magnesium and hearing. Journal of the American Academy of Audiology, 14(4), 202–212.

[855] RUDE, R. K., OLDHAM, S. B., & SINGER, F. R. (1976). FUNCTIONAL HYPOPARATHYROIDISM AND PARATHYROID HORMONE END-ORGAN RESISTANCE IN HUMAN MAGNESIUM DEFICIENCY. Clinical Endocrinology, 5(3), 209–224. doi:10.1111/j.1365-2265.1976.tb01947.x

[856] Agarwal, R., Iezhitsa, I. N., Agarwal, P., & Spasov, A. A. (2013). Mechanisms of cataractogenesis in the presence of magnesium deficiency. Magnesium Research, 26(1), 2–8. doi:10.1684/mrh.2013.0336

[857] Mccoy, J. H., & Kenney, M. A. (1975). Depressed immune response in the magnesium-deficient rat. The Journal of nutrition, 105(6), 791–797. https://doi.org/10.1093/jn/105.6.791

[858] Schmitz, C., & Perraud, A.-L. (2017). Magnesium and the Immune Response. Molecular, Genetic, and Nutritional Aspects of Major and Trace Minerals, 319–331. doi:10.1016/b978-0-12-802168-2.00026-9

[859] Siwek, M., Wróbel, A., Dudek, D., Nowak, G., & Zieba, A. (2005). Udział miedzi i magnezu w patogenezie i terapii zaburzeń afektywnych [The role of copper and magnesium in the pathogenesis and treatment of affective disorders]. Psychiatria polska, 39(5), 911–920.

[860] Bartenstein (2016) 'Magnesium Supplement Guide', Supplement Specs, Accessed Online Feb 04 2021: https://supplementspecs.com/magnesium-supplement-guide/

[861] Slutsky, I., Abumaria, N., Wu, L. J., Huang, C., Zhang, L., Li, B., Zhao, X., Govindarajan, A., Zhao, M. G., Zhuo, M., Tonegawa, S., & Liu, G. (2010). Enhancement of learning and memory by elevating brain magnesium. Neuron, 65(2), 165–177. https://doi.org/10.1016/j.neuron.2009.12.026

[862] Porter et al (2010) 'Alternative Medical Interventions Used in the Treatment and Management of Myalgic Encephalomyelitis/Chronic Fatigue Syndrome and Fibromyalgia', The Journal of Alternative and Complementary MedicineVol. 16, No. 3, https://doi.org/10.1089/acm.2008.0376

[863] Engen et al (2015) 'Effects of transdermal magnesium chloride on quality of life for patients with fibromyalgia: a feasibility study', Journal of Integrative Medicine, Volume 13, Issue 5, September 2015, Pages 306-313.

[864] Rodríguez-Morán, M., & Guerrero-Romero, F. (2003). Oral magnesium supplementation improves insulin sensitivity and metabolic control in type 2 diabetic subjects: a randomized double-blind controlled trial. Diabetes care, 26(4), 1147–1152. https://doi.org/10.2337/diacare.26.4.1147

[865] Houston, M. (2011), The Role of Magnesium in Hypertension and Cardiovascular Disease. The Journal of Clinical Hypertension, 13: 843-847. https://doi.org/10.1111/j.1751-7176.2011.00538.x

[866] Geiss, K. R., Stergiou, N., Jester, Neuenfeld, H. U., & Jester, H. G. (1998). Effects of magnesium orotate on exercise tolerance in patients with coronary heart disease. Cardiovascular drugs and therapy, 12 Suppl 2, 153–156. https://doi.org/10.1023/a:1007796515957

[867] Classen H. G. (2004). Magnesium orotate--experimental and clinical evidence. Romanian journal of internal medicine = Revue roumaine de medecine interne, 42(3), 491–501.

[868] Stepura, O. B., & Martynow, A. I. (2009). Magnesium orotate in severe congestive heart failure (MACH). International journal of cardiology, 134(1), 145–147. https://doi.org/10.1016/j.ijcard.2009.01.047

[869] Gromova, O. A., Torshin, I. Y., Kalacheva, A. G., & Grishina, T. R. (2016). Kardiologiia, 56(3), 73–80. https://doi.org/10.18565/cardio.2016.3.73-80

[870] Garrison et al (2011) 'Magnesium for skeletal muscle cramps', Cochrane Database of Systematic Reviews 2011, Issue 11. Art. No.: CD009402. DOI: 10.1002/14651858.CD009402. Accessed 04 February 2021.

[871] Mertz et al (1988) 'IS CHROMIUM ESSENTIAL FOR HUMANS? Nutrition Reviews, Volume 46, Issue 1, January 1988, Pages 17–20, https://doi.org/10.1111/j.1753-4887.1988.tb05348.x

[872] Liu, L., Cui, W. M., Zhang, S. W., Kong, F. H., Pedersen, M. A., Wen, Y., & Lv, J. P. (2015). Effect of glucose tolerance factor (GTF) from high chromium yeast on glucose metabolism in insulin-resistant 3T3-L1 adipocytes. RSC Advances, 5(5), 3482–3490. doi:10.1039/c4ra10343b

[873] Barrett, J., Brien, P. O., & De Jesus, J. P. (1985). Chromium(III) and the glucose tolerance factor. Polyhedron, 4(1), 1–14. doi:10.1016/s0277-5387(00)84214-x

[874] Bahijiri, S. M., Mira, S. A., Mufti, A. M., & Ajabnoor, M. A. (2000). The effects of inorganic chromium and brewer's yeast supplementation on glucose tolerance, serum lipids and drug dosage in individuals with type 2 diabetes. Saudi medical journal, 21(9), 831–837.

[875] Racek, J., Trefil, L., Rajdl, D., Mudrová, V., Hunter, D., & Senft, V. (2006). Influence of chromium-enriched yeast on blood glucose and insulin variables, blood lipids, and markers of oxidative stress in subjects with type 2 diabetes mellitus. Biological trace element research, 109(3), 215–230. https://doi.org/10.1385/BTER:109:3:215

[876] Li, Y.-C. (1994). Effects of brewer's yeast on glucose tolerance and serum lipids in Chinese adults. Biological Trace Element Research, 41(3), 341–347. doi:10.1007/bf02917434

[877] Schroeder H. A. (1966). Chromium deficiency in rats: a syndrome simulating diabetes mellitus with retarded growth. The Journal of nutrition, 88(4), 439–445. https://doi.org/10.1093/jn/88.4.439

[878] Schroeder, H. A. (1965). Diabetic-like serum glucose levels in chromium deficient rats. Life Sciences, 4(21), 2057–2062. doi:10.1016/0024-3205(65)90322-x

[879] Padmavathi, I. J., Rao, K. R., Venu, L., Ganeshan, M., Kumar, K. A., Rao, C., Harishankar, N., Ismail, A., & Raghunath, M. (2010). Chronic maternal dietary chromium restriction modulates visceral adiposity: probable underlying mechanisms. Diabetes, 59(1), 98–104. https://doi.org/10.2337/db09-0779

[880] NIH (2020) 'Chromium: Fact Sheet for Health Professionals', Dietary Supplement Fact Sheets, Accessed Online Jan 18 2021: https://ods.od.nih.gov/factsheets/Chromium-HealthProfessional/

[881] Doisy et al (1976) 'Chromium Metabolism in Man and Biochemical Effects', in Trace Elements in Human Health and Disease, Volume II: Essential and Toxic Elements, Academic Press, New York, pp 79-80.

[882] Urberg, M., & Zemel, M. B. (1987). Evidence for synergism between chromium and nicotinic acid in the control of glucose tolerance in elderly humans. Metabolism: clinical and experimental, 36(9), 896–899. https://doi.org/10.1016/0026-0495(87)90100-4

[883] Jeejeebhoy, K. N., Chu, R. C., Marliss, E. B., Greenberg, G. R., & Bruce-Robertson, A. (1977). Chromium deficiency, glucose intolerance, and neuropathy reversed by chromium supplementation, in a patient receiving long-term total parenteral nutrition. The American journal of clinical nutrition, 30(4), 531–538. https://doi.org/10.1093/ajcn/30.4.531

[884] Anderson R. A. (1993). Recent advances in the clinical and biochemical effects of chromium deficiency. Progress in clinical and biological research, 380, 221–234.

[885] Stehle, P., Stoffel-Wagner, B., & Kuhn, K. S. (2016). Parenteral trace element provision: recent clinical research and practical conclusions. European journal of clinical nutrition, 70(8), 886–893. https://doi.org/10.1038/ejcn.2016.53

[886] Freund, H., Atamian, S., & Fischer, J. E. (1979). Chromium deficiency during total parenteral nutrition. JAMA, 241(5), 496–498.

[887] Brown, R. O., Forloines-Lynn, S., Cross, R. E., & Heizer, W. D. (1986). Chromium deficiency after long-term total parenteral nutrition. Digestive diseases and sciences, 31(6), 661–664. https://doi.org/10.1007/BF01318699

[888] Fessler T. A. (2013). Trace elements in parenteral nutrition: a practical guide for dosage and monitoring for adult patients. Nutrition in clinical practice : official publication of the American Society for Parenteral and Enteral Nutrition, 28(6), 722–729. https://doi.org/10.1177/0884533613506596

[889] Science Direct (2020) 'Low-Molecular-Weight Chromium-Binding Substance', Biochemistry, Genetics and Molecular Biology, Accessed Online Jan 10 2021: https://www.sciencedirect.com/topics/biochemistry-genetics-and-molecular-biology/low-molecular-weight-chromium-binding-substance

[890] Vincent J. B. (1999). Mechanisms of chromium action: low-molecular-weight chromium-binding substance. Journal of the American College of Nutrition, 18(1), 6–12. https://doi.org/10.1080/07315724.1999.10718821

[891] Vincent J. B. (2015). Is the Pharmacological Mode of Action of Chromium(III) as a Second Messenger?. Biological trace element research, 166(1), 7–12. https://doi.org/10.1007/s12011-015-0231-9

[892] Davis, C. M., & Vincent, J. B. (1997). Chromium oligopeptide activates insulin receptor tyrosine kinase activity. Biochemistry, 36(15), 4382–4385. https://doi.org/10.1021/bi963154t

[893] Salloum, Z, Lehoux, EA, Harper, M-E, Catelas, I. Effects of cobalt and chromium ions on glycolytic flux and the stabilization of hypoxia-inducible factor-1α in macrophages in vitro. J Orthop Res. 2021; 39: 112– 120. https://doi.org/10.1002/jor.24758

[894] Mertz, W. (1981). THE INTERACTION BETWEEN CHROMIUM AND INSULIN. Nutrition, Digestion, Metabolism, 101–105. doi:10.1016/b978-0-08-026825-5.50019-x

[895] Phung et al (2010) 'Improved Glucose Control Associated with i.v. Chromium Administration in Two Patients Receiving Enteral Nutrition', Am J Health Syst Pharm. 2010;67(7):535-541

[896] National Toxicology Program (2018) 'Hexavalent Chromium Factsheet', U.S. Department of Health and Human Services, NIH, Accessed Online Jan 11 2021: https://www.niehs.nih.gov/health/materials/hexavalent_chromium_508.pdf

[897] Wise, S. S., & Wise, J. P., Sr (2012). Chromium and genomic stability. Mutation research, 733(1-2), 78–82. https://doi.org/10.1016/j.mrfmmm.2011.12.002

[898] Agency for Toxic Substances and Disease Registry (2012) 'ToxFAQs™ for Chromium', Toxic Substances Portal, Accessed Online Jan 12 2021: https://web.archive.org/web/20140708162618/http://www.atsdr.cdc.gov/toxfaqs/TF.asp?id=61&tid=17

[899] Indian Council of Medical Research (2009) 'NUTRIENT REQUIREMENTS AND RECOMMENDED DIETARY ALLOWANCES FOR INDIANS', A Report of the Expert Group of the Indian Council of Medical Research, NATIONAL INSTITUTE OF NUTRITION, Accessed Online Jan 12 2021: https://web.archive.org/web/20160615094048/http://icmr.nic.in/final/RDA-2010.pdf#

[900] EFSA NDA Panel (EFSA Panel on Dietetic Products, Nutrition and Allergies), 2014. Scientific Opinion on Dietary Reference Values for chromium. EFSA Journal 2014; 12(10):3845, 25 pp. doi:10.2903/j.efsa.2014.3845

[901] Institute of Medicine (US) Panel on Micronutrients. (2001). Dietary Reference Intakes for Vitamin A, Vitamin K, Arsenic, Boron, Chromium, Copper, Iodine, Iron, Manganese, Molybdenum, Nickel, Silicon, Vanadium, and Zinc. National Academies Press (US).

[902] NIH (2020) 'Chromium: Fact Sheet for Health Professionals', Dietary Supplement Fact Sheets, Accessed Online Jan 18 2021: https://ods.od.nih.gov/factsheets/Chromium-HealthProfessional/

[903] Mertz W. (1969). Chromium occurrence and function in biological systems. Physiological reviews, 49(2), 163–239. https://doi.org/10.1152/physrev.1969.49.2.163

[904] Food and Nutrition Board. Recommended Dietary Allowances. 9th ed National Academy of Sciences; Washington, DC, USA: 1980.

[905] WHO (1996) 'Chromium' In: Trace elements in human nutrition and health, Geneva, 155-60. Accessed Online Jan 11 2021: https://www.who.int/nutrition/publications/micronutrients/9241561734/en/

[906] U. S. Food and Drug Administration (2016) 'Food Labeling: Revision of the Nutrition and Supplement Facts Labels', Docket No. FDA-2012-N-1210, Accessed Online Jan 11 2021: https://www.federalregister.gov/documents/2016/05/27/2016-11867/food-labeling-revision-of-the-nutrition-and-supplement-facts-labels

[907] Trumbo, P. R., & Ellwood, K. C. (2006). Chromium picolinate intake and risk of type 2 diabetes: an evidence-based review by the United States Food and Drug Administration. Nutrition reviews, 64(8), 357–363. https://doi.org/10.1111/j.1753-4887.2006.tb00220.x

[908] Emord (2005) 'Qualified Health Claims: Letter of Enforcement Discretion - Chromium Picolinate and Insulin Resistance(Docket No. 2004Q-0144)', U.S. Food and Drug Administration, Labeling & Nutrition, Accessed Online Jan 12 2021: https://wayback.archive-it.org/7993/20171114183739/https://www.fda.gov/Food/IngredientsPackagingLabeling/LabelingNutrition/ucm073017.htm

[909] American Diabetes Association (2015). (4) Foundations of care: education, nutrition, physical activity, smoking cessation, psychosocial care, and immunization. Diabetes care, 38 Suppl, S20–S30. https://doi.org/10.2337/dc15-S007

[910] American Diabetes Association (2010). Standards of medical care in diabetes--2010. Diabetes care, 33 Suppl 1(Suppl 1), S11–S61. https://doi.org/10.2337/dc10-S011

[911] European Food Safety Authority (EFSA) (2010) 'Scientific Opinion on the substantiation of health claims related to chromium and contribution to normal macronutrient metabolism (ID 260, 401, 4665, 4666, 4667), maintenance of normal blood glucose concentrations (ID 262, 4667), contribution to the maintenance or achievement of a normal body weight (ID 339, 4665, 4666), and reduction of tiredness and fatigue (ID 261) pursuant to Article 13(1) of Regulation (EC) No 1924/2006', EFSA Panel on Dietetic Products, Nutrition and Allergies (NDA), Accessed Online Jan 12 2021: https://efsa.onlinelibrary.wiley.com/doi/epdf/10.2903/j.efsa.2010.1732

[912] Moradi, F., Kooshki, F., Nokhostin, F., Khoshbaten, M., Bazyar, H., & Pourghassem Gargari, B. (2021). A pilot study of the effects of chromium picolinate supplementation on serum fetuin-A, metabolic and inflammatory factors in patients with nonalcoholic fatty liver disease: A double-blind, placebo-controlled trial. Journal of Trace Elements in Medicine and Biology, 63, 126659. doi:10.1016/j.jtemb.2020.126659

[913] Paiva, A. N., Lima, J. G. de, Medeiros, A. C. Q. de, Figueiredo, H. A. O., Andrade, R. L. de, Ururahy, M. A. G., … Almeida, M. das G. (2015). Beneficial effects of oral chromium picolinate supplementation on glycemic control in patients with type 2 diabetes: A randomized clinical study. Journal of Trace Elements in Medicine and Biology, 32, 66–72. doi:10.1016/j.jtemb.2015.05.006

[914] Anderson, R. A., Cheng, N., Bryden, N. A., Polansky, M. M., Cheng, N., Chi, J., & Feng, J. (1997). Elevated intakes of supplemental chromium improve glucose and insulin variables in individuals with type 2 diabetes. Diabetes, 46(11), 1786–1791. https://doi.org/10.2337/diab.46.11.1786

[915] Costello, R. B., Dwyer, J. T., & Bailey, R. L. (2016). Chromium supplements for glycemic control in type 2 diabetes: limited evidence of effectiveness. Nutrition reviews, 74(7), 455–468. https://doi.org/10.1093/nutrit/nuw011

[916] Amato, P., Morales, A. J., & Yen, S. S. C. (2000). Effects of Chromium Picolinate Supplementation on Insulin Sensitivity, Serum Lipids, and Body Composition in Healthy, Nonobese, Older Men and Women. The Journals of Gerontology Series A: Biological Sciences and Medical Sciences, 55(5), M260–M263. doi:10.1093/gerona/55.5.m260

[917] Wilson, B. E., & Gondy, A. (1995). Effects of chromium supplementation on fasting insulin levels and lipid parameters in healthy, non-obese young subjects. Diabetes research and clinical practice, 28(3), 179–184. https://doi.org/10.1016/0168-8227(95)01097-w

[918] Balk, E. M., Tatsioni, A., Lichtenstein, A. H., Lau, J., & Pittas, A. G. (2007). Effect of Chromium Supplementation on Glucose Metabolism and Lipids: A systematic review of randomized controlled trials. Diabetes Care, 30(8), 2154–2163. doi:10.2337/dc06-0996

[919] Piotrowska, A., Pilch, W., Czerwińska-Ledwig, O., Zuziak, R., Siwek, A., Wolak, M., & Nowak, G. (2019). The Possibilities of Using Chromium Salts as an Agent Supporting Treatment of Polycystic Ovary Syndrome. Biological trace element research, 192(2), 91–97. https://doi.org/10.1007/s12011-019-1654-5

[920] Tang, X. L., Sun, Z., & Gong, L. (2018). Chromium supplementation in women with polycystic ovary syndrome: Systematic review and meta-analysis. The journal of obstetrics and gynaecology research, 44(1), 134–143. https://doi.org/10.1111/jog.13462

[921] Maleki, V., Izadi, A., Farsad-Naeimi, A., & Alizadeh, M. (2018). Chromium supplementation does not improve weight loss or metabolic and hormonal variables in patients with polycystic ovary syndrome: A systematic review. Nutrition research (New York, N.Y.), 56, 1–10. https://doi.org/10.1016/j.nutres.2018.04.003

[922] Heshmati, J., Omani-Samani, R., Vesali, S., Maroufizadeh, S., Rezaeinejad, M., Razavi, M., & Sepidarkish, M. (2018). The Effects of Supplementation with Chromium on Insulin Resistance Indices in Women with Polycystic Ovarian Syndrome: A Systematic Review and Meta-Analysis of Randomized Clinical Trials. Hormone and metabolic research = Hormon- und Stoffwechselforschung = Hormones et metabolisme, 50(3), 193–200. https://doi.org/10.1055/s-0044-101835

[923] Fazelian, S., Rouhani, M. H., Bank, S. S., & Amani, R. (2017). Chromium supplementation and polycystic ovary syndrome: A systematic review and meta-analysis. Journal of trace elements in medicine and biology : organ of the Society for Minerals and Trace Elements (GMS), 42, 92–96. https://doi.org/10.1016/j.jtemb.2017.04.008

[924] Gibson, R.S., Scythes, C.A. Chromium, selenium, and other trace element intakes of a selected sample of Canadian premenopausal women. Biol Trace Elem Res 6, 105–116 (1984). https://doi.org/10.1007/BF02916928

[925] Pittler, M. H., Stevinson, C., & Ernst, E. (2003). Chromium picolinate for reducing body weight: meta-analysis of randomized trials. International journal of obesity and related metabolic disorders : journal of the International Association for the Study of Obesity, 27(4), 522–529. https://doi.org/10.1038/sj.ijo.0802262

[926] Onakpoya, I., Posadzki, P., & Ernst, E. (2013). Chromium supplementation in overweight and obesity: a systematic review and meta-analysis of randomized clinical trials. Obesity reviews : an official journal of the International Association for the Study of Obesity, 14(6), 496–507. https://doi.org/10.1111/obr.12026

[927] Willoughby, D., Hewlings, S., & Kalman, D. (2018). Body Composition Changes in Weight Loss: Strategies and Supplementation for Maintaining Lean Body Mass, a Brief Review. Nutrients, 10(12), 1876. https://doi.org/10.3390/nu10121876

[928] Tian, H., Guo, X., Wang, X., He, Z., Sun, R., Ge, S., & Zhang, Z. (2013). Chromium picolinate supplementation for overweight or obese adults. The Cochrane database of systematic reviews, 2013(11), CD010063. https://doi.org/10.1002/14651858.CD010063.pub2

[929] Tsang, C., Taghizadeh, M., Aghabagheri, E., Asemi, Z., & Jafarnejad, S. (2019). A meta-analysis of the effect of chromium supplementation on anthropometric indices of subjects with overweight or obesity. Clinical obesity, 9(4), e12313. https://doi.org/10.1111/cob.12313

[930] Manore M. M. (2012). Dietary supplements for improving body composition and reducing body weight: where is the evidence?. International journal of sport nutrition and exercise metabolism, 22(2), 139–154. https://doi.org/10.1123/ijsnem.22.2.139

[931] Anton, S. D., Morrison, C. D., Cefalu, W. T., Martin, C. K., Coulon, S., Geiselman, P., Han, H., White, C. L., & Williamson, D. A. (2008). Effects of chromium picolinate on food intake and satiety. Diabetes technology & therapeutics, 10(5), 405–412. https://doi.org/10.1089/dia.2007.0292

[932] Kaats, G. R., Blum, K., Fisher, J. A., & Adelman, J. A. (1996). Effects of chromium picolinate supplementation on body composition: a randomized, double-masked, placebo-controlled study. Current Therapeutic Research, 57(10), 747–756. doi:10.1016/s0011-393x(96)80080-4

[933] Hallmark et al (1996) 'Effects of chromium and resistive training on muscle strength and body composition', Medicine & Science in Sports & Exercise: January 1996 - Volume 28 - Issue 1 - p 139-144.

[934] Clancy, S. P., Clarkson, P. M., DeCheke, M. E., Nosaka, K., Freedson, P. S., Cunningham, J. J., & Valentine, B. (1994). Effects of chromium picolinate supplementation on body composition, strength, and urinary chromium loss in football players. International journal of sport nutrition, 4(2), 142–153. https://doi.org/10.1123/ijsn.4.2.142

[935] Thor, M. Y., Harnack, L., King, D., Jasthi, B., & Pettit, J. (2011). Evaluation of the comprehensiveness and reliability of the chromium composition of foods in the literature (). Journal of food composition and analysis : an official publication of the United Nations University, International Network of Food Data Systems, 24(8), 1147–1152. https://doi.org/10.1016/j.jfca.2011.04.006

[936] Toepfer, E. W., Mertz, W., Roginski, E. E., & Polansky, M. M. (1973). Chromium in foods in relation to biological activity. Journal of agricultural and food chemistry, 21(1), 69–71. https://doi.org/10.1021/jf60185a008

[937] Offenbacher, E. G., & Pi-Sunyer, F. X. (1980). Beneficial effect of chromium-rich yeast on glucose tolerance and blood lipids in elderly subjects. Diabetes, 29(11), 919–925. https://doi.org/10.2337/diab.29.11.919

[938] Anderson R. A. (2008). Chromium and polyphenols from cinnamon improve insulin sensitivity. The Proceedings of the Nutrition Society, 67(1), 48–53. https://doi.org/10.1017/S0029665108006010

[939] NIH (2020) 'Chromium: Fact Sheet for Health Professionals', Accessed Online Jan 10 2021: https://ods.od.nih.gov/factsheets/chromium-HealthProfessional/

[940] Anderson, R. A., Bryden, N. A., & Polansky, M. M. (1992). Dietary chromium intake. Freely chosen diets, institutional diet, and individual foods. Biological trace element research, 32, 117–121. https://doi.org/10.1007/BF02784595

[941] Rêczajska et al (2005) 'Determination of chromium content of food and beverages of plant origin', Polish journal of food and nutrition sciences 14, no. 55 (2005): 2.

[942] WebMD (2020) 'Top Foods High in Chromium', Diet & Weight Management, Accessed Online Jan 10 2021: https://www.webmd.com/diet/foods-high-in-chromium#2

[943] Soukaloun, D., et al., Erythrocyte transketolase activity, markers of cardiac dysfunction and the diagnosis of infantile beriberi. PLoS Negl Trop Dis, 2011. 5(2): p. e971.

[944] Wakabayashi, A., Y. Yui, and C. Kawai, A clinical study on thiamine deficiency. Jpn Circ J, 1979. 43(11): p. 995-9.

[945] Cowgill GR. The need for the addition of vitamin B1 to staple american foods. JAMA. 1939.113 (24). 2146-2151.

[946] Cowgill GR. The need for the addition of vitamin B1 to staple american foods. JAMA. 1939.113 (24). 2146-2151.

[947] Cowgill GR. The need for the addition of vitamin B1 to staple american foods. JAMA. 1939.113 (24). 2146-2151.

[948] Sinclair HM. Discussion on the clinical aspects of the vitamin-B complex. Proceedings of the Royal Society of Medicine. 1939. XXXII. 812-817.

[949] Sinclair HM. Discussion on the clinical aspects of the vitamin-B complex. Proceedings of the Royal Society of Medicine. 1939. XXXII. 812-817.

[950] Sinclair HM. Discussion on the clinical aspects of the vitamin-B complex. Proceedings of the Royal Society of Medicine. 1939. XXXII. 812-817.

[951] Williams RD, Mason HL and Smith BF. Induced Vitamin B1 Deficiency in Human Subjects.Proc Staff Meet. Mayo Clin. 1939:14:787-793.

[952] Williams RD. Observations on induced thiamine (vitamin b1) deficiency in man. Arch Intern Med. 1940;66(4):785-799.

[953] Williams RD, Mason HL and Smith BF. Induced Vitamin B1 Deficiency in Human Subjects.Proc Staff Meet. Mayo Clin. 1939:14:787-793.

[954] Williams RD, Mason HL and Smith BF. Induced Vitamin B1 Deficiency in Human Subjects.Proc Staff Meet. Mayo Clin. 1939:14:787-793.

[955] Williams RD, Mason HL and Smith BF. Induced Vitamin B1 Deficiency in Human Subjects.Proc Staff Meet. Mayo Clin. 1939:14:787-793.

[956] Williams RD, Mason HL and Smith BF. Induced Vitamin B1 Deficiency in Human Subjects.Proc Staff Meet. Mayo Clin. 1939:14:787-793.

[957] Williams RD, Mason HL and Smith BF. Induced Vitamin B1 Deficiency in Human Subjects.Proc Staff Meet. Mayo Clin. 1939:14:787-793.

[958] Williams RD. Observations on induced thiamine (vitamin b1) deficiency in man. Arch Intern Med. 1940;66(4):785-799.

[959] Williams RD. Observations on induced thiamine (vitamin b1) deficiency in man. Arch Intern Med. 1940;66(4):785-799.

[960] Williams RD. Observations on induced thiamine (vitamin b1) deficiency in man. Arch Intern Med. 1940;66(4):785-799.

[961] Williams RD. Observations on induced thiamine (vitamin b1) deficiency in man. Arch Intern Med. 1940;66(4):785-799.

[962] Page, G. L., Laight, D., & Cummings, M. H. (2011). Thiamine deficiency in diabetes mellitus and the impact of thiamine replacement on glucose metabolism and vascular disease. International journal of clinical practice, 65(6), 684–690.

[963] Shahzad Alam, S. (2012). Effect of High Dose Thiamine Therapy on Risk Factors in Type 2 Diabetics. Journal of Diabetes & Metabolism, 03(10).

[964] Winkler et al (1999). Effectiveness of different benfotiamine dosage regimens in the treatment of painful diabetic neuropathy. Arzneimittel-Forschung, 49(3), 220–224.

[965] Thornalley P. J. (2005). The potential role of thiamine (vitamin B1) in diabetic complications. Current diabetes reviews, 1(3), 287–298.

[966] Fraser et al (2012). The effects of long-term oral benfotiamine supplementation on peripheral nerve function and inflammatory markers in patients with type 1 diabetes: a 24-month, double-blind, randomized, placebo-controlled trial. Diabetes care, 35(5), 1095–1097.

[967] Haupt et al (2005). Benfotiamine in the treatment of diabetic polyneuropathy--a three-week randomized, controlled pilot study (BEDIP study). International journal of clinical pharmacology and therapeutics, 43(2), 71–77.

[968] Stirban, A., Pop, A., & Tschoepe, D. (2013). A randomized, double-blind, crossover, placebo-controlled trial of 6 weeks benfotiamine treatment on postprandial vascular function and variables of autonomic nerve function in Type 2 diabetes. Diabetic medicine : a journal of the British Diabetic Association, 30(10), 1204–1208.

[969] Ohta T, Ishigaki K: Evaluation of large dose therapy with an active type thiamine (TTFD) in diabetic neuropathy. Shinryo, 1963; 16: 100–9.

[970] Popa et al (2019). Evaluating the Efficacy of the Treatment with Benfotiamine and Alpha-lipoic Acid in Distal Symmetric Painful Diabetic Polyneuropathy. Revista de Chimie.

[971] Hammes et al (2003). Benfotiamine blocks three major pathways of hyperglycemic damage and prevents experimental diabetic retinopathy. Nature medicine, 9(3), 294–299. 4

[972] González-Ortiz, M., et al., Effect of thiamine administration on metabolic profile, cytokines and inflammatory markers in drug-naïve patients with type 2 diabetes. Eur J Nutr, 2011. 50(2): p. 145-9.

[973] Alam, SS, Riaz, S and Akhtar, MW. Effect of high dose thiamine therapy on risk factors in type 2 diabetics. J Diabetes Metab. 2012:3(10):1-9.

[974] Arora, S., et al., Thiamine (vitamin B1) improves endothelium-dependent vasodilatation in the presence of hyperglycemia. Ann Vasc Surg, 2006. 20(5): p. 653-8.

[975] Sambon, M., P. Wins, and L. Bettendorff, Neuroprotective Effects of Thiamine and Precursors with Higher Bioavailability: Focus on Benfotiamine and Dibenzoylthiamine. Int J Mol Sci, 2021. 22(11).

[976] Larkin, J.R., et al., Glucose-induced down regulation of thiamine transporters in the kidney proximal tubular epithelium produces thiamine insufficiency in diabetes. PLoS One, 2012. 7(12): p. e53175.

[977] Nixon, P.F., R.J. Diefenbach, and R.G. Duggleby, Inhibition of transketolase and pyruvate decarboxylase by omeprazole. Biochem Pharmacol, 1992. 44(1): p. 177-9.

[978] Liang, X., et al., Metformin is a Substrate and Inhibitor of the Human Thiamine Transporter, THTR-2 (SLC19A3). Mol Pharm, 2015. 12(12): p. 4301-10.

[979] Alston, T.A. and R.H. Abeles, Enzymatic conversion of the antibiotic metronidazole to an analog of thiamine. Arch Biochem Biophys, 1987. 257(2): p. 357-62.

[980] Giacomini, M.M., et al., Interaction of 2,4-Diaminopyrimidine-Containing Drugs Including Fedratinib and Trimethoprim with Thiamine Transporters. Drug Metab Dispos, 2017. 45(1): p. 76-85.

[981] Karadima, V., et al., Drug-micronutrient interactions: food for thought and thought for action. Epma j, 2016. 7(1): p. 10.

[982] Onishi, H., et al., High proportion of thiamine deficiency in referred cancer patients with delirium: a retrospective descriptive study. Eur J Clin Nutr, 2021. 75(10): p. 1499-1505.

[983] Macrotrends (2023) 'Japan Life Expectancy 1950-2023', Accessed Online March 2nd 2023: https://www.macrotrends.net/countries/JPN/japan/life-expectancy

[984] Wikipedia (2023) 'Sumo', Life as a professional sumo wrestler, Accessed Online March 2nd 2023: https://en.wikipedia.org/wiki/Sumo#Life_as_a_professional_sumo_wrestler

[985] Hoshi, A., & Inaba, Y. (1995). Nihon eiseigaku zasshi. Japanese journal of hygiene, 50(3), 730–736. https://doi.org/10.1265/jjh.50.730

[986] Shipley (2022) 'Please sir, I want Sumo: How Sumo wrestlers fuel up for fights', Sliced, Accessed Online March 2nd 2023: https://fedfedfed.com/sliced/please-sir-i-want-sumo-how-sumo-wrestlers-fuel-up-for-fights

[987] Mullur et al (2014). Thyroid Hormone Regulation of Metabolism. Physiological Reviews, 94(2), 355–382.

[988] Moeller, L. C., & Broecker-Preuss, M. (2011). Transcriptional regulation by nonclassical action of thyroid hormone. Thyroid research, 4 Suppl 1(Suppl 1), S6. https://doi.org/10.1186/1756-6614-4-S1-S6

[989] Yen P. M. (2001). Physiological and molecular basis of thyroid hormone action. Physiological reviews, 81(3), 1097–1142. https://doi.org/10.1152/physrev.2001.81.3.1097

[990] Nishi M. (2018). Diabetes mellitus and thyroid diseases. Diabetology international, 9(2), 108–112.

[991] Wang C. (2013). The Relationship between Type 2 Diabetes Mellitus and Related Thyroid Diseases. Journal of diabetes research, 2013, 390534.

[992] Ray S, Ghosh S (2016) Thyroid Disorders and Diabetes Mellitus: Double Trouble J Dia Res Ther 2(1): doi http://dx.doi.org/10.16966/2380-5544.113

[993] Ogbonna SU, Ezeani IU, Okafor CI, Chinenye S. Association between glycemic status and thyroid dysfunction in patients with type 2 diabetes mellitus. Diabetes Metab Syndr Obes. 2019;12:1113-1122

[994] Nishi M. (2018). Diabetes mellitus and thyroid diseases. Diabetology international, 9(2), 108–112.

[995] Donckier (2003) "Endocrine diseases and diabetes," in Text Book of Diabetes Mellitus, J. C. Pickup and G. Williams, Eds., vol. 27, pp. 21–27, Blackwell Publishing Company, Chichester, UK, 2003.

[996] Stanická et al (2005). Insulin sensitivity and counter-regulatory hormones in hypothyroidism and during thyroid hormone replacement therapy. Clinical chemistry and laboratory medicine, 43(7), 715–720.

[997] Brenta G. (2011). Why can insulin resistance be a natural consequence of thyroid dysfunction?. Journal of thyroid research, 2011, 152850. https://doi.org/10.4061/2011/152850

[998] Mitrou et al (2010). Insulin action in hyperthyroidism: a focus on muscle and adipose tissue. Endocrine reviews, 31(5), 663–679.

[999] Dimitriadis, G., Baker, B., Marsh, H., Mandarino, L., Rizza, R., Bergman, R., Haymond, M., & Gerich, J. (1985). Effect of thyroid hormone excess on action, secretion, and metabolism of insulin in humans. American Journal of Physiology-Endocrinology and Metabolism, 248(5), E593–E601. https://doi.org/10.1152/ajpendo.1985.248.5.e593

[1000] CAVALLO-PERIN, P., BRUNO, A., BOINE, L., CASSADER, M., LENTI, G. and PAGANO, G. (1988), Insulin resistance in Graves' disease: a quantitative in-vivo evaluation. European Journal of Clinical Investigation, 18: 607-613. https://doi.org/10.1111/j.1365-2362.1988.tb01275.x

[1001] Beylot M. (1996). Regulation of in vivo ketogenesis: role of free fatty acids and control by epinephrine, thyroid hormones, insulin and glucagon. Diabetes & metabolism, 22(5), 299–304.

[1002] Knudsen, N., Laurberg, P., Rasmussen, L. B., Bülow, I., Perrild, H., Ovesen, L., & Jørgensen, T. (2005). Small Differences in Thyroid Function May Be Important for Body Mass Index and the Occurrence of Obesity in the Population. The Journal of Clinical Endocrinology & Metabolism, 90(7), 4019–4024. doi:10.1210/jc.2004-2225

[1003] Fox, C. S., Pencina, M. J., D'Agostino, R. B., Murabito, J. M., Seely, E. W., Pearce, E. N., & Vasan, R. S. (2008). Relations of thyroid function to body weight: cross-sectional and longitudinal observations in a community-based sample. Archives of internal medicine, 168(6), 587–592. https://doi.org/10.1001/archinte.168.6.587

[1004] Mory et al (1981). Effects of hypothyroidism on the brown adipose tissue of adult rats: comparison with the effects of adaptation to cold. The Journal of endocrinology, 91(3), 515–524.

[1005] Wang, C. (2013). The Relationship between Type 2 Diabetes Mellitus and Related Thyroid Diseases. Journal of Diabetes Research, 2013, 1–9.

[1006] Kapadia et al (2012). Association between altered thyroid state and insulin resistance. Journal of pharmacology & pharmacotherapeutics, 3(2), 156–160.

[1007] Maratou et al (2010). Studies of insulin resistance in patients with clinical and subclinical hyperthyroidism. European journal of endocrinology, 163(4), 625–630.

[1008] Chen et al (2010) 'Associations between cardiovascular risk, insulin resistance, β-cell function and thyroid dysfunction: a cross-sectional study in She ethnic minority group of Fujian Province in China', European Journal of Endocrinology, Volume 163: Issue 5, pp 775-782.

[1009] Brenta et al (2009). Acute thyroid hormone withdrawal in athyreotic patients results in a state of insulin resistance. Thyroid : official journal of the American Thyroid Association, 19(6), 665–669.

[1010] Choi, Y.M., Kim, M.K., Kwak, M.K. et al. Association between thyroid hormones and insulin resistance indices based on the Korean National Health and Nutrition Examination Survey. Sci Rep 11, 21738 (2021).

[1011] Peppa et al (2011). Lipid abnormalities and cardiometabolic risk in patients with overt and subclinical thyroid disease. Journal of lipids, 2011, 575840.

[1012] Wang, C. C., & Reusch, J. E. (2012). Diabetes and cardiovascular disease: changing the focus from glycemic control to improving long-term survival. The American journal of cardiology, 110(9 Suppl), 58B–68B.

[1013] Rezzonico et al (2011). The association of insulin resistance with subclinical thyrotoxicosis. Thyroid : official journal of the American Thyroid Association, 21(9), 945–949.

[1014] Tang et al (2017). Correlation between Insulin Resistance and Thyroid Nodule in Type 2 Diabetes Mellitus. International journal of endocrinology, 2017, 1617458.

[1015] Fang et al (2018). Cancer risk in Chinese diabetes patients: a retrospective cohort study based on management data. Endocrine connections, 7(12), 1415–1423.

[1016] Yeo et al (2014). Diabetes mellitus and risk of thyroid cancer: a meta-analysis. PloS one, 9(6), e98135.

[1017] Li, H., & Qian, J. (2017). Association of diabetes mellitus with thyroid cancer risk: A meta-analysis of cohort studies. Medicine, 96(47), e8230.

[1018] Bakker et al (2001). The relationship between thyrotropin and low density lipoprotein cholesterol is modified by insulin sensitivity in healthy euthyroid subjects. The Journal of clinical endocrinology and metabolism, 86(3), 1206–1211.

[1019] Tayal et al (2008). Evaluation of lipid profile in hypothyroid patients-our experience. Thyroid Research and Practice, 5(2), 43.

[1020] Khan et al (2017). Study of Thyroid Disorders among Type 2 Diabetic Patients Attending a Tertiary Care Hospital. Mymensingh medical journal : MMJ, 26(4), 874–878.

[1021] Khatiwada et al (2015). Thyroid Dysfunction and Associated Risk Factors among Nepalese Diabetes Mellitus Patients. International journal of endocrinology, 2015, 570198.

[1022] Han et al (2015). Subclinical Hypothyroidism and Type 2 Diabetes: A Systematic Review and Meta-Analysis. PloS one, 10(8), e0135233.

[1023] Wu et al (2015). Relationship between Diabetic Retinopathy and Subclinical Hypothyroidism: a meta-analysis. Scientific reports, 5, 12212.

[1024] Wang et al (2019). Association between thyroid function and diabetic nephropathy in euthyroid subjects with type 2 diabetes mellitus: a cross-sectional study in China. Oncotarget, 10(2), 88–97.

[1025] Centeno Maxzud et al (2016). Prevalencia de disfunción tiroidea en pacientes con diabetes mellitus tipo 2 [Prevalence of thyroid dysfunction in patients with type 2 diabetes mellitus]. Medicina, 76(6), 355–358.

[1026] Ozair et al (2018). Prevalence of thyroid disorders in North Indian Type 2 diabetic subjects: A cross sectional study. Diabetes & metabolic syndrome, 12(3), 301–304.

[1027] Palma et al (2013). Prevalence of thyroid dysfunction in patients with diabetes mellitus. Diabetology & metabolic syndrome, 5(1), 58.

[1028] Kalra, S., Aggarwal, S., & Khandelwal, D. (2019). Thyroid Dysfunction and Type 2 Diabetes Mellitus: Screening Strategies and Implications for Management. Diabetes therapy : research, treatment and education of diabetes and related disorders, 10(6), 2035–2044.

[1029] Kadiyala et al (2010), Thyroid dysfunction in patients with diabetes: clinical implications and screening strategies. International Journal of Clinical Practice, 64: 1130-1139.

[1030] Perros et al (1995). Frequency of thyroid dysfunction in diabetic patients: value of annual screening. Diabetic medicine : a journal of the British Diabetic Association, 12(7), 622–627.

[1031] Orzan et al (2016). Type 1 Diabetes and Thyroid Autoimmunity in Children. Maedica, 11(4), 308–312.

[1032] Solá et al (2002). Association between diabetic ketoacidosis and thyrotoxicosis. Acta diabetologica, 39(4), 235–237.

[1033] Le Moli et al (2015). Type 2 diabetic patients with Graves' disease have more frequent and severe Graves' orbitopathy. Nutrition, metabolism, and cardiovascular diseases : NMCD, 25(5), 452–457.

[1034] Farishta F, Farishta S (2015) Insulin resistance and thyroid hypofunction in obese women – A cross sectional study. Integr Obesity Diabetes . 1: doi: 10.15761/IOD.1000013

[1035] Sisk, J. (2004). Thyroid Disease in Women-Diagnostic Conundrum. Today's Dietitian. The Magazine for nutritional professionals, 6, 42.

[1036] Safian et al (2020). Thyroid Dysfunction in Pregnant Women with Gestational Diabetes Mellitus. Current diabetes reviews, 16(8), 895–899.

[1037] Knight et al (2016). Maternal hypothyroxinaemia in pregnancy is associated with obesity and adverse maternal metabolic parameters. European journal of endocrinology, 174(1), 51–57.

[1038] Cai et al (2016). The Influence of Gestational Diabetes on Neurodevelopment of Children in the First Two Years of Life: A Prospective Study. PloS one, 11(9), e0162113.

[1039] Pop et al (2003). Maternal hypothyroxinaemia during early pregnancy and subsequent child development: a 3-year follow-up study. Clinical endocrinology, 59(3), 282–288.

[1040] Yang et al (2015). Thyroid antibodies and gestational diabetes mellitus: a meta-analysis. Fertility and sterility, 104(3), 665–71.e3.

[1041] Männistö et al (2010). Thyroid dysfunction and autoantibodies during pregnancy as predictive factors of pregnancy complications and maternal morbidity in later life. The Journal of clinical endocrinology and metabolism, 95(3), 1084–1094.

[1042] Ortega, E., Koska, J., Pannacciulli, N., Bunt, J. C., & Krakoff, J. (2008). Free triiodothyronine plasma concentrations are positively associated with insulin secretion in euthyroid individuals. European Journal of Endocrinology, 158(2), 217–221. https://doi.org/10.1530/eje-07-0592

[1043] Ren, R., Jiang, X., Zhang, X., Guan, Q., Yu, C., Li, Y., Gao, L., Zhang, H. and Zhao, J. (2014), Association between thyroid hormones and body fat in euthyroid subjects. Clin Endocrinol, 80: 585-590. https://doi.org/10.1111/cen.12311

[1044] Roos et al (2007) 'Thyroid Function Is Associated with Components of the Metabolic Syndrome in Euthyroid Subjects ', The Journal of Clinical Endocrinology & Metabolism, Volume 92, Issue 2, 1 February 2007, Pages 491–496, https://doi.org/10.1210/jc.2006-1718

[1045] Prats-Puig, A., Sitjar, C., Ribot, R., Calvo, M., Clausell-Pomés, N., Soler-Roca, M., Soriano-Rodríguez, P., Osiniri, I., Ros-Miquel, M., Bassols, J., de Zegher, F., Ibáñez, L. and López-Bermejo, A. (2012), Relative Hypoadiponectinemia, Insulin Resistance, and Increased Visceral Fat in Euthyroid Prepubertal Girls With Low-Normal Serum Free Thyroxine. Obesity, 20: 1455-1461. https://doi.org/10.1038/oby.2011.206

[1046] Kouidhi, S., Berhouma, R., Ammar, M., Rouissi, K., Jarboui, S., Clerget-Froidevaux, M.-S., Seugnet, I., Abid, H., Bchir, F., Demeneix, B., Guissouma, H., & Elgaaied, A. B. (2012). Relationship of Thyroid Function with Obesity and Type 2 Diabetes in Euthyroid Tunisian Subjects. Endocrine Research, 38(1), 15–23. https://doi.org/10.3109/07435800.2012.699987

[1047] Lin, Y. and Sun, Z. (2011), Thyroid hormone potentiates insulin signaling and attenuates hyperglycemia and insulin resistance in a mouse model of type 2 diabetes. British Journal of Pharmacology, 162: 597-610. https://doi.org/10.1111/j.1476-5381.2010.01056.x

[1048] Bollinger, S. S., Weltman, N. Y., Gerdes, A. M., & Schlenker, E. H. (2015). T3 supplementation affects ventilatory timing & glucose levels in type 2 diabetes mellitus model. Respiratory Physiology & Neurobiology, 205, 92–98. https://doi.org/10.1016/j.resp.2014.10.020

[1049] Luna-Vazquez, F., Cruz-Lumbreras, R., Rodríguez-Castelán, J., Cervantes-Rodríguez, M., Rodríguez-Antolín, J., Arroyo-Helguera, O., Castelán, F., Martínez-Gómez, M., & Cuevas, E. (2014). Association between the serum concentration of triiodothyronine with components of metabolic syndrome, cardiovascular risk, and diet in euthyroid post-menopausal women without and with metabolic syndrome. SpringerPlus, 3(1). https://doi.org/10.1186/2193-1801-3-266

[1050] Kapadia, K. B., Bhatt, P. A., & Shah, J. S. (2012). Association between altered thyroid state and insulin resistance. Journal of pharmacology & pharmacotherapeutics, 3(2), 156–160. https://doi.org/10.4103/0976-500X.95517

[1051] Bilgin, H., & Pirgon, Ö. (2014). Thyroid Function in Obese Children with Non-Alcoholic Fatty Liver Disease. Journal of Clinical Research in Pediatric Endocrinology, 152–157. https://doi.org/10.4274/jcrpe.1488

[1052] De Pergola, G., Ciampolillo, A., Paolotti, S., Trerotoli, P., & Giorgino, R. (2007). Free triiodothyronine and thyroid stimulating hormone are directly associated with waist circumference, independently of insulin resistance, metabolic parameters and blood pressure in overweight and obese women. Clinical endocrinology, 67(2), 265–269. https://doi.org/10.1111/j.1365-2265.2007.02874.x

[1053] Iacobellis, G., Ribaudo, M. C., Zappaterreno, A., Iannucci, C. V., & Leonetti, F. (2005). Relationship of thyroid function with body mass index, leptin, insulin sensitivity and adiponectin in euthyroid obese women. Clinical endocrinology, 62(4), 487–491. https://doi.org/10.1111/j.1365-2265.2005.02247.x

[1054] Radetti, G., Kleon, W., Buzi, F., Crivellaro, C., Pappalardo, L., di Iorgi, N., & Maghnie, M. (2008). Thyroid function and structure are affected in childhood obesity. The Journal of clinical endocrinology and metabolism, 93(12), 4749–4754. https://doi.org/10.1210/jc.2008-0823

[1055] Moulin de Moraes, C. M., Mancini, M. C., de Melo, M. E., Figueiredo, D. A., Villares, S. M., Rascovski, A., Zilberstein, B., & Halpern, A. (2005). Prevalence of subclinical hypothyroidism in a morbidly obese population and improvement after weight loss induced by Roux-en-Y gastric bypass. Obesity surgery, 15(9), 1287–1291. https://doi.org/10.1381/096089205774512537

[1056] Bastemir, M., Akin, F., Alkis, E., & Kaptanoglu, B. (2007). Obesity is associated with increased serum TSH level, independent of thyroid function. Swiss medical weekly, 137(29-30), 431–434.

[1057] Nyrnes, A., Jorde, R., & Sundsfjord, J. (2005). Serum TSH is positively associated with BMI. International Journal of Obesity, 30(1), 100–105. https://doi.org/10.1038/sj.ijo.0803112

[1058] Fox, C. S., Pencina, M. J., D'Agostino, R. B., Murabito, J. M., Seely, E. W., Pearce, E. N., & Vasan, R. S. (2008). Relations of thyroid function to body weight: cross-sectional and longitudinal observations in a community-based sample. Archives of internal medicine, 168(6), 587–592. https://doi.org/10.1001/archinte.168.6.587

[1059] Alevizaki, M., Saltiki, K., Voidonikola, P., Mantzou, E., Papamichael, C., & Stamatelopoulos, K. (2009). Free thyroxine is an independent predictor of subcutaneous fat in euthyroid individuals. European journal of endocrinology, 161(3), 459–465. https://doi.org/10.1530/EJE-09-0441

[1060] Knudsen, N., Laurberg, P., Rasmussen, L. B., Bülow, I., Perrild, H., Ovesen, L., & Jørgensen, T. (2005). Small differences in thyroid function may be important for body mass index and the occurrence of obesity in the population. The Journal of clinical endocrinology and metabolism, 90(7), 4019–4024. https://doi.org/10.1210/jc.2004-2225

[1061] Wang, F., Tan, Y., Wang, C., Zhang, X., Zhao, Y., Song, X., … Zhao, J. (2012). Thyroid-Stimulating Hormone Levels within the Reference Range Are Associated with Serum Lipid Profiles Independent of Thyroid Hormones. The Journal of Clinical Endocrinology & Metabolism, 97(8), 2724–2731. doi:10.1210/jc.2012-1133

[1062] Wang, F., Tan, Y., Wang, C., Zhang, X., Zhao, Y., Song, X., … Zhao, J. (2012). Thyroid-Stimulating Hormone Levels within the Reference Range Are Associated with Serum Lipid Profiles Independent of Thyroid Hormones. The Journal of Clinical Endocrinology & Metabolism, 97(8), 2724–2731. doi:10.1210/jc.2012-1133

[1063] Gavin, L. A., McMahon, F., & Moeller, M. (1985). Modulation of Adipose Lipoprotein Lipase by Thyroid Hormone and Diabetes: The Significance of the Low T3 State. Diabetes, 34(12), 1266–1271. doi:10.2337/diab.34.12.1266

[1064] Rodondi, N., den Elzen, W. P., Bauer, D. C., Cappola, A. R., Razvi, S., Walsh, J. P., Asvold, B. O., Iervasi, G., Imaizumi, M., Collet, T. H., Bremner, A., Maisonneuve, P., Sgarbi, J. A., Khaw, K. T., Vanderpump, M. P., Newman, A. B., Cornuz, J., Franklyn, J. A., Westendorp, R. G., Vittinghoff, E., … Thyroid Studies Collaboration (2010). Subclinical hypothyroidism and the risk of coronary heart disease and mortality. JAMA, 304(12), 1365–1374. https://doi.org/10.1001/jama.2010.1361

[1065] Dons, Robert F.; Jr, Frank H. Wians (2009). Endocrine and metabolic disorders clinical lab testing manual (4th ed.). Boca Raton: CRC Press. p. 10. ISBN 9781420079364.

[1066] Biondi (2013) 'The Normal TSH Reference Range: What Has Changed in the Last Decade?', The Journal of Clinical Endocrinology & Metabolism, Volume 98, Issue 9, 1 September 2013, Pages 3584–3587, https://doi.org/10.1210/jc.2013-2760

[1067] Hollowell, J. G., Staehling, N. W., Flanders, W. D., Hannon, W. H., Gunter, E. W., Spencer, C. A., & Braverman, L. E. (2002). Serum TSH, T(4), and thyroid antibodies in the United States population (1988 to 1994): National Health and Nutrition Examination Survey (NHANES III). The Journal of clinical endocrinology and metabolism, 87(2), 489–499. https://doi.org/10.1210/jcem.87.2.8182

[1068] Vadiveloo, T., Donnan, P. T., Murphy, M. J., & Leese, G. P. (2013). Age- and Gender-Specific TSH Reference Intervals in People With No Obvious Thyroid Disease in Tayside, Scotland: The Thyroid Epidemiology, Audit, and Research Study (TEARS). The Journal of Clinical Endocrinology & Metabolism, 98(3), 1147–1153. doi:10.1210/jc.2012-3191

[1069] Laurberg, P., Knudsen, N., Andersen, S., Carlé, A., Pedersen, I. B., & Karmisholt, J. (2012). Thyroid Function and Obesity. European Thyroid Journal, 1(3), 159–167. doi:10.1159/000342994

[1070] Samuels, M. H. (2014). Psychiatric and cognitive manifestations of hypothyroidism. Current Opinion in Endocrinology & Diabetes and Obesity, 21(5), 377–383. doi:10.1097/med.0000000000000089

[1071] Bennett, W. E., & Heuckeroth, R. O. (2012). Hypothyroidism Is a Rare Cause of Isolated Constipation. Journal of Pediatric Gastroenterology and Nutrition, 54(2), 285–287. doi:10.1097/mpg.0b013e318239714f

[1072] Joffe, R.T., Pearce, E.N., Hennessey, J.V., Ryan, J.J. and Stern, R.A. (2013), Subclinical hypothyroidism, mood, and cognition in older adults: a review. Int J Geriatr Psychiatry, 28: 111-118. doi:10.1002/gps.3796

[1073] Taylor, P. N., Albrecht, D., Scholz, A., Gutierrez-Buey, G., Lazarus, J. H., Dayan, C. M., & Okosieme, O. E. (2018). Global epidemiology of hyperthyroidism and hypothyroidism. Nature reviews. Endocrinology, 14(5), 301–316. https://doi.org/10.1038/nrendo.2018.18

[1074] Garmendia Madariaga, A., Santos Palacios, S., Guillén-Grima, F., & Galofré, J. C. (2014). The Incidence and Prevalence of Thyroid Dysfunction in Europe: A Meta-Analysis. The Journal of Clinical Endocrinology & Metabolism, 99(3), 923–931. doi:10.1210/jc.2013-2409

[1075] Bülow Pedersen, I., Laurberg, P., Knudsen, N., Jørgensen, T., Perrild, H., Ovesen, L., & Rasmussen, L. B. (2007). An Increased Incidence of Overt Hypothyroidism after Iodine Fortification of Salt in Denmark: A Prospective Population Study. The Journal of Clinical Endocrinology & Metabolism, 92(8), 3122–3127. doi:10.1210/jc.2007-0732

[1076] Boelaert, K., Newby, P. R., Simmonds, M. J., Holder, R. L., Carr-Smith, J. D., Heward, J. M., Manji, N., Allahabadia, A., Armitage, M., Chatterjee, K. V., Lazarus, J. H., Pearce, S. H., Vaidya, B., Gough, S. C., & Franklyn, J. A. (2010). Prevalence and relative risk of other autoimmune diseases in subjects with autoimmune thyroid disease. The American journal of medicine, 123(2), 183.e1–183.e1839. https://doi.org/10.1016/j.amjmed.2009.06.030

[1077] Schultheiss, U. T., Teumer, A., Medici, M., Li, Y., Daya, N., Chaker, L., Homuth, G., Uitterlinden, A. G., Nauck, M., Hofman, A., Selvin, E., Völzke, H., Peeters, R. P., & Köttgen, A. (2015). A genetic risk score for thyroid peroxidase antibodies associates with clinical thyroid disease in community-based populations. The Journal of clinical endocrinology and metabolism, 100(5), E799–E807. https://doi.org/10.1210/jc.2014-4352

[1078] Marinò, M., Latrofa, F., Menconi, F., Chiovato, L., & Vitti, P. (2015). Role of genetic and non-genetic factors in the etiology of Graves' disease. Journal of endocrinological investigation, 38(3), 283–294. https://doi.org/10.1007/s40618-014-0214-2

[1079] Bülow Pedersen, I., Knudsen, N., Carlé, A., Schomburg, L., Köhrle, J., Jørgensen, T., … Laurberg, P. (2013). Serum selenium is low in newly diagnosed Graves' disease: a population-based study. Clinical Endocrinology, 79(4), 584–590. doi:10.1111/cen.12185

[1080] Tomer, Y. & Davies, T. F. (1993) Infection, thyroid disease, and autoimmunity. Endocr. Rev. 14, 107–120.

[1081] Hennemann, G., Docter, R., Friesema, E. C. H., de Jong, M., Krenning, E. P., & Visser, T. J. (2001). Plasma Membrane Transport of Thyroid Hormones and Its Role inThyroid Hormone Metabolism and Bioavailability. Endocrine Reviews, 22(4), 451–476. doi:10.1210/edrv.22.4.0435

[1082] Krenning, E., Docter, R., Bernard, B., Visser, T., & Hennemann, G. (1981). Characteristics of active transport of thyroid hormone into rat hepatocytes. Biochimica et biophysica acta, 676(3), 314–320. https://doi.org/10.1016/0304-4165(81)90165-3

[1083] Centanni, M., & Robbins, J. (1987). Role of sodium in thyroid hormone uptake by rat skeletal muscle. The Journal of clinical investigation, 80(4), 1068–1072. https://doi.org/10.1172/JCI113162

[1084] de Jong, M., Visser, T. J., Bernard, B., Docter, R., Vos, R. A., Hennemann, G., & Krenning, E. P. (1993). Transport and metabolism of iodothyronines in cultured human hepatocytes. The journal of clinical endocrinology and metabolism, 77(1), 139–143. https://doi.org/10.1210/jcem.77.1.8392080

[1085] Krenning, E., Docter, R., Bernard, B., Visser, T., & Hennemann, G. (1980). Regulation of the active transport of 3,3',5-triiodothyronine (T3) into primary cultured rat hepatocytes by ATP. FEBS letters, 119(2), 279–282. https://doi.org/10.1016/0014-5793(80)80271-7

[1086] Osty, J., Valensi, P., Samson, M., Francon, J., & Blondeau, J. P. (1990). Transport of thyroid hormones by human erythrocytes: kinetic characterization in adults and newborns. The Journal of clinical endocrinology and metabolism, 71(6), 1589–1595. https://doi.org/10.1210/jcem-71-6-1589

[1087] Knudsen, N., Laurberg, P., Perrild, H., Bülow, I., Ovesen, L., & Jørgensen, T. (2002). Risk factors for goiter and thyroid nodules. Thyroid : official journal of the American Thyroid Association, 12(10), 879–888. https://doi.org/10.1089/105072502761016502

[1088] Venturi (2015) 'Iodine, PUFAs and Iodolipids in Health and Diseases: An Evolutionary Perspective', Human Evolution. 29 (1–3): 185–205. ISSN 0393-9375.

[1089] Cocchi and Venturi (2000) 'Iodide, antioxidant function and omega-6 and omega-3 fatty acids: A new hypothesis of biochemical cooperation?', Progress in Nutrition 2:15-19.

[1090] NIH (2020) 'Iodine: Fact Sheet for Health Professionals', Dietary Supplement Fact Sheets, Accessed Online Dec 20 2020: https://ods.od.nih.gov/factsheets/Iodine-HealthProfessional/

[1091] World Health Organization & Food and Agriculture Organization of the United Nations. (2004). 'Vitamin and mineral requirements in human nutrition'. Geneva, Switzerland: WHO. Accessed Online Dec 20 2020: https://www.who.int/nutrition/publications/micronutrients/9241546123/en/

[1092] de Benoist et al (2008) 'Iodine deficiency in 2007: Global progress since 2003', Food and Nutrition Bulletin, vol. 29, no. 3 © 2008, The United Nations University, Accessed Online Dec 21 2020: https://www.who.int/nutrition/publications/micronutrients/FNBvol29N3sep08.pdf

[1093] Leung, A. M., & Braverman, L. E. (2014). Consequences of excess iodine. Nature reviews. Endocrinology, 10(3), 136–142. https://doi.org/10.1038/nrendo.2013.251

[1094] Laurberg, P., Cerqueira, C., Ovesen, L., Rasmussen, L. B., Perrild, H., Andersen, S., Pedersen, I. B., & Carlé, A. (2010). Iodine intake as a determinant of thyroid disorders in populations. Best practice & research. Clinical endocrinology & metabolism, 24(1), 13–27. https://doi.org/10.1016/j.beem.2009.08.013

[1095] Teng, W., Shan, Z., Teng, X., Guan, H., Li, Y., Teng, D., … Li, C. (2006). Effect of Iodine Intake on Thyroid Diseases in China. New England Journal of Medicine, 354(26), 2783–2793. doi:10.1056/nejmoa054022

[1096] Farebrother, J., Zimmermann, M. B., & Andersson, M. (2019). Excess iodine intake: sources, assessment, and effects on thyroid function. Annals of the New York Academy of Sciences, 1446(1), 44–65. https://doi.org/10.1111/nyas.14041

[1097] Flores-Rebollar, A., Moreno-Castañeda, L., Vega-Servín, N. S., López-Carrasco, G., & Ruiz-Juvera, A. (2015). PREVALENCE OF AUTOIMMUNE THYROIDITIS AND THYROID DYSFUNCTION IN HEALTHY ADULT MEXICANS WITH A SLIGHTLY EXCESSIVE IODINE INTAKE. Nutricion hospitalaria, 32(2), 918–924. https://doi.org/10.3305/nh.2015.32.2.9246

[1098] Luo, Y., Kawashima, A., Ishido, Y., Yoshihara, A., Oda, K., Hiroi, N., Ito, T., Ishii, N., & Suzuki, K. (2014). Iodine excess as an environmental risk factor for autoimmune thyroid disease. International journal of molecular sciences, 15(7), 12895–12912. https://doi.org/10.3390/ijms150712895

[1099] Institute of Medicine (US) Panel on Micronutrients (2001) 'Dietary Reference Intakes for Vitamin A, Vitamin K, Arsenic, Boron, Chromium, Copper, Iodine, Iron, Manganese, Molybdenum, Nickel, Silicon, Vanadium, and Zinc', Washington (DC): National Academies Press (US); 2001.

[1100] Gardner, D. F., Centor, R. M., & Utiger, R. D. (1988). Effects of low dose oral iodide supplementation on thyroid function in normal men. Clinical endocrinology, 28(3), 283–288. https://doi.org/10.1111/j.1365-2265.1988.tb01214.x

[1101] Chow, C. C., Phillips, D. I., Lazarus, J. H., & Parkes, A. B. (1991). Effect of low dose iodide supplementation on thyroid function in potentially susceptible subjects: are dietary iodide levels in Britain acceptable?. Clinical endocrinology, 34(5), 413–416. https://doi.org/10.1111/j.1365-2265.1991.tb00314.x

[1102] World Health Organization. 1989. Toxological evaluation of certain food additives and contaminants. WHO Food Additives Series 24. Prepared by: The 33rd Meeting of the Joint FAO/WHO Expert Committee on Food Additives (JECFA). Geneva, Switzerland: World Health Organization.

[1103] Patrick L. (2008). Iodine: deficiency and therapeutic considerations. Alternative medicine review : a journal of clinical therapeutic, 13(2), 116–127.

[1104] Nagataki S. (2008). The average of dietary iodine intake due to the ingestion of seaweeds is 1.2 mg/day in Japan. Thyroid : official journal of the American Thyroid Association, 18(6), 667–668. https://doi.org/10.1089/thy.2007.0379

[1105] Zava, T. T., & Zava, D. T. (2011). Assessment of Japanese iodine intake based on seaweed consumption in Japan: A literature-based analysis. Thyroid research, 4, 14. https://doi.org/10.1186/1756-6614-4-14

[1106] Pearce et al (2004) 'Sources of Dietary Iodine: Bread, Cows' Milk, and Infant Formula in the Boston Area', The Journal of Clinical Endocrinology & Metabolism, Volume 89, Issue 7, 1 July 2004, Pages 3421–3424, https://doi.org/10.1210/jc.2003-032002

[1107] Thomson, B. M., Vannoort, R. W., & Haslemore, R. M. (2008). Dietary exposure and trends of exposure to nutrient elements iodine, iron, selenium and sodium from the 2003-4 New Zealand Total Diet Survey. The British journal of nutrition, 99(3), 614–625. https://doi.org/10.1017/S0007114507812001

[1108] Pennington JAT, Schoen SA, Salmon GD, Young B, Johnson RD, Marts RW. Composition of Core Foods of the U.S. Food Supply, 1982-1991. III. Copper, Manganese, Selenium, and Iodine. J Food Comp Anal. 1995;8(2):171-217.

[1109] Barikmo, I., Henjum, S., Dahl, L., Oshaug, A., & Torheim, L. E. (2011). Environmental implication of iodine in water, milk and other foods used in Saharawi refugees camps in Tindouf, Algeria. Journal of Food Composition and Analysis, 24(4-5), 637–641. doi:10.1016/j.jfca.2010.10.003

[1110] Ershow, A. G., Skeaff, S. A., Merkel, J. M., & Pehrsson, P. R. (2018). Development of Databases on Iodine in Foods and Dietary Supplements. Nutrients, 10(1), 100. https://doi.org/10.3390/nu10010100

[1111] NIH (2020) 'Iodine: Health Professional Fact Sheet', Dietary Supplement Fact Sheets, Accessed Online Dec 21 2020: https://ods.od.nih.gov/factsheets/Iodine-HealthProfessional/

[1112] USDA (2020) 'USDA, FDA and ODS-NIH Database for the Iodine Content of Common Foods Release 1.0 (2020)', Iodine, Accessed Online Dec 21 2020: https://www.ars.usda.gov/northeast-area/beltsville-md-bhnrc/beltsville-human-nutrition-research-center/methods-and-application-of-food-composition-laboratory/mafcl-site-pages/iodine/

[1113] Pehrsson, P. R., Patterson, K. Y., Spungen, J. H., Wirtz, M. S., Andrews, K. W., Dwyer, J. T., & Swanson, C. A. (2016). Iodine in food-and dietary supplement-composition databases. The American journal of clinical nutrition, 104 Suppl 3(Suppl 3), 868S–76S. https://doi.org/10.3945/ajcn.115.110064

[1114] College of Agriculture and Life Sciences (2019) 'Glucosinolates (Goitrogenic Glycosides)', Department of Animal Science - Plants Poisonous to Livestock, Accessed Online Dec 23 2020: http://poisonousplants.ansci.cornell.edu/toxicagents/glucosin.html

[1115] Petre (2017) 'Are Goitrogens in Foods Harmful?', Healthline, Accessed Online Dec 23 2020: https://www.healthline.com/nutrition/goitrogens-in-foods

[1116] Rungapamestry, V., Duncan, A. J., Fuller, Z., & Ratcliffe, B. (2007). Effect of cooking brassica vegetables on the subsequent hydrolysis and metabolic fate of glucosinolates. The Proceedings of the Nutrition Society, 66(1), 69–81. https://doi.org/10.1017/S0029665107005319

[1117] McMillan, M., Spinks, E. A., & Fenwick, G. R. (1986). Preliminary Observations on the Effect of Dietary Brussels Sprouts on Thyroid Function. Human Toxicology, 5(1), 15–19. https://doi.org/10.1177/096032718600500104

[1118] National Cancer Institute (2012) 'Cruciferous Vegetables and Cancer Prevention', Cancer Causes and Prevention, NIH, Accessed Online Dec 23 2020: https://www.cancer.gov/about-cancer/causes-prevention/risk/diet/cruciferous-vegetables-fact-sheet

[1119] Hecht, S. S. (2000). Inhibition of carcinogenesis by isothiocyanates. Drug metabolism reviews, 32(3-4), 395–411. https://doi.org/10.1081/dmr-100102342

[1120] Murillo, G., & Mehta, R. G. (2001). Cruciferous vegetables and cancer prevention. Nutrition and cancer, 41(1-2), 17–28. https://doi.org/10.1080/01635581.2001.9680607

[1121] Dai, G., Levy, O., & Carrasco, N. (1996). Cloning and characterization of the thyroid iodide transporter. Nature, 379(6564), 458–460. https://doi.org/10.1038/379458a0

[1122] Dohán, O., De la Vieja, A., Paroder, V., Riedel, C., Artani, M., Reed, M., Ginter, C. S., & Carrasco, N. (2003). The sodium/iodide Symporter (NIS): characterization, regulation, and medical significance. Endocrine reviews, 24(1), 48–77. https://doi.org/10.1210/er.2001-0029

[1123] Hennemann, G., Docter, R., Friesema, E. C. H., de Jong, M., Krenning, E. P., & Visser, T. J. (2001). Plasma Membrane Transport of Thyroid Hormones and Its Role inThyroid Hormone Metabolism and Bioavailability. Endocrine Reviews, 22(4), 451–476. doi:10.1210/edrv.22.4.0435

[1124] Krenning, E., Docter, R., Bernard, B., Visser, T., & Hennemann, G. (1981). Characteristics of active transport of thyroid hormone into rat hepatocytes. Biochimica et biophysica acta, 676(3), 314–320. https://doi.org/10.1016/0304-4165(81)90165-3

[1125] Centanni, M., & Robbins, J. (1987). Role of sodium in thyroid hormone uptake by rat skeletal muscle. The Journal of clinical investigation, 80(4), 1068–1072. https://doi.org/10.1172/JCI113162

[1126] de Jong, M., Visser, T. J., Bernard, B. F., Docter, R., Vos, R. A., Hennemann, G., & Krenning, E. P. (1993). Transport and metabolism of iodothyronines in cultured human hepatocytes. The Journal of clinical endocrinology and metabolism, 77(1), 139–143. https://doi.org/10.1210/jcem.77.1.8392080

[1127] Krenning, E., Docter, R., Bernard, B., Visser, T., & Hennemann, G. (1980). Regulation of the active transport of 3,3',5-triiodothyronine (T3) into primary cultured rat hepatocytes by ATP. FEBS letters, 119(2), 279–282. https://doi.org/10.1016/0014-5793(80)80271-7

[1128] Osty, J., Valensi, P., Samson, M., Francon, J., & Blondeau, J. P. (1990). Transport of thyroid hormones by human erythrocytes: kinetic characterization in adults and newborns. The Journal of clinical endocrinology and metabolism, 71(6), 1589–1595. https://doi.org/10.1210/jcem-71-6-1589

[1129] Ergin AB, Bena J, Nasr CE (2017) Hypothyroidism and Hyponatremia: Simple Association or True Causation. Open J Thyroid Res 1(1): 012-016.

[1130] Bates, J. M., Spate, V. L., Morris, J. S., St Germain, D. L., & Galton, V. A. (2000). Effects of selenium deficiency on tissue selenium content, deiodinase activity, and thyroid hormone economy in the rat during development. Endocrinology, 141(7), 2490–2500. https://doi.org/10.1210/endo.141.7.7571

[1131] Contempre, B., Dumont, J. E., Ngo, B., Thilly, C. H., Diplock, A. T., & Vanderpas, J. (1991). Effect of selenium supplementation in hypothyroid subjects of an iodine and selenium deficient area: the possible danger of indiscriminate supplementation of iodine-deficient subjects with selenium. The Journal of clinical endocrinology and metabolism, 73(1), 213–215. https://doi.org/10.1210/jcem-73-1-213

[1132] https://www.ncbi.nlm.nih.gov/pubmed/21036373

[1133] Iwaoka, T., Umeda, T., Inoue, J., Naomi, S., Sasaki, M., Fujimoto, Y., Gui, C., Ideguchi, Y., & Sato, T. (1994). Dietary NaCl restriction deteriorates oral glucose tolerance in hypertensive patients with impairment of glucose tolerance. American journal of hypertension, 7(5), 460–463. https://doi.org/10.1093/ajh/7.5.460

[1134] Iwaoka, T., Umeda, T., Ohno, M., Inoue, J., Naomi, S., Sato, T., & Kawakami, I. (1988). The effect of low and high NaCl diets on oral glucose tolerance. Klinische Wochenschrift, 66(16), 724–728. https://doi.org/10.1007/BF01726415

[1135] Garg, R., Williams, G. H., Hurwitz, S., Brown, N. J., Hopkins, P. N., & Adler, G. K. (2011). Low-salt diet increases insulin resistance in healthy subjects. Metabolism: clinical and experimental, 60(7), 965–968. https://doi.org/10.1016/j.metabol.2010.09.005

[1136] Garg, R., Sun, B., & Williams, J. (2014). Effect of low salt diet on insulin resistance in salt-sensitive versus salt-resistant hypertension. Hypertension (Dallas, Tex. : 1979), 64(6), 1384–1387. https://doi.org/10.1161/HYPERTENSIONAHA.114.03880

[1137] Gomi, T., Shibuya, Y., Sakurai, J., Hirawa, N., Hasegawa, K., & Ikeda, T. (1998). Strict dietary sodium reduction worsens insulin sensitivity by increasing sympathetic nervous activity in patients with primary hypertension. American journal of hypertension, 11(9), 1048–1055. https://doi.org/10.1016/s0895-7061(98)00126-5

[1138] Townsend, R. R., Kapoor, S., & McFadden, C. B. (2007). Salt intake and insulin sensitivity in healthy human volunteers. Clinical science (London, England : 1979), 113(3), 141–148. https://doi.org/10.1042/CS20060361

[1139] Perry, C. G., Palmer, T., Cleland, S. J., Morton, I. J., Salt, I. P., Petrie, J. R., Gould, G. W., & Connell, J. M. (2003). Decreased insulin sensitivity during dietary sodium restriction is not mediated by effects of angiotensin II on insulin action. Clinical science (London, England : 1979), 105(2), 187–194. https://doi.org/10.1042/CS20020320

[1140] Egan, B. M., Weder, A. B., Petrin, J., & Hoffman, R. G. (1991). Neurohumoral and metabolic effects of short-term dietary NaCl restriction in men. Relationship to salt-sensitivity status. American journal of hypertension, 4(5 Pt 1), 416–421. https://doi.org/10.1093/ajh/4.5.416

[1141] Ruppert, M., Diehl, J., Kolloch, R., Overlack, A., Kraft, K., Göbel, B., Hittel, N., & Stumpe, K. O. (1991). Short-term dietary sodium restriction increases serum lipids and insulin in salt-sensitive and salt-resistant normotensive adults. Klinische Wochenschrift, 69 Suppl 25, 51–57.

[1142] Weder, A. B., & Egan, B. M. (1991). Potential deleterious impact of dietary salt restriction on cardiovascular risk factors. Klinische Wochenschrift, 69 Suppl 25, 45–50.

[1143] Egan, B. M., Stepniakowski, K., & Goodfriend, T. L. (1994). Renin and aldosterone are higher and the hyperinsulinemic effect of salt restriction greater in subjects with risk factors clustering. American journal of hypertension, 7(10 Pt 1), 886–893. https://doi.org/10.1016/0895-7061(94)P1710-H

[1144] Del Río, A., & Rodríguez-Villamil, J. L. (1993). Metabolic effects of strict salt restriction in essential hypertensive patients. Journal of internal medicine, 233(5), 409–414. https://doi.org/10.1111/j.1365-2796.1993.tb00692.x

[1145] Meland, E., Laerum, E., Aakvaag, A., & Ulvik, R. J. (1994). Salt restriction and increased insulin production in hypertensive patients. Scandinavian journal of clinical and laboratory investigation, 54(5), 405–409. https://doi.org/10.3109/00365519409088441

[1146] Feldman, R. D., & Schmidt, N. D. (1999). Moderate dietary salt restriction increases vascular and systemic insulin resistance. American journal of hypertension, 12(6), 643–647. https://doi.org/10.1016/s0895-7061(99)00016-3

[1147] https://www.ncbi.nlm.nih.gov/pubmed/20226958

[1148] Yatabe, M. S., Yatabe, J., Yoneda, M., Watanabe, T., Otsuki, M., Felder, R. A., Jose, P. A., & Sanada, H. (2010). Salt sensitivity is associated with insulin resistance, sympathetic overactivity, and decreased suppression of circulating renin activity in lean patients with essential hypertension. The American journal of clinical nutrition, 92(1), 77–82. https://doi.org/10.3945/ajcn.2009.29028

[1149] Ongphiphadhanakul, B., Fang, S. L., Tang, K.-T., Patwardhan, N. A., & Braverman, L. E. (1994). Tumor necrosis factor-α decreases thyrotropin-induced 5′-deiodinase activity in FRTL-5 thyroid cells. European Journal of Endocrinology, 130(5), 502–507. doi:10.1530/eje.0.1300502

[1150] Abdullatif, H. D., & Ashraf, A. P. (2006). REVERSIBLE SUBCLINICAL HYPOTHYROIDISM IN THE PRESENCE OF ADRENAL INSUFFICIENCY. Endocrine Practice, 12(5), 572–575. doi:10.4158/ep.12.5.572

[1151] Wadden, T. A., Mason, G., Foster, G. D., Stunkard, A. J., & Prange, A. J. (1990). Effects of a very low calorie diet on weight, thyroid hormones and mood. International journal of obesity, 14(3), 249–258.

[1152] Fliers, E., Kalsbeek, A., & Boelen, A. (2014). MECHANISMS IN ENDOCRINOLOGY: Beyond the fixed setpoint of the hypothalamus–pituitary–thyroid axis. European Journal of Endocrinology, 171(5), R197–R208. doi:10.1530/eje-14-0285

[1153] Chan, J. L., Heist, K., DePaoli, A. M., Veldhuis, J. D., & Mantzoros, C. S. (2003). The role of falling leptin levels in the neuroendocrine and metabolic adaptation to short-term starvation in healthy men. Journal of Clinical Investigation, 111(9), 1409–1421. doi:10.1172/jci200317490

[1154] CARLSON, H. E., DRENICK, E. J., CHOPRA, I. J., & HERSHMAN, J. M. (1977). Alterations in Basal and TRH-Stimulated Serum Levels of Thyrotropin, Prolactin, and Thyroid Hormones in Starved Obese Men. The Journal of Clinical Endocrinology & Metabolism, 45(4), 707–713. doi:10.1210/jcem-45-4-707

[1155] Anita Boelen, Wilmar Maarten Wiersinga, and Eric Fliers.Thyroid.Feb 2008.123-129.http://doi.org/10.1089/thy.2007.0253

1156 Friedman, J. M., & Halaas, J. L. (1998). Leptin and the regulation of body weight in mammals. Nature, 395(6704), 763–770. doi:10.1038/27376

1157 Margetic, S., Gazzola, C., Pegg, G. G., & Hill, R. A. (2002). Leptin: a review of its peripheral actions and interactions. International journal of obesity and related metabolic disorders : journal of the International Association for the Study of Obesity, 26(11), 1407–1433. https://doi.org/10.1038/sj.ijo.0802142

1158 Montague, C. T., Farooqi, I. S., Whitehead, J. P., Soos, M. A., Rau, H., Wareham, N. J., Sewter, C. P., Digby, J. E., Mohammed, S. N., Hurst, J. A., Cheetham, C. H., Earley, A. R., Barnett, A. H., Prins, J. B., & O'Rahilly, S. (1997). Congenital leptin deficiency is associated with severe early-onset obesity in humans. Nature, 387(6636), 903–908. https://doi.org/10.1038/43185

1159 Farooqi, I. S., Matarese, G., Lord, G. M., Keogh, J. M., Lawrence, E., Agwu, C., Sanna, V., Jebb, S. A., Perna, F., Fontana, S., Lechler, R. I., DePaoli, A. M., & O'Rahilly, S. (2002). Beneficial effects of leptin on obesity, T cell hyporesponsiveness, and neuroendocrine/metabolic dysfunction of human congenital leptin deficiency. The Journal of clinical investigation, 110(8), 1093–1103. https://doi.org/10.1172/JCI15693

1160 Gibson, W. T., Farooqi, I. S., Moreau, M., DePaoli, A. M., Lawrence, E., O'Rahilly, S., & Trussell, R. A. (2004). Congenital leptin deficiency due to homozygosity for the Delta133G mutation: report of another case and evaluation of response to four years of leptin therapy. The Journal of clinical endocrinology and metabolism, 89(10), 4821–4826. https://doi.org/10.1210/jc.2004-0376

1161 Farooqi, I. S., Jebb, S. A., Langmack, G., Lawrence, E., Cheetham, C. H., Prentice, A. M., Hughes, I. A., McCamish, M. A., & O'Rahilly, S. (1999). Effects of recombinant leptin therapy in a child with congenital leptin deficiency. The New England journal of medicine, 341(12), 879–884. https://doi.org/10.1056/NEJM199909163411204

1162 Knight, Z. A., Hannan, K. S., Greenberg, M. L., & Friedman, J. M. (2010). Hyperleptinemia Is Required for the Development of Leptin Resistance. PLoS ONE, 5(6), e11376. doi:10.1371/journal.pone.0011376

1163 Haas, V. K., Gaskin, K. J., Kohn, M. R., Clarke, S. D., & Müller, M. J. (2010). Different thermic effects of leptin in adolescent females with varying body fat content. Clinical nutrition (Edinburgh, Scotland), 29(5), 639–645. https://doi.org/10.1016/j.clnu.2010.03.013

1164 Maffei, M., Halaas, J., Ravussin, E., Pratley, R. E., Lee, G. H., Zhang, Y., … Friedman, J. M. (1995). Leptin levels in human and rodent: Measurement of plasma leptin and ob RNA in obese and weight-reduced subjects. Nature Medicine, 1(11), 1155–1161. doi:10.1038/nm1195-1155

1165 Lindqvist, A., de la Cour, C. D., Stegmark, A., Håkanson, R., & Erlanson-Albertsson, C. (2005). Overeating of palatable food is associated with blunted leptin and ghrelin responses. Regulatory Peptides, 130(3), 123–132. doi:10.1016/j.regpep.2005.05.002

1166 Jung, C. H., & Kim, M. S. (2013). Molecular mechanisms of central leptin resistance in obesity. Archives of pharmacal research, 36(2), 201–207. https://doi.org/10.1007/s12272-013-0020-y

1167 Santini, F., Galli, G., Maffei, M., Fierabracci, P., Pelosini, C., Marsili, A., Giannetti, M., Castagna, M. G., Checchi, S., Molinaro, E., Piaggi, P., Pacini, F., Elisei, R., Vitti, P., & Pinchera, A. (2010). Acute exogenous TSH administration stimulates leptin secretion in vivo. European journal of endocrinology, 163(1), 63–67. https://doi.org/10.1530/EJE-10-0138

1168 Oge, A., Bayraktar, F., Saygili, F., Guney, E., & Demir, S. (2005). TSH influences serum leptin levels independent of thyroid hormones in hypothyroid and hyperthyroid patients. Endocrine journal, 52(2), 213–217. https://doi.org/10.1507/endocrj.52.213

1169 Menendez, C., Baldelli, R., Camiña, J. P., Escudero, B., Peino, R., Dieguez, C., & Casanueva, F. F. (2003). TSH stimulates leptin secretion by a direct effect on adipocytes. The Journal of endocrinology, 176(1), 7–12. https://doi.org/10.1677/joe.0.1760007

1170 Iacobellis, G., Ribaudo, M. C., Zappaterreno, A., Iannucci, C. V., & Leonetti, F. (2005). Relationship of thyroid function with body mass index, leptin, insulin sensitivity and adiponectin in euthyroid obese women. Clinical endocrinology, 62(4), 487–491. https://doi.org/10.1111/j.1365-2265.2005.02247.x

1171 Zimmermann-Belsing, T., Brabant, G., Holst, J. J., & Feldt-Rasmussen, U. (2003). Circulating leptin and thyroid dysfunction. European journal of endocrinology, 149(4), 257–271. https://doi.org/10.1530/eje.0.1490257

1172 Reinehr T. (2010). Obesity and thyroid function. Molecular and cellular endocrinology, 316(2), 165–171. https://doi.org/10.1016/j.mce.2009.06.005

1173 Reinehr, T., de Sousa, G., & Andler, W. (2006). Hyperthyrotropinemia in obese children is reversible after weight loss and is not related to lipids. The Journal of clinical endocrinology and metabolism, 91(8), 3088–3091. https://doi.org/10.1210/jc.2006-0095

1174 Nannipieri, M., Cecchetti, F., Anselmino, M., Camastra, S., Niccolini, P., Lamacchia, M., Rossi, M., Iervasi, G., & Ferrannini, E. (2009). Expression of thyrotropin and thyroid hormone receptors in adipose tissue of patients with morbid obesity and/or type 2 diabetes: effects of weight loss. International journal of obesity (2005), 33(9), 1001–1006. https://doi.org/10.1038/ijo.2009.140

1175 De Pergola, G., Ciampolillo, A., Paolotti, S., Trerotoli, P., & Giorgino, R. (2007). Free triiodothyronine and thyroid stimulating hormone are directly associated with waist circumference, independently of insulin resistance, metabolic parameters and blood pressure in overweight and obese women. Clinical endocrinology, 67(2), 265–269. https://doi.org/10.1111/j.1365-2265.2007.02874.x

1176 Cusin, I., Rouru, J., Visser, T., Burger, A. G., & Rohner-Jeanrenaud, F. (2000). Involvement of thyroid hormones in the effect of intracerebroventricular leptin infusion on uncoupling protein-3 expression in rat muscle. Diabetes, 49(7), 1101–1105. https://doi.org/10.2337/diabetes.49.7.1101

1177 Gong, D. W., He, Y., Karas, M., & Reitman, M. (1997). Uncoupling protein-3 is a mediator of thermogenesis regulated by thyroid hormone, beta3-adrenergic agonists, and leptin. The Journal of biological chemistry, 272(39), 24129–24132. https://doi.org/10.1074/jbc.272.39.24129

1178 Nannipieri, M., Cecchetti, F., Anselmino, M., Camastra, S., Niccolini, P., Lamacchia, M., Rossi, M., Iervasi, G., & Ferrannini, E. (2009). Expression of thyrotropin and thyroid hormone receptors in adipose tissue of patients with morbid obesity and/or type 2 diabetes: effects of weight loss. International journal of obesity (2005), 33(9), 1001–1006. https://doi.org/10.1038/ijo.2009.140

1179 Kok, P., Roelfsema, F., Langendonk, J. G., Frölich, M., Burggraaf, J., Meinders, A. E., & Pijl, H. (2005). High circulating thyrotropin levels in obese women are reduced after body weight loss induced by caloric restriction. The Journal of clinical endocrinology and metabolism, 90(8), 4659–4663. https://doi.org/10.1210/jc.2005-0920

1180 Bray, G. A., Fisher, D. A., & Chopra, I. J. (1976). Relation of thyroid hormones to body-weight. Lancet (London, England), 1(7971), 1206–1208. https://doi.org/10.1016/s0140-6736(76)92158-9

1181 Doucet, E., St-Pierre, S., Alméras, N., Després, J. P., Bouchard, C., & Tremblay, A. (2001). Evidence for the existence of adaptive thermogenesis during weight loss. The British journal of nutrition, 85(6), 715–723. https://doi.org/10.1079/bjn2001348

1182 Dulloo, A. G., & Jacquet, J. (1998). Adaptive reduction in basal metabolic rate in response to food deprivation in humans: a role for feedback signals from fat stores. The American Journal of Clinical Nutrition, 68(3), 599–606. doi:10.1093/ajcn/68.3.599

1183 Bevilacqua, L., Ramsey, J. J., Hagopian, K., Weindruch, R., & Harper, M.-E. (2004). Effects of short- and medium-term calorie restriction on muscle mitochondrial proton leak and reactive oxygen species production. American Journal of Physiology-Endocrinology and Metabolism, 286(5), E852–E861. doi:10.1152/ajpendo.00367.2003

1184 Esterbauer, H., Oberkofler, H., Dallinger, G., Breban, D., Hell, E., Krempler, F., & Patsch, W. (1999). Uncoupling protein-3 gene expression: reduced skeletal muscle mRNA in obese humans during pronounced weight loss. Diabetologia, 42(3), 302–309. doi:10.1007/s001250051155

1185 Fothergill, E., Guo, J., Howard, L., Kerns, J. C., Knuth, N. D., Brychta, R., … Hall, K. D. (2016). Persistent metabolic adaptation 6 years after "The Biggest Loser" competition. Obesity, 24(8), 1612–1619. doi:10.1002/oby.21538

1186 Mäestu, J., Jürimäe, J., Valter, I., & Jürimäe, T. (2008). Increases in ghrelin and decreases in leptin without altering adiponectin during extreme weight loss in male competitive bodybuilders. Metabolism, 57(2), 221–225. doi:10.1016/j.metabol.2007.09.004

1187 Byrne, N. M., Sainsbury, A., King, N. A., Hills, A. P., & Wood, R. E. (2017). Intermittent energy restriction improves weight loss efficiency in obese men: the MATADOR study. International Journal of Obesity, 42(2), 129–138. doi:10.1038/ijo.2017.206

1188 Byrne, N. M., Sainsbury, A., King, N. A., Hills, A. P., & Wood, R. E. (2017). Intermittent energy restriction improves weight loss efficiency in obese men: the MATADOR study. International Journal of Obesity, 42(2), 129–138. doi:10.1038/ijo.2017.206

1189 Chin-Chance, C., Polonsky, K. S., & Schoeller, D. A. (2000). Twenty-four-hour leptin levels respond to cumulative short-term energy imbalance and predict subsequent intake. The Journal of clinical endocrinology and metabolism, 85(8), 2685–2691. https://doi.org/10.1210/jcem.85.8.6755

1190 Dirlewanger, M., di Vetta, V., Guenat, E., Battilana, P., Seematter, G., Schneiter, P., Jéquier, E., & Tappy, L. (2000). Effects of short-term carbohydrate or fat overfeeding on energy expenditure and plasma leptin concentrations in healthy female subjects. International journal of obesity and related metabolic disorders : journal of the International Association for the Study of Obesity, 24(11), 1413–1418. https://doi.org/10.1038/sj.ijo.0801395

1191 Spaulding, S. W., Chopra, I. J., Sherwin, R. S., & Lyall, S. S. (1976). EFFECT OF CALORIC RESTRICTION AND DIETARY COMPOSITION ON SERUM T3 AND REVERSE T3 IN MAN. The Journal of Clinical Endocrinology & Metabolism, 42(1), 197–200. doi:10.1210/jcem-42-1-197

1192 Jenkins, A. B., Markovic, T. P., Fleury, A., & Campbell, L. V. (1997). Carbohydrate intake and short-term regulation of leptin in humans. Diabetologia, 40(3), 348–351. https://doi.org/10.1007/s001250050686

[1193] Azizi, F. (1978). Effect of dietary composition on fasting-induced changes in serum thyroid hormones and thyrotropin. Metabolism, 27(8), 935–942. doi:10.1016/0026-0495(78)90137-3

[1194] Spaulding, S. W., Chopra, I. J., Sherwin, R. S., & Lyall, S. S. (1976). EFFECT OF CALORIC RESTRICTION AND DIETARY COMPOSITION ON SERUM T3 AND REVERSE T3 IN MAN. The Journal of Clinical Endocrinology & Metabolism, 42(1), 197–200. doi:10.1210/jcem-42-1-197

[1195] Paz-Filho, G., Wong, M.-L., Licinio, J., & Mastronardi, C. (2012). Leptin therapy, insulin sensitivity, and glucose homeostasis. Indian Journal of Endocrinology and Metabolism, 16(9), 549. doi:10.4103/2230-8210.105571

[1196] Berglund, E. D., Vianna, C. R., Donato, J., Kim, M. H., Chuang, J.-C., Lee, C. E., … Elmquist, J. K. (2012). Direct leptin action on POMC neurons regulates glucose homeostasis and hepatic insulin sensitivity in mice. Journal of Clinical Investigation, 122(3), 1000–1009. doi:10.1172/jci59816

[1197] Fery et al (1982) 'Hormonal and metabolic changes induced by an isocaloric isoproteinic ketogenic diet in healthy subjects', Diabete Metab. 1982 Dec;8(4):299-305.

[1198] Kinzig, K. P., Honors, M. A., & Hargrave, S. L. (2010). Insulin sensitivity and glucose tolerance are altered by maintenance on a ketogenic diet. Endocrinology, 151(7), 3105–3114. https://doi.org/10.1210/en.2010-0175

[1199] Boden et al (2005). Effect of a low-carbohydrate diet on appetite, blood glucose levels, and insulin resistance in obese patients with type 2 diabetes. Annals of internal medicine, 142(6), 403–411. https://doi.org/10.7326/0003-4819-142-6-200503150-00006

[1200] Ellis, Amy C; Hyatt, Tanya C; Gower, Barbara A; Hunter, Gary R (2017-05-02). "Respiratory Quotient Predicts Fat Mass Gain in Premenopausal Women". Obesity (Silver Spring, Md.). 18 (12): 2255–2259.

[1201] al-Saady et al (1989) 'High fat, low carbohydrate, enteral feeding lowers PaCO2 and reduces the period of ventilation in artificially ventilated patients', Intensive Care Med. 1989;15(5):290-5.

[1202] Bohr et al (1904) 'Concerning a Biologically Important Relationship - The Influence of the Carbon Dioxide Content of Blood on its Oxygen Binding', Skand. Arch. Physiol. 16, 401-412 (1904) by Ulf Marquardt for CHEM-342, January 1997, Accessed Online: https://www1.udel.edu/chem/white/C342/Bohr(1904).html

[1203] Lee and Levine (1999) 'Acute respiratory alkalosis associated with low minute ventilation in a patient with severe hypothyroidism', Can J Anaesth. 1999 Feb;46(2):185-9.

[1204] De Jong, M., Docter, R., Bernard, B. F., van der Heijden, J. T., van Toor, H., Krenning, E. P., & Hennemann, G. (1994). T4 uptake into the perfused rat liver and liver T4 uptake in humans are inhibited by fructose. The American journal of physiology, 266(5 Pt 1), E768–E775. https://doi.org/10.1152/ajpendo.1994.266.5.E768

[1205] De Jong, M., Docter, R., Van Der Hoek, H. J., Vos, R. A., Krenning, E. P., & Hennemann, G. (1992). Transport of 3,5,3'-triiodothyronine into the perfused rat liver and subsequent metabolism are inhibited by fasting. Endocrinology, 131(1), 463–470. https://doi.org/10.1210/endo.131.1.1612027

[1206] Bodoky, G., Yang, Z. J., Meguid, M. M., Laviano, A., & Szeverenyi, N. (1995). Effects of fasting, intermittent feeding, or continuous parenteral nutrition on rat liver and brain energy metabolism as assessed by 31P-NMR. Physiology & behavior, 58(3), 521–527. https://doi.org/10.1016/0031-9384(95)00078-w

[1207] De Jong, M., Docter, R., Bernard, B. F., van der Heijden, J. T., van Toor, H., Krenning, E. P., & Hennemann, G. (1994). T4 uptake into the perfused rat liver and liver T4 uptake in humans are inhibited by fructose. The American journal of physiology, 266(5 Pt 1), E768–E775. https://doi.org/10.1152/ajpendo.1994.266.5.E768

[1208] Greene, H. L., Wilson, F. A., Hefferan, P., Terry, A. B., Moran, J. R., Slonim, A. E., Claus, T. H., & Burr, I. M. (1978). ATP depletion, a possible role in the pathogenesis of hyperuricemia in glycogen storage disease type I. The Journal of clinical investigation, 62(2), 321–328. https://doi.org/10.1172/JCI109132

[1209] Birdsong, W. T., Fierro, L., Williams, F. G., Spelta, V., Naves, L. A., Knowles, M., … McCleskey, E. W. (2010). Sensing Muscle Ischemia: Coincident Detection of Acid and ATP via Interplay of Two Ion Channels. Neuron, 68(4), 739–749. doi:10.1016/j.neuron.2010.09.029

[1210] Kalra et al (2019). Thyroid Dysfunction and Type 2 Diabetes Mellitus: Screening Strategies and Implications for Management. Diabetes therapy : research, treatment and education of diabetes and related disorders, 10(6), 2035–2044.

[1211] Krysiak, R., Gilowska, M., Szkróbka, W., & Okopień, B. (2016). The effect of metformin on the hypothalamic-pituitary-thyroid axis in patients with type 2 diabetes and amiodarone-induced hypothyroidism. Pharmacological Reports, 68(2), 490–494. https://doi.org/10.1016/j.pharep.2015.11.010

[1212] Nishi M. (2018). Diabetes mellitus and thyroid diseases. Diabetology international, 9(2), 108–112.

[1213] Gutch et al (2017) 'Unusual antithyroid drug-induced hypoglycemia', Chrismed Journal of Health and Research, 4:3, 198-200.

[1214] Bilic-Komarica et al (2012). Effects of treatment with L-thyroxin on glucose regulation in patients with subclinical hypothyroidism. Medical archives (Sarajevo, Bosnia and Herzegovina), 66(6), 364–368.

[1215] Fuchs, F. D., & Whelton, P. K. (2020). High Blood Pressure and Cardiovascular Disease. Hypertension, 75(2), 285–292. doi:10.1161/hypertensionaha.119.14240

[1216] Franklin, S. S., & Wong, N. D. (2013). Hypertension and Cardiovascular Disease: Contributions of the Framingham Heart Study. Global Heart, 8(1), 49. doi:10.1016/j.gheart.2012.12.004

[1217] Lopez, A. D., & Mathers, C. D. (2006). Measuring the global burden of disease and epidemiological transitions: 2002-2030. Annals of tropical medicine and parasitology, 100(5-6), 481–499. https://doi.org/10.1179/136485906X97417

[1218] World Health Organization (2019) 'Hypertension', Health Topics, Fact Sheets, Accessed Online Dec 28 2020: https://www.who.int/news-room/fact-sheets/detail/hypertension

[1219] Rigaud and Forette (2001) 'Hypertension in Older Adults', The Journals of Gerontology: Series A, Volume 56, Issue 4, 1 April 2001, Pages M217–M225, https://doi.org/10.1093/gerona/56.4.M217

[1220] Roger, V. L., Go, A. S., Lloyd-Jones, D. M., Benjamin, E. J., Berry, J. D., Borden, W. B., Bravata, D. M., Dai, S., Ford, E. S., Fox, C. S., Fullerton, H. J., Gillespie, C., Hailpern, S. M., Heit, J. A., Howard, V. J., Kissela, B. M., Kittner, S. J., Lackland, D. T., Lichtman, J. H., Lisabeth, L. D., ... American Heart Association Statistics Committee and Stroke Statistics Subcommittee (2012). Executive summary: heart disease and stroke statistics--2012 update: a report from the American Heart Association. Circulation, 125(1), 188–197. https://doi.org/10.1161/CIR.0b013e3182456d46

[1221] Hall, J. E., do Carmo, J. M., da Silva, A. A., Wang, Z., & Hall, M. E. (2015). Obesity-Induced Hypertension. Circulation Research, 116(6), 991–1006. doi:10.1161/circresaha.116.305697

[1222] Dimeo, F., Pagonas, N., Seibert, F., Arndt, R., Zidek, W., & Westhoff, T. H. (2012). Aerobic Exercise Reduces Blood Pressure in Resistant Hypertension. Hypertension, 60(3), 653–658. doi:10.1161/hypertensionaha.112.197780

[1223] Beilin, L. J., & Puddey, I. B. (2006). Alcohol and Hypertension. Hypertension, 47(6), 1035–1038. doi:10.1161/01.hyp.0000218586.21932.3c

[1224] Primatesta, P., Falaschetti, E., Gupta, S., Marmot, M. G., & Poulter, N. R. (2001). Association Between Smoking and Blood Pressure. Hypertension, 37(2), 187–193. doi:10.1161/01.hyp.37.2.187

[1225] Samiee Rad et al (2020). Association between hypertension and insulin resistance in non-diabetic adult populations: a community-based study from the Iran. Arterial Hypertension, 24(4), 159–166.

[1226] Babu, G. R., Murthy, G., Ana, Y., Patel, P., Deepa, R., Neelon, S., Kinra, S., & Reddy, K. S. (2018). Association of obesity with hypertension and type 2 diabetes mellitus in India: A meta-analysis of observational studies. World journal of diabetes, 9(1), 40–52. https://doi.org/10.4239/wjd.v9.i1.40

[1227] Saad, M. F., Rewers, M., Selby, J., Howard, G., Jinagouda, S., Fahmi, S., ... Haffner, S. M. (2004). Insulin Resistance and Hypertension. Hypertension, 43(6), 1324–1331. doi:10.1161/01.hyp.0000128019.19363.f9

[1228] Lastra et al (2010). Salt, aldosterone, and insulin resistance: impact on the cardiovascular system. Nature reviews. Cardiology, 7(10), 577–584.

[1229] Zhou, MS., Wang, A. & Yu, H. Link between insulin resistance and hypertension: What is the evidence from evolutionary biology?. Diabetol Metab Syndr 6, 12 (2014).

[1230] Fournier et al (1986). Blood pressure, insulin, and glycemia in nondiabetic subjects. The American journal of medicine, 80(5), 861–864.

[1231] Falkner et al (1990). Insulin resistance and blood pressure in young black men. Hypertension (Dallas, Tex. : 1979), 16(6), 706–711.

[1232] Manolio et al (1990). Association of fasting insulin with blood pressure and lipids in young adults. The CARDIA study. Arteriosclerosis: An Official Journal of the American Heart Association, Inc., 10(3), 430–436.

[1233] Young, D. B., Lin, H., & McCabe, R. D. (1995). Potassium's cardiovascular protective mechanisms. The American journal of physiology, 268(4 Pt 2), R825–R837. https://doi.org/10.1152/ajpregu.1995.268.4.R825

[1234] Haddy, F. J., Vanhoutte, P. M., & Feletou, M. (2006). Role of potassium in regulating blood flow and blood pressure. American journal of physiology. Regulatory, integrative and comparative physiology, 290(3), R546–R552. https://doi.org/10.1152/ajpregu.00491.2005

[1235] Houston M. C. (2011). The importance of potassium in managing hypertension. Current hypertension reports, 13(4), 309–317. https://doi.org/10.1007/s11906-011-0197-8

[1236] SAGILD, U., ANDERSEN, V., & ANDREASEN, P. B. (1961). Glucose tolerance and insulin responsiveness in experimental potassium depletion. Acta medica Scandinavica, 169, 243–251. https://doi.org/10.1111/j.0954-6820.1961.tb07829.x

[1237] Rowe, J. W., Tobin, J. D., Rosa, R. M., & Andres, R. (1980). Effect of experimental potassium deficiency on glucose and insulin metabolism. Metabolism, 29(6), 498–502. doi:10.1016/0026-0495(80)90074-8

[1238] Ekmekcioglu, C., Elmadfa, I., Meyer, A. L., & Moeslinger, T. (2016). The role of dietary potassium in hypertension and diabetes. Journal of physiology and biochemistry, 72(1), 93–106. https://doi.org/10.1007/s13105-015-0449-1

[1239] Chatterjee, R., Yeh, H. C., Shafi, T., Selvin, E., Anderson, C., Pankow, J. S., Miller, E., & Brancati, F. (2010). Serum and dietary potassium and risk of incident type 2 diabetes mellitus: The Atherosclerosis Risk in Communities (ARIC) study. Archives of internal medicine, 170(19), 1745–1751. https://doi.org/10.1001/archinternmed.2010.362

[1240] DeFronzo, R. A., Felig, P., Ferrannini, E., & Wahren, J. (1980). Effect of graded doses of insulin on splanchnic and peripheral potassium metabolism in man. The American journal of physiology, 238(5), E421–E427. https://doi.org/10.1152/ajpendo.1980.238.5.E421

[1241] Sterns, R. H., Grieff, M., & Bernstein, P. L. (2016). Treatment of hyperkalemia: something old, something new. Kidney international, 89(3), 546–554. https://doi.org/10.1016/j.kint.2015.11.018

[1242] Oria-Hernández, J., Cabrera, N., Pérez-Montfort, R., & Ramírez-Silva, L. (2005). Pyruvate kinase revisited: the activating effect of K+. The Journal of biological chemistry, 280(45), 37924–37929. https://doi.org/10.1074/jbc.M508490200

[1243] Lee, H., Lee, J., Hwang, S. S., Kim, S., Chin, H. J., Han, J. S., & Heo, N. J. (2013). Potassium intake and the prevalence of metabolic syndrome: the Korean National Health and Nutrition Examination Survey 2008-2010. PloS one, 8(1), e55106. https://doi.org/10.1371/journal.pone.0055106

[1244] Colditz, G. A., Manson, J. E., Stampfer, M. J., Rosner, B., Willett, W. C., & Speizer, F. E. (1992). Diet and risk of clinical diabetes in women. The American journal of clinical nutrition, 55(5), 1018–1023. https://doi.org/10.1093/ajcn/55.5.1018

[1245] Chatterjee, R., Colangelo, L. A., Yeh, H. C., Anderson, C. A., Daviglus, M. L., Liu, K., & Brancati, F. L. (2012). Potassium intake and risk of incident type 2 diabetes mellitus: the Coronary Artery Risk Development in Young Adults (CARDIA) Study. Diabetologia, 55(5), 1295–1303. https://doi.org/10.1007/s00125-012-2487-3

[1246] Scherrer et al (1994). Nitric oxide release accounts for insulin's vascular effects in humans. The Journal of clinical investigation, 94(6), 2511–2515.

[1247] Schulman, I. H., & Zhou, M. S. (2009). Vascular insulin resistance: a potential link between cardiovascular and metabolic diseases. Current hypertension reports, 11(1), 48–55.

[1248] Zhou et al (2010). Vascular inflammation, insulin resistance, and endothelial dysfunction in salt-sensitive hypertension: role of nuclear factor kappa B activation. Journal of hypertension, 28(3), 527–535.

[1249] Muniyappa et al (2007). Cardiovascular actions of insulin. Endocrine reviews, 28(5), 463–491.

[1250] Horita et al (2011). Insulin resistance, obesity, hypertension, and renal sodium transport. International journal of hypertension, 2011, 391762.

[1251] Manhiani, M. M., Cormican, M. T., & Brands, M. W. (2011). Chronic sodium-retaining action of insulin in diabetic dogs. American journal of physiology. Renal physiology, 300(4), F957–F965.

[1252] Schulman, I. H., & Zhou, M. S. (2009). Vascular insulin resistance: a potential link between cardiovascular and metabolic diseases. Current hypertension reports, 11(1), 48–55.

[1253] Cooper et al (2007). Renin-angiotensin-aldosterone system and oxidative stress in cardiovascular insulin resistance. American journal of physiology. Heart and circulatory physiology, 293(4), H2009–H2023.

[1254] Prisant, L. M., Gujral, J. S., & Mulloy, A. L. (2006). Hyperthyroidism: a secondary cause of isolated systolic hypertension. Journal of clinical hypertension (Greenwich, Conn.), 8(8), 596–599.

[1255] Cappola, A. R., & Ladenson, P. W. (2003). Hypothyroidism and atherosclerosis. The Journal of clinical endocrinology and metabolism, 88(6), 2438–2444.

[1256] Berta et al (2019). Hypertension in Thyroid Disorders. Frontiers in endocrinology, 10, 482.

[1257] Cai, Y., Ren, Y., & Shi, J. (2011). Blood pressure levels in patients with subclinical thyroid dysfunction: a meta-analysis of cross-sectional data. Hypertension Research, 34(10), 1098–1105.

[1258] Berta et al (2019). Hypertension in Thyroid Disorders. Frontiers in endocrinology, 10, 482.

[1259] Saito, I., Ito, K., & Saruta, T. (1983). Hypothyroidism as a cause of hypertension. Hypertension (Dallas, Tex. : 1979), 5(1), 112–115.

[1260] Gu, Y, Zheng, L, Zhang, Q, et al. Relationship between thyroid function and elevated blood pressure in euthyroid adults. J Clin Hypertens. 2018; 20: 1541–1549.

[1261] Ittermann et al (2012). Serum thyroid-stimulating hormone levels are associated with blood pressure in children and adolescents. The Journal of clinical endocrinology and metabolism, 97(3), 828–834.

[1262] Ittermann et al (2013). High serum thyrotropin levels are associated with current but not with incident hypertension. Thyroid : official journal of the American Thyroid Association, 23(8), 955–963.

[1263] He et al (2018). Effect of Levothyroxine on Blood Pressure in Patients With Subclinical Hypothyroidism: A Systematic Review and Meta-Analysis. Frontiers in endocrinology, 9, 454.

[1264] Tian et al (2014). Effects of TSH on the function of human umbilical vein endothelial cells. Journal of molecular endocrinology, 52(2), 215–222.

[1265] Cai et al (2015). Thyroid hormone affects both endothelial and vascular smooth muscle cells in rat arteries. European journal of pharmacology, 747, 18–28.

[1266] Arnett et al (1994). Arterial stiffness: a new cardiovascular risk factor?. American journal of epidemiology, 140(8), 669–682.

[1267] Owen et al (2006). Subclinical hypothyroidism, arterial stiffness, and myocardial reserve. The Journal of clinical endocrinology and metabolism, 91(6), 2126–2132.

[1268] Obuobie et al (2002). Increased central arterial stiffness in hypothyroidism. The Journal of clinical endocrinology and metabolism, 87(10), 4662–4666.

[1269] Zhang, Z., Cogswell, M. E., Gillespie, C., Fang, J., Loustalot, F., Dai, S., Carriquiry, A. L., Kuklina, E. V., Hong, Y., Merritt, R., & Yang, Q. (2013). Association between usual sodium and potassium intake and blood pressure and hypertension among U.S. adults: NHANES 2005-2010. PloS one, 8(10), e75289. https://doi.org/10.1371/journal.pone.0075289

[1270] Whelton, P. K., & He, J. (2014). Health effects of sodium and potassium in humans. Current opinion in lipidology, 25(1), 75–79. https://doi.org/10.1097/MOL.0000000000000033

[1271] Graudal et al (2020). Effects of low sodium diet versus high sodium diet on blood pressure, renin, aldosterone, catecholamines, cholesterol, and triglyceride. The Cochrane database of systematic reviews, 12(12), CD004022.

[1272] Graudal et al (1998). Effects of sodium restriction on blood pressure, renin, aldosterone, catecholamines, cholesterols, and triglyceride: a meta-analysis. JAMA, 279(17), 1383–1391.

[1273] Feldman, R. D., & Schmidt, N. D. (1999). Moderate dietary salt restriction increases vascular and systemic insulin resistance. American journal of hypertension, 12(6), 643–647.

[1274] Omvik, P., & Lund-Johansen, P. (1986). Is Sodium Restriction Effective Treatment of Borderline and Mild Essential Hypertension? A Long-Term Haemodynamic Study at Rest and During Exercise. Journal of Hypertension, 4(5), 535–541.

[1275] Poulter, N. (1998). Dietary sodium intake and mortality: NHANES. The Lancet, 352(9132), 987–988. https://doi.org/10.1016/s0140-6736(05)61542-5

[1276] Cohen et al (2006). Sodium Intake and Mortality in the NHANES II Follow-up Study. The American Journal of Medicine, 119(3), 275.e7-275.e14.

[1277] Cohen et al (2008). Sodium intake and mortality follow-up in the Third National Health and Nutrition Examination Survey (NHANES III). Journal of general internal medicine, 23(9), 1297–1302.

[1278] Alderman et al (1995). Low urinary sodium is associated with greater risk of myocardial infarction among treated hypertensive men. Hypertension (Dallas, Tex. : 1979), 25(6), 1144–1152.

[1279] Feldman, R. D., & Schmidt, N. D. (1999). Moderate dietary salt restriction increases vascular and systemic insulin resistance. American journal of hypertension, 12(6), 643–647.

[1280] Iwaoka et al (1994). Dietary NaCl restriction deteriorates oral glucose tolerance in hypertensive patients with impairment of glucose tolerance. American journal of hypertension, 7(5), 460–463.

[1281] DiNicolantonio and O'Keefe (2023) 'Sodium restriction and insulin resistance: A review of 23 clinical trials', Journal of Insulin Resistance, 6(1), a78.

[1282] Zhou et al (2014). Link between insulin resistance and hypertension: What is the evidence from evolutionary biology?. Diabetology & metabolic syndrome, 6(1), 12.

[1283] Laffer, C. L., & Elijovich, F. (2013). Differential predictors of insulin resistance in nondiabetic salt-resistant and salt-sensitive subjects. Hypertension (Dallas, Tex. : 1979), 61(3), 707–715.

[1284] Shen et al (1988). Resistance to insulin-stimulated-glucose uptake in patients with hypertension. The Journal of clinical endocrinology and metabolism, 66(3), 580–583.

[1285] Lind L, Lithell H, Gustafsson IB, Pollare T, Ljunghall S. Metabolic cardiovascular risk factors and sodium sensitivity in hypertensive subjects. American Journal of Hypertension. 1992 Aug;5(8):502-505.

[1286] Sharma, A. M., Schorr, U., & Distler, A. (1993). Insulin resistance in young salt-sensitive normotensive subjects. Hypertension (Dallas, Tex. : 1979), 21(3), 273–279.

[1287] Facchini et al (1999). Blood pressure, sodium intake, insulin resistance, and urinary nitrate excretion. Hypertension (Dallas, Tex. : 1979), 33(4), 1008–1012.

[1288] DiBona G. F. (1977). Neurogenic regulation of renal tubular sodium reabsorption. The American journal of physiology, 233(2), F73–F81.

[1289] John W Rowe, James B Young, Kenneth L Minaker, Arthur L Stevens, Johanna Pallotta, Lewis Landsberg; Effect of Insulin and Glucose Infusions on Sympathetic Nervous System Activity in Normal Man. Diabetes 1 March 1981; 30 (3): 219–225.

[1290] Hollenberg N. K. (1984). The renin-angiotensin system and sodium homeostasis. Journal of cardiovascular pharmacology, 6 Suppl 1, S176–S183.

308

[1291] DeFronzo R. A. (1981). The effect of insulin on renal sodium metabolism. A review with clinical implications. Diabetologia, 21(3), 165–171.

[1292] Christopher D Saudek, Philip R Boulter, Robert H Knopp, Ronald A Arky; Sodium Retention Accompanying Insulin Treatment of Diabetes Mellitus. Diabetes 1 March 1974; 23 (3): 240–246.

[1293] Hoffmann, I., Alfieri, A. & Cubeddu, L. Effects of lifestyle changes and metformin on salt sensitivity and nitric oxide metabolism in obese salt-sensitive Hispanics. J Hum Hypertens 21, 571–578 (2007).

[1294] Muntzel, M. S., Nyeduala, B., & Barrett, S. (1999). High dietary salt enhances acute depressor responses to metformin. American journal of hypertension, 12(12 Pt 1-2), 1256–1259.

[1295] Muntzel et al (1999). Metformin attenuates salt-induced hypertension in spontaneously hypertensive rats. Hypertension (Dallas, Tex. : 1979), 33(5), 1135–1140.

[1296] Rocchini et al (1989). The effect of weight loss on the sensitivity of blood pressure to sodium in obese adolescents. The New England journal of medicine, 321(9), 580–585.

[1297] DiNicolantonio, J. J., & O'Keefe, J. H. (2022). Added Sugars Drive Insulin Resistance, Hyperinsulinemia, Hypertension, Type 2 Diabetes and Coronary Heart Disease. Missouri medicine, 119(6), 519–523.

[1298] DiNicolantonio, J. J., & O'Keefe, J. H. (2016). Hypertension Due to Toxic White Crystals in the Diet: Should We Blame Salt or Sugar?. Progress in cardiovascular diseases, 59(3), 219–225.

[1299] Beck-Nielsen, H., Pedersen, O., & Lindskov, H.O. (1980). Impaired cellular insulin binding and insulin sensitivity induced by high-fructose feeding in normal subjects. The American journal of clinical nutrition, 33 2, 273-8 .

[1300] Lastra et al (2010). Salt, aldosterone, and insulin resistance: impact on the cardiovascular system. Nature reviews. Cardiology, 7(10), 577–584.

[1301] Chen et al (2009). Metabolic syndrome and salt sensitivity of blood pressure in non-diabetic people in China: a dietary intervention study. Lancet (London, England), 373(9666), 829–835.

[1302] Nesbitt S. D. (2005). Hypertension in black patients: special issues and considerations. Current hypertension reports, 7(4), 244–248.

[1303] Weder A. B. (2007). Evolution and hypertension. Hypertension (Dallas, Tex. : 1979), 49(2), 260–265.

[1304] Young J. H. (2007). Evolution of blood pressure regulation in humans. Current hypertension reports, 9(1), 13–18.

[1305] Mente, A., O'Donnell, M. J., Rangarajan, S., McQueen, M. J., Poirier, P., Wielgosz, A., Morrison, H., Li, W., Wang, X., Di, C., Mony, P., Devanath, A., Rosengren, A., Oguz, A., Zatonska, K., Yusufali, A. H., Lopez-Jaramillo, P., Avezum, A., Ismail, N., Lanas, F., ... PURE Investigators (2014). Association of urinary sodium and potassium excretion with blood pressure. The New England journal of medicine, 371(7), 601–611. https://doi.org/10.1056/NEJMoa1311989

[1306] Jackson, S. L., Cogswell, M. E., Zhao, L., Terry, A. L., Wang, C. Y., Wright, J., Coleman King, S. M., Bowman, B., Chen, T. C., Merritt, R., & Loria, C. M. (2018). Association Between Urinary Sodium and Potassium Excretion and Blood Pressure Among Adults in the United States: National Health and Nutrition Examination Survey, 2014. Circulation, 137(3), 237–246. https://doi.org/10.1161/CIRCULATIONAHA.117.029193

[1307] Rosário, R., Santos, R., Lopes, L., Agostinis-Sobrinho, C., Moreira, C., Mota, J., ... Abreu, S. (2018). Fruit, vegetable consumption and blood pressure in healthy adolescents: A longitudinal analysis from the LabMed study. Nutrition, Metabolism and Cardiovascular Diseases, 28(10), 1075–1080. doi:10.1016/j.numecd.2018.05.014

[1308] Utsugi, M. T., Ohkubo, T., Kikuya, M., Kurimoto, A., Sato, R. I., Suzuki, K., Metoki, H., Hara, A., Tsubono, Y., & Imai, Y. (2008). Fruit and vegetable consumption and the risk of hypertension determined by self measurement of blood pressure at home: the Ohasama study. Hypertension research : official journal of the Japanese Society of Hypertension, 31(7), 1435–1443. https://doi.org/10.1291/hypres.31.1435

[1309] Borgi, L., Muraki, I., Satija, A., Willett, W. C., Rimm, E. B., & Forman, J. P. (2016). Fruit and Vegetable Consumption and the Incidence of Hypertension in Three Prospective Cohort Studies. Hypertension, 67(2), 288–293. doi:10.1161/hypertensionaha.115.06497

[1310] Wang, L., Manson, J. E., Gaziano, J. M., Buring, J. E., & Sesso, H. D. (2012). Fruit and Vegetable Intake and the Risk of Hypertension in Middle-Aged and Older Women. American Journal of Hypertension, 25(2), 180–189. doi:10.1038/ajh.2011.186

[1311] Roger, V. L., Go, A. S., Lloyd-Jones, D. M., Benjamin, E. J., Berry, J. D., Borden, W. B., Bravata, D. M., Dai, S., Ford, E. S., Fox, C. S., Fullerton, H. J., Gillespie, C., Hailpern, S. M., Heit, J. A., Howard, V. J., Kissela, B. M., Kittner, S. J., Lackland, D. T., Lichtman, J. H., Lisabeth, L. D., ... American Heart Association Statistics Committee and Stroke Statistics Subcommittee (2012). Executive summary: heart disease and stroke statistics--2012 update: a report from the American Heart Association. Circulation, 125(1), 188–197. https://doi.org/10.1161/CIR.0b013e3182456d46

[1312] Panel on Dietary Reference Intakes for Electrolytes and Water; Standing Committee on the Scientific Evaluation of Dietary Reference Intakes; Food and Nutrition Board; Institute of Medicine. Dietary Reference Intakes for Water, Potassium, Sodium, Chloride, and Sulfate; The National Academies Press: Washington, DC, USA, 2005.

[1313] World Health Organization (WHO). Guideline: Potassium Intake for Adults and Children; WHO: Geneva, Switzerland, 2012.

[1314] Chobanian, A. V., Bakris, G. L., Black, H. R., Cushman, W. C., Green, L. A., Izzo, J. L., Jr, Jones, D. W., Materson, B. J., Oparil, S., Wright, J. T., Jr, Roccella, E. J., Joint National Committee on Prevention, Detection, Evaluation, and Treatment of High Blood Pressure. National Heart, Lung, and Blood Institute, & National High Blood Pressure Education Program Coordinating Committee (2003). Seventh report of the Joint National Committee on Prevention, Detection, Evaluation, and Treatment of High Blood Pressure. Hypertension (Dallas, Tex. : 1979), 42(6), 1206–1252. https://doi.org/10.1161/01.HYP.0000107251.49515.c2

[1315] NIH (2021) 'Potassium', Fact Sheet for Health Professionals, Accessed Online March 30th 2022: https://ods.od.nih.gov/factsheets/Potassium-HealthProfessional/

[1316] Fulgoni, V. L., 3rd, Keast, D. R., Bailey, R. L., & Dwyer, J. (2011). Foods, fortificants, and supplements: Where do Americans get their nutrients?. The Journal of nutrition, 141(10), 1847–1854. https://doi.org/10.3945/jn.111.142257

[1317] DeSalvo, K. B., Olson, R., & Casavale, K. O. (2016). Dietary Guidelines for Americans. JAMA, 315(5), 457–458. https://doi.org/10.1001/jama.2015.18396

[1318] Khaw, K. T., & Rose, G. (1982). Population study of blood pressure and associated factors in St Lucia, West Indies. International journal of epidemiology, 11(4), 372–377. https://doi.org/10.1093/ije/11.4.372

[1319] Khaw, K. T., & Barrett-Connor, E. (1987). Dietary potassium and stroke-associated mortality. A 12-year prospective population study. The New England journal of medicine, 316(5), 235–240. https://doi.org/10.1056/NEJM198701293160502

[1320] He, J., Tell, G. S., Tang, Y. C., Mo, P. S., & He, G. Q. (1991). Relation of electrolytes to blood pressure in men. The Yi people study. Hypertension, 17(3), 378–385. doi:10.1161/01.hyp.17.3.378

[1321] Reed, D., McGee, D., Yano, K., & Hankin, J. (1985). Diet, blood pressure, and multicollinearity. Hypertension (Dallas, Tex. : 1979), 7(3 Pt 1), 405–410.

[1322] D'Elia, L., Barba, G., Cappuccio, F. P., & Strazzullo, P. (2011). Potassium intake, stroke, and cardiovascular disease a meta-analysis of prospective studies. Journal of the American College of Cardiology, 57(10), 1210–1219. https://doi.org/10.1016/j.jacc.2010.09.070

[1323] Aburto, N. J., Hanson, S., Gutierrez, H., Hooper, L., Elliott, P., & Cappuccio, F. P. (2013). Effect of increased potassium intake on cardiovascular risk factors and disease: systematic review and meta-analyses. BMJ (Clinical research ed.), 346, f1378. https://doi.org/10.1136/bmj.f1378

[1324] NIH (2020) 'Potassium: Fact Sheet for Health Professionals', Dietary Supplement Fact Sheets, Accessed Online Dec 26 2020: https://ods.od.nih.gov/factsheets/Potassium-HealthProfessional/

[1325] U.S. Department of Agriculture, Agricultural Research Service. FoodData Centralexternal link disclaimer, 2019.

[1326] USDA (2015) '2015-2020 Dietary Guidelines for Americans', December 2015. Available at http://health.gov/dietaryguidelines/2015/guidelines/.

[1327] SELF Nutrition Data (2018) 'Foods highest in Potassium', Accessed Online Dec 26 2020: https://nutritiondata.self.com/foods-00012200000000000000-w.html

[1328] Eaton, S. B., & Konner, M. (1985). Paleolithic nutrition. A consideration of its nature and current implications. The New England journal of medicine, 312(5), 283–289. https://doi.org/10.1056/NEJM198501313120505

[1329] Denton D (1982) Hunger for salt, an anthropological, physiological and medical analysis. Springer Berlin, Heidelberg, New York, pp 573–575

[1330] Ben-Dor et al (2021) 'The evolution of the human trophic level during the Pleistocene', American Journal of Physical Anthropology 175(325).

[1331] Konner, M., & Eaton, S. B. (2010). Paleolithic nutrition: twenty-five years later. Nutrition in clinical practice : official publication of the American Society for Parenteral and Enteral Nutrition, 25(6), 594–602. https://doi.org/10.1177/0884533610385702

[1332] Eaton, S. B., & Konner, M. (1985). Paleolithic Nutrition. New England Journal of Medicine, 312(5), 283–289. doi:10.1056/nejm198501313120505

[1333] Khaw, K. T., & Barrett-Connor, E. (1984). Dietary potassium and blood pressure in a population. The American Journal of Clinical Nutrition, 39(6), 963–968. doi:10.1093/ajcn/39.6.963

[1334] Langford H. G. (1983). Dietary potassium and hypertension: epidemiologic data. Annals of internal medicine, 98(5 Pt 2), 770–772. https://doi.org/10.7326/0003-4819-98-5-770

[1335] FDA (2020) 'Sodium in Your Diet: Use the Nutrition Facts Label and Reduce Your Intake', Nutrition Education Resources & Materials, Accessed Online Dec 30 2020: https://www.fda.gov/food/nutrition-education-resources-materials/sodium-your-diet

[1336] Lewis (2020) 'Overview of Electrolytes', MSD Manual Consumer Version, Accessed Online Feb 18 2021: https://www.msdmanuals.com/home/hormonal-and-metabolic-disorders/electrolyte-balance/overview-of-electrolytes

[1337] Lee J. W. (2010). Fluid and electrolyte disturbances in critically ill patients. Electrolyte & blood pressure : E & BP, 8(2), 72–81. https://doi.org/10.5049/EBP.2010.8.2.72

[1338] Weglicki, W., Quamme, G., Tucker, K., Haigney, M., & Resnick, L. (2005). Potassium, magnesium, and electrolyte imbalance and complications in disease management. Clinical and experimental hypertension (New York, N.Y. : 1993), 27(1), 95–112. https://doi.org/10.1081/ceh-200044275

[1339] Tello, L., & Perez-Freytes, R. (2017). Fluid and Electrolyte Therapy During Vomiting and Diarrhea. The Veterinary clinics of North America. Small animal practice, 47(2), 505–519. https://doi.org/10.1016/j.cvsm.2016.09.013

[1340] Dhondup, T., & Qian, Q. (2017). Electrolyte and Acid-Base Disorders in Chronic Kidney Disease and End-Stage Kidney Failure. Blood Purification, 43(1-3), 179–188. doi:10.1159/000452725

[1341] Winston A. P. (2012). The clinical biochemistry of anorexia nervosa. Annals of clinical biochemistry, 49(Pt 2), 132–143. https://doi.org/10.1258/acb.2011.011185

[1342] Hauhouot-Attoungbre, M. L., Mlan, W. C., Edjeme, N. A., Ahibo, H., Vilasco, B., & Monnet, D. (2005). Intérêt du ionogramme chez le brûlé thermique grave [Disturbances of electrolytes in severe thermal burns]. Annales de biologie clinique, 63(4), 417–421.

[1343] Olivero J. J., Sr (2016). Cardiac Consequences Of Electrolyte Imbalance. Methodist DeBakey cardiovascular journal, 12(2), 125–126. https://doi.org/10.14797/mdcj-12-2-125

[1344] Bara, M., Guiet-Bara, A., & Durlach, J. (1993). Regulation of sodium and potassium pathways by magnesium in cell membranes. Magnesium research, 6(2), 167–177.

[1345] NISHIMUTA, M., KODAMA, N., YOSHITAKE, Y., SHIMADA, M., & SERIZAWA, N. (2018). Dietary Salt (Sodium Chloride) Requirement and Adverse Effects of Salt Restriction in Humans. Journal of Nutritional Science and Vitaminology, 64(2), 83–89. doi:10.3177/jnsv.64.83

[1346] NISHIMUTA, M., KODAMA, N., MORIKUNI, E., YOSHIOKA, Y. H., MATSUZAKI, N., TAKEYAMA, H., … KITAJIMA, H. (2005). Positive Correlation between Dietary Intake of Sodium and Balances of Calcium and Magnesium in Young Japanese Adults-Low Sodium Intake Is a Risk Factor for Loss of Calcium and Magnesium-. Journal of Nutritional Science and Vitaminology, 51(4), 265–270. doi:10.3177/jnsv.51.265

[1347] KODAMA, N., NISHIMUTA, M., & SUZUKI, K. (2003). Negative Balance of Calcium and Magnesium under Relatively Low Sodium Intake in Humans. Journal of Nutritional Science and Vitaminology, 49(3), 201–209. doi:10.3177/jnsv.49.201

[1348] DiNicolantonio, J. J., O'Keefe, J. H., & Wilson, W. (2018). Subclinical magnesium deficiency: a principal driver of cardiovascular disease and a public health crisis. Open Heart, 5(1), e000668. doi:10.1136/openhrt-2017-000668

[1349] Ahmad, A., & Bloom, S. (1989). Sodium pump and calcium channel modulation of Mg-deficiency cardiomyopathy. The American journal of cardiovascular pathology, 2(4), 277–283.

[1350] Dyckner, T., & Wester, P. O. (1979). Ventricular extrasystoles and intracellular electrolytes before and after potassium and magnesium infusions in patients on diuretic treatment. American Heart Journal, 97(1), 12–18. doi:10.1016/0002-8703(79)90108-x

[1351] Dyckner, T., & Wester, P. O. (2009). Relation between Potassium, Magnesium and Cardiac Arrhythmias. Acta Medica Scandinavica, 209(S647), 163–169. doi:10.1111/j.0954-6820.1981.tb02652.x

[1352] Boyd, J. C., Bruns, D. E., DiMarco, J. P., Sugg, N. K., & Wills, M. R. (1984). Relationship of potassium and magnesium concentrations in serum to cardiac arrhythmias. Clinical Chemistry, 30(5), 754–757. doi:10.1093/clinchem/30.5.754

[1353] Riddell, D. R., & Owen, J. S. (1997). Nitric Oxide and Platelet Aggregation. Vitamins & Hormones, 25–48. doi:10.1016/s0083-6729(08)60639-1

[1354] Hobbs, D. A., George, T. W., & Lovegrove, J. A. (2013). The effects of dietary nitrate on blood pressure and endothelial function: a review of human intervention studies. Nutrition Research Reviews, 26(2), 210–222. doi:10.1017/s0954422413000188

[1355] Park, J. W., Piknova, B., Nghiem, N., Lozier, J. N., & Schechter, A. N. (2014). Inhibitory effect of nitrite on coagulation processes demonstrated by thrombelastography. Nitric oxide : biology and chemistry, 40, 45–51. https://doi.org/10.1016/j.niox.2014.05.006

[1356] Matsushita, K., Morrell, C. N., Cambien, B., Yang, S.-X., Yamakuchi, M., Bao, C., … Lowenstein, C. J. (2003). Nitric Oxide Regulates Exocytosis by S-Nitrosylation of N-ethylmaleimide-Sensitive Factor. Cell, 115(2), 139–150. doi:10.1016/s0092-8674(03)00803-1

[1357] O'Donnell, V. B., & Freeman, B. A. (2001). Interactions Between Nitric Oxide and Lipid Oxidation Pathways. Circulation Research, 88(1), 12–21. doi:10.1161/01.res.88.1.12

[1358] Davies, K. P. (2015). Development and therapeutic applications of nitric oxide releasing materials to treat erectile dysfunction. Future Science OA, 1(1). doi:10.4155/fso.15.53

[1359] Bivalacqua, T., Champion, H., Mehta, Y., Abdel-Mageed, A., Sikka, S., Ignarro, L., … Hellstrom, W. (2000). Adenoviral gene transfer of endothelial nitric oxide synthase (eNOS) to the penis improves age-related erectile dysfunction in the rat. International Journal of Impotence Research, 12(S3), S8–S17. doi:10.1038/sj.ijir.3900556

[1360] Mayo Clinic Stafff (2019) 'High blood pressure and sex: Overcome the challenges', Mayo Clinic, Accessed Online Nov 11 2020: https://www.mayoclinic.org/diseases-conditions/high-blood-pressure/in-depth/high-blood-pressure-and-sex/art-20044209

[1361] McIntyre, M., & Dominiczak, A. F. (1997). Nitric oxide and cardiovascular disease. Postgraduate Medical Journal, 73(864), 630–634. doi:10.1136/pgmj.73.864.630

[1362] Houston, M., & Hays, L. (2014). Acute Effects of an Oral Nitric Oxide Supplement on Blood Pressure, Endothelial Function, and Vascular Compliance in Hypertensive Patients. The Journal of Clinical Hypertension, n/a–n/a. doi:10.1111/jch.12352

[1363] Zhang, S., Yang, T., Xu, X., Wang, M., Zhong, L., Yang, Y., … Wang, C. (2015). Oxidative stress and nitric oxide signaling related biomarkers in patients with pulmonary hypertension: a case control study. BMC Pulmonary Medicine, 15(1). doi:10.1186/s12890-015-0045-8

[1364] Wu, G., & Meininger, C. J. (2002). REGULATION OFNITRICOXIDESYNTHESIS BYDIETARYFACTORS. Annual Review of Nutrition, 22(1), 61–86. doi:10.1146/annurev.nutr.22.110901.145329

[1365] Ochiai, M., Hayashi, T., Morita, M., Ina, K., Maeda, M., Watanabe, F., & Morishita, K. (2012). Short-term effects of l-citrulline supplementation on arterial stiffness in middle-aged men. International Journal of Cardiology, 155(2), 257–261. doi:10.1016/j.ijcard.2010.10.004

[1366] Cormio, L., De Siati, M., Lorusso, F., Selvaggio, O., Mirabella, L., Sanguedolce, F., & Carrieri, G. (2011). Oral L-citrulline supplementation improves erection hardness in men with mild erectile dysfunction. Urology, 77(1), 119–122. https://doi.org/10.1016/j.urology.2010.08.028

[1367] Gonzales, J. U., Raymond, A., Ashley, J., & Kim, Y. (2017). Does l-citrulline supplementation improve exercise blood flow in older adults?. Experimental physiology, 102(12), 1661–1671. https://doi.org/10.1113/EP086587

[1368] Bailey et al (2010) 'Acute l-arginine supplementation reduces the O2 cost of moderate-intensity exercise and enhances high-intensity exercise tolerance', Journal of Applied Physiology, Volume 109 Issue 5, Pages 1394-1403.

[1369] Orozco-Gutiérrez, J. J., Castillo-Martínez, L., Orea-Tejeda, A., Vázquez-Díaz, O., Valdespino-Trejo, A., Narváez-David, R., Keirns-Davis, C., Carrasco-Ortiz, O., Navarro-Navarro, A., & Sánchez-Santillán, R. (2010). Effect of L-arginine or L-citrulline oral supplementation on blood pressure and right ventricular function in heart failure patients with preserved ejection fraction. Cardiology journal, 17(6), 612–618.

[1370] McKinley-Barnard, S., Andre, T., Morita, M., & Willoughby, D. S. (2015). Combined L-citrulline and glutathione supplementation increases the concentration of markers indicative of nitric oxide synthesis. Journal of the International Society of Sports Nutrition, 12, 27. https://doi.org/10.1186/s12970-015-0086-7

[1371] Ghigo, D., Geromin, D., Franchino, C., Todde, R., Priotto, C., Costamagna, C., Arese, M., Garbarino, G., Pescarmona, G. P., & Bosia, A. (1996). Correlation between nitric oxide synthase activity and reduced glutathione level in human and murine endothelial cells. Amino acids, 10(3), 277–281. https://doi.org/10.1007/BF00807330

[1372] Andrew, P. (1999). Enzymatic function of nitric oxide synthases. Cardiovascular Research, 43(3), 521–531. doi:10.1016/s0008-6363(99)00115-7

[1373] Chen, G., Dunbar, R. L., Gao, W., & Ebner, T. J. (2001). Role of Calcium, Glutamate Neurotransmission, and Nitric Oxide in Spreading Acidification and Depression in the Cerebellar Cortex. The Journal of Neuroscience, 21(24), 9877–9887. doi:10.1523/jneurosci.21-24-09877.2001

[1374] Okuda, Y., Kawashima, K., Sawada, T., Tsurumaru, K., Asano, M., Suzuki, S., … Yamashita, K. (1997). Eicosapentaenoic Acid Enhances Nitric Oxide Production by Cultured Human Endothelial Cells. Biochemical and Biophysical Research Communications, 232(2), 487–491. doi:10.1006/bbrc.1997.6328

[1375] Swartz-Basile, D. A., Goldblatt, M. I., Blaser, C., Decker, P. A., Ahrendt, S. A., Sarna, S. K., & Pitt, H. A. (2000). Iron Deficiency Diminishes Gallbladder Neuronal Nitric Oxide Synthase. Journal of Surgical Research, 90(1), 26–31. doi:10.1006/jsre.2000.5827

[1376] Goldblatt, M. (2001). Iron deficiency suppresses ileal nitric oxide synthase activity,. Journal of Gastrointestinal Surgery, 5(4), 393–400. doi:10.1016/s1091-255x(01)80068-8

[1377] ALDERTON, W. K., COOPER, C. E., & KNOWLES, R. G. (2001). Nitric oxide synthases: structure, function and inhibition. Biochemical Journal, 357(3), 593. doi:10.1042/0264-6021:3570593

[1378] Persechini, A., McMillan, K., & Masters, B. S. S. (1995). Inhibition of Nitric Oxide Synthase Activity by Zn2+ Ion. Biochemistry, 34(46), 15091–15095. doi:10.1021/bi00046a015

[1379] Kim, D.-H., Meza, C. A., Clarke, H., Kim, J.-S., & Hickner, R. C. (2020). Vitamin D and Endothelial Function. Nutrients, 12(2), 575. doi:10.3390/nu12020575

[1380] Dawes M, Ritter JM. (2000). 'Mg2+-induced vasodilation in human vasculature is inhibited by NG-monomethyl-L-arginine but not by indomethacin'. J. Vasc. Res. 37:276–81

[1381] Pearson, P. J., Evora, P. R. B., Seccombe, J. F., & Schaff, H. V. (1998). Hypomagnesemia Inhibits Nitric Oxide Release From Coronary Endothelium: Protective Role of Magnesium Infusion After Cardiac Operations11This article has been selected for the open discussion forum on the STS Web site: http://www.sts.org/annals. The Annals of Thoracic Surgery, 65(4), 967–972. doi:10.1016/s0003-4975(98)00020-4

[1382] Wu, G., Haynes, T. E., Li, H., Yan, W., & Meininger, C. J. (2001). Glutamine metabolism to glucosamine is necessary for glutamine inhibition of endothelial nitric oxide synthesis. The Biochemical journal, 353(Pt 2), 245–252. https://doi.org/10.1042/0264-6021:3530245

[1383] Williams, S. B., Goldfine, A. B., Timimi, F. K., Ting, H. H., Roddy, M. A., Simonson, D. C., & Creager, M. A. (1998). Acute hyperglycemia attenuates endothelium-dependent vasodilation in humans in vivo. Circulation, 97(17), 1695–1701. https://doi.org/10.1161/01.cir.97.17.1695

[1384] Grundy, S. M., Benjamin, I. J., Burke, G. L., Chait, A., Eckel, R. H., Howard, B. V., … Sowers, J. R. (1999). Diabetes and Cardiovascular Disease. Circulation, 100(10), 1134–1146. doi:10.1161/01.cir.100.10.1134

[1385] Weksler-Zangen, S., Jörns, A., Tarsi-Chen, L., Vernea, F., Aharon-Hananel, G., Saada, A., … Raz, I. (2013). Dietary copper supplementation restores β-cell function of Cohen diabetic rats: a link between mitochondrial function and glucose-stimulated insulin secretion. American Journal of Physiology-Endocrinology and Metabolism, 304(10), E1023–E1034. doi:10.1152/ajpendo.00036.2013

[1386] A scientific review: the role of chromium in insulin resistance. (2004). The Diabetes educator, Suppl, 2–14.

[1387] Prabodh, S., Prakash, D. S. R. S., Sudhakar, G., Chowdary, N. V. S., Desai, V., & Shekhar, R. (2010). Status of Copper and Magnesium Levels in Diabetic Nephropathy Cases: a Case-Control Study from South India. Biological Trace Element Research, 142(1), 29–35. doi:10.1007/s12011-010-8750-x

[1388] DiNicolantonio, J. J., O'Keefe, J. H., & Wilson, W. (2018). Subclinical magnesium deficiency: a principal driver of cardiovascular disease and a public health crisis. Open Heart, 5(1), e000668. doi:10.1136/openhrt-2017-000668

[1389] DiNicolantonio, J. J., Mangan, D., & O'Keefe, J. H. (2018). The fructose–copper connection: Added sugars induce fatty liver and insulin resistance via copper deficiency. Journal of Insulin Resistance, 3(1). doi:10.4102/jir.v3i1.43

[1390] Takagawa, Y., Berger, M. E., Hori, M. T., Tuck, M. L., & Golub, M. S. (2001). Long-term fructose feeding impairs vascular relaxation in rat mesenteric arteries. American Journal of Hypertension, 14(8), 811–817. doi:10.1016/s0895-7061(01)01298-5

[1391] Beauchamp (2016). Why do we like sweet taste: A bitter tale?. Physiology & behavior, 164(Pt B), 432–437.

[1392] Rowland HM, Rockwell Parker M, Jiang P, Reed DR, Beauchamp GK. Comparative Taste Biology with Special Focus on Birds and Reptiles. In: Doty RL, editor. Handbook of Olfaction and Gustation. John Wiley & Sons, Inc; 2015. pp. 957–982.

[1393] Jiang et al (2012). Major taste loss in carnivorous mammals. Proceedings of the National Academy of Sciences of the United States of America, 109(13), 4956–4961.

[1394] Huffman M. A. (2003). Animal self-medication and ethno-medicine: exploration and exploitation of the medicinal properties of plants. The Proceedings of the Nutrition Society, 62(2), 371–381.

[1395] Cowart BJ, Beauchamp GK, Mennella JA. Development of Taste and Smell in the Neonate. In: Polin RA, Fox WW, Abman SH, editors. Fetal and Neonatal Physiology. Elsevier Saunders; Philadelphia: 2011. pp. 1899–1907.

[1396] Harrison et al (2010). Efficacy of sweet solutions for analgesia in infants between 1 and 12 months of age: a systematic review. Archives of disease in childhood, 95(6), 406–413.

[1397] Blass, E. M., & Watt, L. B. (1999). Suckling- and sucrose-induced analgesia in human newborns. Pain, 83(3), 611–623.

[1398] Niki et al (2015). Modulation of sweet taste sensitivities by endogenous leptin and endocannabinoids in mice. The Journal of physiology, 593(11), 2527–2545.

[1399] Cui et al (2006). The heterodimeric sweet taste receptor has multiple potential ligand binding sites. Current pharmaceutical design, 12(35), 4591–4600.

[1400] Hoon et al (1999). Putative mammalian taste receptors: a class of taste-specific GPCRs with distinct topographic selectivity. Cell, 96(4), 541–551.

[1401] Sainz et al (2001). Identification of a novel member of the T1R family of putative taste receptors. Journal of neurochemistry, 77(3), 896–903.

[1402] Zhao et al (2003). The receptors for mammalian sweet and umami taste. Cell, 115(3), 255–266.

[1403] Damak et al (2003). Detection of sweet and umami taste in the absence of taste receptor T1r3. Science (New York, N.Y.), 301(5634), 850–853.

[1404] Yee et al (2011). Glucose transporters and ATP-gated K+ (KATP) metabolic sensors are present in type 1 taste receptor 3 (T1r3)-expressing taste cells. Proceedings of the National Academy of Sciences of the United States of America, 108(13), 5431–5436.

[1405] ACS (2019) 'Saccharin', Accessed Online March 27th 2023: https://www.acs.org/molecule-of-the-week/archive/s/saccharin

[1406] Anon. (July 17, 1886). "The inventor of saccharine". Scientific American. new series. 60 (3): 36.

[1407] Goldhaber (2021) 'The Long, Tortured History Of Artificial Sweeteners', American Council on Science and Health, Accessed Online March 27th 2023: https://www.acsh.org/news/2021/08/18/long-tortured-history-artificial-sweeteners-15738#:~:text=The%20search%20for%20sweet%2Dtasting,an%20illegal%20substitution%20for%20sugar.

[1408] FDA (2018) 'Additional Information about High-Intensity Sweeteners Permitted for Use in Food in the United States', Accessed Online March 27th 2023: https://www.fda.gov/food/food-additives-petitions/additional-information-about-high-intensity-sweeteners-permitted-use-food-united-states

[1409] Weihrauch, M. R., & Diehl, V. (2004). Artificial sweeteners--do they bear a carcinogenic risk?. Annals of oncology : official journal of the European Society for Medical Oncology, 15(10), 1460–1465.

[1410] EFSA Panel on Food Additives and Nutrient Sources added to Food (ANS). (2013). Scientific Opinion on the re-evaluation of aspartame (E 951) as a food additive [JB]. EFSA Journal, 11(12).

[1411] EFSA (European Food Safety Authority) 2020. Outcome of thepublic consultation on a draft protocolfor the assessment of hazard identification and characterisation of sweeteners. EFSA supporting publication 2020: 17(2): EN-1803. 25 pp.doi: 10.2903/sp.efsa.2020.EN-1803

[1412] FDA US Food and Drug Administration. High-Intensity Sweeteners. (2014). Available online at: https://www.fda.gov/food/food-additives-petitions/high-intensity-sweeteners

[1413] Food Standards Agency Current EU Approved Additives and their E Numbers. (2016). Available online at: https://www.food.gov.uk/business-guidance/approved-additives-and-e-numbers

[1414] Revised Opinion of the Scientific Committee on Food on Cyclamic Acid and its Sodium and Calcium Salts (expressed on 9 March 2000). Scientific Committee on Food; (2000). Available online at: https://ec.europa.eu/food/sites/food/files/safety/docs/sci-com_scf_out53_en.pdf

[1415] Mortensen A. Sweeteners permitted in the European Union: safety aspects. Scand J Food Nutr. (2006) 50:104–16. 10.1080/17482970600982719

[1416] FDA (2018) 'Additional Information about High-Intensity Sweeteners Permitted for Use in Food in the United States', Accessed Online April 11th 2023: https://www.fda.gov/food/food-additives-petitions/additional-information-about-high-intensity-sweeteners-permitted-use-food-united-states#Luo_Han_Guo_fruit_extracts

[1417] FDA Agency Response Letter GRAS Notice No. GRN 000738 [THAUMATIN sweetener and food flavor modifier] (2018).

[1418] Fitch et al (2012). Position of the Academy of Nutrition and Dietetics: use of nutritive and nonnutritive sweeteners. Journal of the Academy of Nutrition and Dietetics, 112(5), 739–758.

[1419] Sylvetsky et al (2017). Consumption of Low-Calorie Sweeteners among Children and Adults in the United States. Journal of the Academy of Nutrition and Dietetics, 117(3), 441–448.e2.

[1420] Miller, P. E., & Perez, V. (2014). Low-calorie sweeteners and body weight and composition: a meta-analysis of randomized controlled trials and prospective cohort studies. The American journal of clinical nutrition, 100(3), 765–777.

[1421] Shankar, P., Ahuja, S., & Sriram, K. (2013). Non-nutritive sweeteners: review and update. Nutrition (Burbank, Los Angeles County, Calif.), 29(11-12), 1293–1299.

[1422] Rogers et al (2016). Does low-energy sweetener consumption affect energy intake and body weight? A systematic review, including meta-analyses, of the evidence from human and animal studies. International journal of obesity (2005), 40(3), 381–394.

[1423] Lohner, S., Toews, I., & Meerpohl, J. J. (2017). Health outcomes of non-nutritive sweeteners: analysis of the research landscape. Nutrition journal, 16(1), 55.

[1424] Brown, R. J., de Banate, M. A., & Rother, K. I. (2010). Artificial sweeteners: a systematic review of metabolic effects in youth. International journal of pediatric obesity : IJPO : an official journal of the International Association for the Study of Obesity, 5(4), 305–312.

[1425] Azad et al (2017). Nonnutritive sweeteners and cardiometabolic health: a systematic review and meta-analysis of randomized controlled trials and prospective cohort studies. CMAJ : Canadian Medical Association journal = journal de l'Association medicale canadienne, 189(28), E929–E939.

[1426] Christofides E. A. (2021). POINT: Artificial Sweeteners and Obesity-Not the Solution and Potentially a Problem. Endocrine practice : official journal of the American College of Endocrinology and the American Association of Clinical Endocrinologists, 27(10), 1052–1055.

[1427] Pearlman, M., Obert, J., & Casey, L. (2017). The Association Between Artificial Sweeteners and Obesity. Current gastroenterology reports, 19(12), 64.

[1428] Young et al (2019). Low-calorie sweetener use, weight, and metabolic health among children: A mini-review. Pediatric obesity, 14(8), e12521.

[1429] Rogers et al (2016). Does low-energy sweetener consumption affect energy intake and body weight? A systematic review, including meta-analyses, of the evidence from human and animal studies. International journal of obesity (2005), 40(3), 381–394.

[1430] Rogers et al (2016). Does low-energy sweetener consumption affect energy intake and body weight? A systematic review, including meta-analyses, of the evidence from human and animal studies. International journal of obesity (2005), 40(3), 381–394.

[1431] Toews et al (2019). Association between intake of non-sugar sweeteners and health outcomes: systematic review and meta-analyses of randomised and non-randomised controlled trials and observational studies. BMJ, k4718.

[1432] Mejia, E., & Pearlman, M. (2019). Natural Alternative Sweeteners and Diabetes Management. *Current Diabetes Reports*, *19*(12). https://doi.org/10.1007/s11892-019-1273-8

[1433] Suez et al (2014). Artificial sweeteners induce glucose intolerance by altering the gut microbiota. Nature, 514(7521), 181–186.

[1434] Suez et al (2022). Personalized microbiome-driven effects of non-nutritive sweeteners on human glucose tolerance. Cell, 185(18), 3307–3328.e19.

[1435] Suez et al (2022). Personalized microbiome-driven effects of non-nutritive sweeteners on human glucose tolerance. Cell, 185(18), 3307–3328.e19.

[1436] Pang, M. D., Goossens, G. H., & Blaak, E. E. (2021). The Impact of Artificial Sweeteners on Body Weight Control and Glucose Homeostasis. Frontiers in nutrition, 7, 598340.

[1437] Mace, O. J., Affleck, J., Patel, N., & Kellett, G. L. (2007). Sweet taste receptors in rat small intestine stimulate glucose absorption through apical GLUT2. The Journal of physiology, 582(Pt 1), 379–392.

[1438] Margolskee et al (2007). T1R3 and gustducin in gut sense sugars to regulate expression of Na+-glucose cotransporter 1. Proceedings of the National Academy of Sciences of the United States of America, 104(38), 15075–15080.

[1439] Ma et al (2010). Effect of the artificial sweetener, sucralose, on small intestinal glucose absorption in healthy human subjects. The British journal of nutrition, 104(6), 803–806.

[1440] Imamura et al (2015). Consumption of sugar sweetened beverages, artificially sweetened beverages, and fruit juice and incidence of type 2 diabetes: systematic review, meta-analysis, and estimation of population attributable fraction. BMJ (Clinical research ed.), 351, h3576.

[1441] Daher, M. I., Matta, J. M., & Abdel Nour, A. M. (2019). Non-nutritive sweeteners and type 2 diabetes: Should we ring the bell?. Diabetes research and clinical practice, 155, 107786.

[1442] Sun, Z., Wang, W., Li, L., Zhang, X., Ning, Z., Mayne, J., Walker, K., Stintzi, A., & Figeys, D. (2022). Comprehensive Assessment of Functional Effects of Commonly Used Sugar Substitute Sweeteners on *Ex Vivo* Human Gut Microbiome. *Microbiology Spectrum*, *10*(4). https://doi.org/10.1128/spectrum.00412-22

[1443] Watanabe, A., Tochio, T., Kadota, Y., Takahashi, M., Kitaura, Y., Ishikawa, H., Yasutake, T., Nakano, M., Shinohara, H., Kudo, T., Nishimoto, Y., Mizuguchi, Y., Endo, A., & Shimomura, Y. (2021). Supplementation of 1-Kestose Modulates the Gut Microbiota Composition to Ameliorate Glucose Metabolism in Obesity-Prone Hosts. *Nutrients*, *13*(9), 2983. https://doi.org/10.3390/nu13092983

[1444] Ruiz-Ojeda, F. J., Plaza-Díaz, J., Sáez-Lara, M. J., & Gil, A. (2019). Effects of Sweeteners on the Gut Microbiota: A Review of Experimental Studies and Clinical Trials. *Advances in Nutrition*, *10*, S31–S48. https://doi.org/10.1093/advances/nmy037

[1445] Tandon, D., Haque, M. M., Gote, M., Jain, M., Bhaduri, A., Dubey, A. K., & Mande, S. S. (2019). A prospective randomized, double-blind, placebo-controlled, dose-response relationship study to investigate efficacy of fructo-oligosaccharides (FOS) on human gut microflora. *Scientific Reports*, *9*(1). https://doi.org/10.1038/s41598-019-41837-3

[1446] Suez et al (2014). Artificial sweeteners induce glucose intolerance by altering the gut microbiota. Nature, 514(7521), 181–186.

[1447] Santos et al (2018). Artificial sweetener saccharin disrupts intestinal epithelial cells' barrier function in vitro. Food & function, 9(7), 3815–3822.

[1448] de La Serre et al (2010). Propensity to high-fat diet-induced obesity in rats is associated with changes in the gut microbiota and gut inflammation. American journal of physiology. Gastrointestinal and liver physiology, 299(2), G440–G448.

[1449] Bleau et al (2015). Crosstalk between intestinal microbiota, adipose tissue and skeletal muscle as an early event in systemic low-grade inflammation and the development of obesity and diabetes. Diabetes/metabolism research and reviews, 31(6), 545–561.

[1450] André, P., Laugerette, F., & Féart, C. (2019). Metabolic Endotoxemia: A Potential Underlying Mechanism of the Relationship between Dietary Fat Intake and Risk for Cognitive Impairments in Humans?. Nutrients, 11(8), 1887.

[1451] Stienstra et al (2012). The inflammasome puts obesity in the danger zone. Cell metabolism, 15(1), 10–18.

[1452] Jager et al (2007). Interleukin-1beta-induced insulin resistance in adipocytes through down-regulation of insulin receptor substrate-1 expression. Endocrinology, 148(1), 241–251.

[1453] Bian et al (2017). Gut Microbiome Response to Sucralose and Its Potential Role in Inducing Liver Inflammation in Mice. Frontiers in physiology, 8, 487.

[1454] Cui et al (2006). The heterodimeric sweet taste receptor has multiple potential ligand binding sites. Current pharmaceutical design, 12(35), 4591–4600.

[1455] Laffitte, A., Neiers, F., & Briand, L. (2014). Functional roles of the sweet taste receptor in oral and extraoral tissues. Current opinion in clinical nutrition and metabolic care, 17(4), 379–385.

[1456] van Opstal et al (2019). Dietary sugars and non-caloric sweeteners elicit different homeostatic and hedonic responses in the brain. Nutrition (Burbank, Los Angeles County, Calif.), 60, 80–86.

[1457] Smeets et al (2005). Functional magnetic resonance imaging of human hypothalamic responses to sweet taste and calories. The American journal of clinical nutrition, 82(5), 1011–1016.

[1458] Holst J. J. (2004). On the physiology of GIP and GLP-1. Hormone and metabolic research = Hormon- und Stoffwechselforschung = Hormones et metabolisme, 36(11-12), 747–754.

[1459] Han, P., Bagenna, B., & Fu, M. (2019). The sweet taste signalling pathways in the oral cavity and the gastrointestinal tract affect human appetite and food intake: a review. International journal of food sciences and nutrition, 70(2), 125–135.

[1460] Steinert et al (2011). Effects of carbohydrate sugars and artificial sweeteners on appetite and the secretion of gastrointestinal satiety peptides. The British journal of nutrition, 105(9), 1320–1328.

313

1461 Kojima, I., & Nakagawa, Y. (2011). The Role of the Sweet Taste Receptor in Enteroendocrine Cells and Pancreatic β-Cells. Diabetes & metabolism journal, 35(5), 451–457.

1462 Heijboer et al (2006). Gut-brain axis: regulation of glucose metabolism. Journal of neuroendocrinology, 18(12), 883–894.

1463 Ford et al (2011). Effects of oral ingestion of sucralose on gut hormone response and appetite in healthy normal-weight subjects. European journal of clinical nutrition, 65(4), 508–513.

1464 Maersk, M., Belza, A., Holst, J. J., Fenger-Grøn, M., Pedersen, S. B., Astrup, A., & Richelsen, B. (2012). Satiety scores and satiety hormone response after sucrose-sweetened soft drink compared with isocaloric semi-skimmed milk and with non-caloric soft drink: a controlled trial. European journal of clinical nutrition, 66(4), 523–529.

1465 Dalenberg et al (2020). Short-Term Consumption of Sucralose with, but Not without, Carbohydrate Impairs Neural and Metabolic Sensitivity to Sugar in Humans. Cell metabolism, 31(3), 493–502.e7.

1466 Butchko et al (2002). Aspartame: review of safety. Regulatory toxicology and pharmacology : RTP, 35(2 Pt 2), S1–S93.

1467 Magnuson et al (2007). Aspartame: a safety evaluation based on current use levels, regulations, and toxicological and epidemiological studies. Critical reviews in toxicology, 37(8), 629–727.

1468 Picard (2013) 'The complicated truth behind aspartame', Accessed Online March 29th 2023: https://www.theglobeandmail.com/life/health-and-fitness/health/the-complicated-truth-behind-aspartame/article16069158/

1469 Prodolliet, J., & Bruelhart, M. (1993). Determination of aspartame and its major decomposition products in foods. Journal of AOAC International, 76(2), 275–282.

1470 Magnuson et al (2007). Aspartame: a safety evaluation based on current use levels, regulations, and toxicological and epidemiological studies. Critical reviews in toxicology, 37(8), 629–727.

1471 Azad et al (2017). Nonnutritive sweeteners and cardiometabolic health: a systematic review and meta-analysis of randomized controlled trials and prospective cohort studies. CMAJ : Canadian Medical Association journal = journal de l'Association medicale canadienne, 189(28), E929–E939.

1472 Rogers et al (2016). Does low-energy sweetener consumption affect energy intake and body weight? A systematic review, including meta-analyses, of the evidence from human and animal studies. International journal of obesity (2005), 40(3), 381–394.

1473 Rodin J. (1990). Comparative effects of fructose, aspartame, glucose, and water preloads on calorie and macronutrient intake. The American journal of clinical nutrition, 51(3), 428–435.

1474 Colagiuri, S., Miller, J. J., & Edwards, R. A. (1989). Metabolic effects of adding sucrose and aspartame to the diet of subjects with noninsulin-dependent diabetes mellitus. The American journal of clinical nutrition, 50(3), 474–478.

1475 Nehrling, J. K., Kobe, P., McLane, M. P., Olson, R. E., Kamath, S., & Horwitz, D. L. (1985). Aspartame use by persons with diabetes. Diabetes care, 8(5), 415–417.

1476 Okuno et al (1986). Glucose tolerance, blood lipid, insulin and glucagon concentration after single or continuous administration of aspartame in diabetics. Diabetes research and clinical practice, 2(1), 23–27.

1477 Ahmad, S. Y., Friel, J. K., & MacKay, D. S. (2020). The effect of the artificial sweeteners on glucose metabolism in healthy adults: a randomized, double-blinded, crossover clinical trial. Applied physiology, nutrition, and metabolism = Physiologie appliquee, nutrition et metabolisme, 45(6), 606–612.

1478 Hall, W. L., Millward, D. J., Rogers, P. J., & Morgan, L. M. (2003). Physiological mechanisms mediating aspartame-induced satiety. Physiology & behavior, 78(4-5), 557–562.

1479 Horwitz, D. L., McLane, M., & Kobe, P. (1988). Response to single dose of aspartame or saccharin by NIDDM patients. Diabetes care, 11(3), 230–234.

1480 Business Wire (31 March 2017). "Sweetener Market Projected to Be Worth USD 2.84 Billion by 2021: Technavio". Yahoo Finance. Archived from the original on 25 April 2017.

1481 de Oliveira et al (2015). Thermal degradation of sucralose: a combination of analytical methods to determine stability and chlorinated byproducts. Scientific reports, 5, 9598.

1482 Magnuson, B. A., Roberts, A., & Nestmann, E. R. (2017). Critical review of the current literature on the safety of sucralose. Food and chemical toxicology : an international journal published for the British Industrial Biological Research Association, 106(Pt A), 324–355.

1483 Berry, C., Brusick, D., Cohen, S. M., Hardisty, J. F., Grotz, V. L., & Williams, G. M. (2016). Sucralose Non-Carcinogenicity: A Review of the Scientific and Regulatory Rationale. Nutrition and cancer, 68(8), 1247–1261.

1484 FDA (1999) 'Food Additives Permitted for Direct Addition to Food for Human Consumption; Sucralose', Federal Register / Vol. 64, No. 155, Accessed Online March 27th 2023: https://www.govinfo.gov/content/pkg/FR-1999-08-12/pdf/99-20888.pdf

1485 Knight I. (1994). The development and applications of sucralose, a new high-intensity sweetener. Canadian journal of physiology and pharmacology, 72(4), 435–439.

1486 Sims, J., Roberts, A., Daniel, J. W., & Renwick, A. G. (2000). The metabolic fate of sucralose in rats. Food and chemical toxicology : an international journal published for the British Industrial Biological Research Association, 38 Suppl 2, S115–S121.

1487 [USFDA] US Food and Drug Administration (1999) Food additives permitted for direct addition to food for human consumption: sucralose. Fed Reg 64:43908–43909. http://www.fda.gov/ohrms/dockets/98fr/081299b.txt.

1488 Miller, P. E., & Perez, V. (2014). Low-calorie sweeteners and body weight and composition: a meta-analysis of randomized controlled trials and prospective cohort studies. The American journal of clinical nutrition, 100(3), 765–777.

1489 Glendinning et al (2020). Low-calorie sweeteners cause only limited metabolic effects in mice. American journal of physiology. Regulatory, integrative and comparative physiology, 318(1), R70–R80.

1490 Iizuka K. (2022). Is the Use of Artificial Sweeteners Beneficial for Patients with Diabetes Mellitus? The Advantages and Disadvantages of Artificial Sweeteners. Nutrients, 14(21), 4446.

1491 Suez et al (2022). Personalized microbiome-driven effects of non-nutritive sweeteners on human glucose tolerance. Cell, 185(18), 3307–3328.e19.

1492 Uebanso et al (2017). Effects of Low-Dose Non-Caloric Sweetener Consumption on Gut Microbiota in Mice. Nutrients, 9(6), 560.

1493 Wang, Q. P., Browman, D., Herzog, H., & Neely, G. G. (2018). Non-nutritive sweeteners possess a bacteriostatic effect and alter gut microbiota in mice. PloS one, 13(7), e0199080.

1494 Grotz et al (2003). Lack of effect of sucralose on glucose homeostasis in subjects with type 2 diabetes. Journal of the American Dietetic Association, 103(12), 1607–1612.

1495 Ma et al (2010). Effect of the artificial sweetener, sucralose, on small intestinal glucose absorption in healthy human subjects. The British journal of nutrition, 104(6), 803–806.

1496 Wu et al (2012). Effects of different sweet preloads on incretin hormone secretion, gastric emptying, and postprandial glycemia in healthy humans. The American journal of clinical nutrition, 95(1), 78–83.

1497 Temizkan et al (2015). Sucralose enhances GLP-1 release and lowers blood glucose in the presence of carbohydrate in healthy subjects but not in patients with type 2 diabetes. European journal of clinical nutrition, 69(2), 162–166.

[1498] Ma et al (2009). Effect of the artificial sweetener, sucralose, on gastric emptying and incretin hormone release in healthy subjects. American journal of physiology. Gastrointestinal and liver physiology, 296(4), G735–G739.

[1499] Steinert, R. E., Frey, F., Töpfer, A., Drewe, J., & Beglinger, C. (2011). Effects of carbohydrate sugars and artificial sweeteners on appetite and the secretion of gastrointestinal satiety peptides. The British journal of nutrition, 105(9), 1320–1328.

[1500] Thomson et al (2019). Short-term impact of sucralose consumption on the metabolic response and gut microbiome of healthy adults. The British journal of nutrition, 122(8), 856–862.

[1501] Temizkan et al (2015). Sucralose enhances GLP-1 release and lowers blood glucose in the presence of carbohydrate in healthy subjects but not in patients with type 2 diabetes. European journal of clinical nutrition, 69(2), 162–166

[1502] Wu et al (2012). Effects of different sweet preloads on incretin hormone secretion, gastric emptying, and postprandial glycemia in healthy humans. The American journal of clinical nutrition, 95(1), 78–83.

[1503] Brown et al (2011). Short-term consumption of sucralose, a nonnutritive sweetener, is similar to water with regard to select markers of hunger signaling and short-term glucose homeostasis in women. Nutrition research (New York, N.Y.), 31(12), 882–888.

[1504] Ma et al (2009). Effect of the artificial sweetener, sucralose, on gastric emptying and incretin hormone release in healthy subjects. American journal of physiology. Gastrointestinal and liver physiology, 296(4), G735–G739.

[1505] Pepino et al (2013). Sucralose affects glycemic and hormonal responses to an oral glucose load. Diabetes care, 36(9), 2530–2535.

[1506] Lertrit et al (2018). Effects of sucralose on insulin and glucagon-like peptide-1 secretion in healthy subjects: a randomized, double-blind, placebo-controlled trial. Nutrition (Burbank, Los Angeles County, Calif.), 55-56, 125–130.

[1507] Sylvetsky, A. C., Brown, R. J., Blau, J. E., Walter, M., & Rother, K. I. (2016). Hormonal responses to non-nutritive sweeteners in water and diet soda. Nutrition & metabolism, 13, 71.

[1508] von Rymon Lipinski, G.-W. (1985). The new intense sweetener Acesulfame K. Food Chemistry, 16(3–4), 259–269.

[1509] Joint FAO/WHO Expert Committee on Food Additives 555: Acesulfame Potassium. Food Additives Series. Geneva: World Health Organization; (1983).

[1510] Magnuson et al (2016). Biological fate of low-calorie sweeteners. Nutrition reviews, 74(11), 670–689.

[1511] Renwick A. G. (1986). The metabolism of intense sweeteners. Xenobiotica; the fate of foreign compounds in biological systems, 16(10-11), 1057–1071.

[1512] von Rymon Lipinski G, Klug C, Acesulfame K. In: O'Brien NL. editor. Alternative Sweeteners. 4th ed Boca Raton, FL: CRC Press; (2012). p. 13–30.

[1513] Bian et al (2017). The artificial sweetener acesulfame potassium affects the gut microbiome and body weight gain in CD-1 mice. PloS one, 12(6), e0178426.

[1514] Uebanso et al (2017). Effects of Low-Dose Non-Caloric Sweetener Consumption on Gut Microbiota in Mice. Nutrients, 9(6), 560.

[1515] Pearson R. Saccharin. In: O'Brien Nabors L e. editor. Alternative Sweeteners. 4th ed Boca Raton, FL: CRC Press; (2012). p. 147–66.

[1516] Sweatman, T. W., & Renwick, A. G. (1980). The tissue distribution and pharmacokinetics of saccharin in the rat. Toxicology and applied pharmacology, 55(1), 18–31.

[1517] Renwick A. G. (1985). The disposition of saccharin in animals and man--a review. Food and chemical toxicology : an international journal published for the British Industrial Biological Research Association, 23(4-5), 429–435.

[1518] Bian et al (2017). Saccharin induced liver inflammation in mice by altering the gut microbiota and its metabolic functions. Food and chemical toxicology : an international journal published for the British Industrial Biological Research Association, 107(Pt B), 530–539.

[1519] Ghosh, S., & Sudha, M. L. (2012). A review on polyols: new frontiers for health-based bakery products. International journal of food sciences and nutrition, 63(3), 372–379.

[1520] Alfarouk et al (2020). The Pentose Phosphate Pathway Dynamics in Cancer and Its Dependency on Intracellular pH. Metabolites, 10(7), 285.

[1521] Ge et al (2020). The Role of the Pentose Phosphate Pathway in Diabetes and Cancer. Frontiers in Endocrinology, 11.

[1522] Wang et al (2012). Activated glucose-6-phosphate dehydrogenase is associated with insulin resistance by upregulating pentose and pentosidine in diet-induced obesity of rats. Hormone and metabolic research = Hormon- und Stoffwechselforschung = Hormones et metabolisme, 44(13), 938–942.

[1523] MONTAGUE, W., & TAYLOR, K. W. (1970). THE ROLE OF THE PENTOSE PHOSPHATE PATHWAY IN INSULIN SECRETION. The Structure and Metabolism of the Pancreatic Islets, 263–273.

[1524] Witkowski et al (2023). The artificial sweetener erythritol and cardiovascular event risk. Nature Medicine, 29(3), 710–718.

[1525] Wen et al (2018). Erythritol Attenuates Postprandial Blood Glucose by Inhibiting α-Glucosidase. Journal of agricultural and food chemistry, 66(6), 1401–1407.

[1526] Flint et al (2014). Effects of erythritol on endothelial function in patients with type 2 diabetes mellitus: a pilot study. Acta diabetologica, 51(3), 513–516.

[1527] Goyal, S. K., Samsher, & Goyal, R. K. (2010). Stevia (Stevia rebaudiana) a bio-sweetener: a review. International journal of food sciences and nutrition, 61(1), 1–10.

[1528] Cardello et al (1999). Measurement of the relative sweetness of stevia extract, aspartame and cyclamate/saccharin blend as compared to sucrose at different concentrations. Plant foods for human nutrition (Dordrecht, Netherlands), 54(2), 119–130.

[1529] Ashwell M. (2015). Stevia, Nature's Zero-Calorie Sustainable Sweetener: A New Player in the Fight Against Obesity. Nutrition today, 50(3), 129–134.

[1530] Gardana et al (2003). Metabolism of stevioside and rebaudioside A from Stevia rebaudiana extracts by human microflora. Journal of agricultural and food chemistry, 51(22), 6618–6622.

[1531] Hutapea A, Toskulkao C, Buddhasukh D, Wilairat P, Glinsukon T. Digestion of stevioside, a natural sweetener, by various digestive enzymes. J Clin Biochem Nutr. (1997) 23:177–86. 10.3164/jcbn.23.177

[1532] Purkayastha et al (2014). In vitro metabolism of rebaudioside B, D, and M under anaerobic conditions: comparison with rebaudioside A. Regulatory toxicology and pharmacology : RTP, 68(2), 259–268.

[1533] Wingard et al (1980). Intestinal degradation and absorption of the glycosidic sweeteners stevioside and rebaudioside A. Experientia, 36(5), 519–520.

[1534] Roberts, A., & Renwick, A. G. (2008). Comparative toxicokinetics and metabolism of rebaudioside A, stevioside, and steviol in rats. Food and chemical toxicology : an international journal published for the British Industrial Biological Research Association, 46 Suppl 7, S31–S39.

[1535] Wheeler et al (2008). Pharmacokinetics of rebaudioside A and stevioside after single oral doses in healthy men. Food and chemical toxicology : an international journal published for the British Industrial Biological Research Association, 46 Suppl 7, S54–S60.

[1536] Koyama et al (2003). In vitro metabolism of the glycosidic sweeteners, stevia mixture and enzymatically modified stevia in human intestinal microflora. Food and chemical toxicology : an international journal published for the British Industrial Biological Research Association, 41(3), 359–374.

[1537] Bundgaard Anker et al (2019). Effect of Steviol Glycosides on Human Health with Emphasis on Type 2 Diabetic Biomarkers: A Systematic Review and Meta-Analysis of Randomized Controlled Trials. Nutrients, 11(9), 1965.

[1538] EFSA Panel on Food Additives and Flavourings (FAF) et al (2019). Safety of use of Monk fruit extract as a food additive in different food categories [JB]. EFSA Journal, 17(12).

[1539] FDA (2018) 'Additional Information about High-Intensity Sweeteners Permitted for Use in Food in the United States', Accessed Online March 29th 2023: https://www.fda.gov/food/food-additives-petitions/additional-information-about-high-intensity-sweeteners-permitted-use-food-united-states#Luo_Han_Guo_fruit_extracts

[1540] Liu et al (2018). Antiglycation and antioxidant activities of mogroside extract from Siraitia grosvenorii (Swingle) fruits. Journal of food science and technology, 55(5), 1880–1888.

[1541] Xu et al (2013). Antioxidant effect of mogrosides against oxidative stress induced by palmitic acid in mouse insulinoma NIT-1 cells. Brazilian journal of medical and biological research = Revista brasileira de pesquisas medicas e biologicas, 46(11), 949–955.

[1542] Di, R., Huang, M.-T., & Ho, C.-T. (2011). Anti-inflammatory Activities of Mogrosides from Momordica grosvenori in Murine Macrophages and a Murine Ear Edema Model. Journal of Agricultural and Food Chemistry, 59(13), 7474–7481.

[1543] Roberfroid M. B. (2005). Introducing inulin-type fructans. The British journal of nutrition, 93 Suppl 1, S13–S25.

[1544] Roberfroid M. B. (2007). Inulin-type fructans: functional food ingredients. The Journal of nutrition, 137(11 Suppl), 2493S–2502S.

[1545] Slavin J. (2013). Fiber and prebiotics: mechanisms and health benefits. Nutrients, 5(4), 1417–1435.

[1546] Kalyani Nair et al (2010). Inulin Dietary Fiber with Functional and Health Attributes—A Review. Food Reviews International, 26(2), 189–203.

[1547] Niness K. R. (1999). Inulin and oligofructose: what are they?. The Journal of nutrition, 129(7 Suppl), 1402S–6S.

[1548] Coulthard, M. G., & Ruddock, V. (1983). Validation of inulin as a marker for glomerular filtration in preterm babies. Kidney international, 23(2), 407–409.

[1549] Rao et al (2019). Effect of Inulin-Type Carbohydrates on Insulin Resistance in Patients with Type 2 Diabetes and Obesity: A Systematic Review and Meta-Analysis. Journal of Diabetes Research, 2019, 1–13.

[1550] Wang et al (2019). Inulin-type fructans supplementation improves glycemic control for the prediabetes and type 2 diabetes populations: results from a GRADE-assessed systematic review and dose–response meta-analysis of 33 randomized controlled trials. Journal of Translational Medicine, 17(1).

[1551] Dehghan et al (2013). Effects of high performance inulin supplementation on glycemic status and lipid profile in women with type 2 diabetes: a randomized, placebo-controlled clinical trial. Health promotion perspectives, 3(1), 55–63.

[1552] Causey et al (2000). Effects of dietary inulin on serum lipids, blood glucose and the gastrointestinal environment in hypercholesterolemic men. Nutrition Research, 20(2), 191–201.

[1553] Liu et al (2017). Effect of inulin-type fructans on blood lipid profile and glucose level: a systematic review and meta-analysis of randomized controlled trials. European journal of clinical nutrition, 71(1), 9–20.

[1554] Russo et al (2008). Inulin-enriched pasta affects lipid profile and Lp(a) concentrations in Italian young healthy male volunteers. European journal of nutrition, 47(8), 453–459.

[1555] Lightowler et al (2017). Replacement of glycaemic carbohydrates by inulin-type fructans from chicory (oligofructose, inulin) reduces the postprandial blood glucose and insulin response to foods: report of two double-blind, randomized, controlled trials. European Journal of Nutrition, 57(3), 1259–1268.

[1556] Cai et al (2018). Milk Powder Co-Supplemented with Inulin and Resistant Dextrin Improves Glycemic Control and Insulin Resistance in Elderly Type 2 Diabetes Mellitus: A 12-Week Randomized, Double-Blind, Placebo-Controlled Trial. Molecular nutrition & food research, 62(24), e1800865.

[1557] Jackson et al (1999). The effect of the daily intake of inulin on fasting lipid, insulin and glucose concentrations in middle-aged men and women. The British journal of nutrition, 82(1), 23–30.

[1558] Coudray, C., Demigné, C., & Rayssiguier, Y. (2003). Effects of dietary fibers on magnesium absorption in animals and humans. The Journal of nutrition, 133(1), 1–4.

[1559] Griffin et al (2003). Enriched chicory inulin increases calcium absorption mainly in girls with lower calcium absorption. Nutrition Research, 23(7), 901–909.

[1560] Abrams et al (2005). A combination of prebiotic short- and long-chain inulin-type fructans enhances calcium absorption and bone mineralization in young adolescents. The American Journal of Clinical Nutrition, 82(2), 471–476.

[1561] Greer, J. B., & O'Keefe, S. J. (2011). Microbial induction of immunity, inflammation, and cancer. Frontiers in physiology, 1, 168.

[1562] Andoh et al (2003). Role of dietary fiber and short-chain fatty acids in the colon. Current pharmaceutical design, 9(4), 347–358.

[1563] Makharia, A., Catassi, C., & Makharia, G. K. (2015). The Overlap between Irritable Bowel Syndrome and Non-Celiac Gluten Sensitivity: A Clinical Dilemma. Nutrients, 7(12), 10417–10426.

[1564] Spiller R. (2017). How do FODMAPs work?. Journal of gastroenterology and hepatology, 32 Suppl 1, 36–39.

[1565] Bacchetta et al (2008). 'Renal hypersensitivity' to inulin and IgA nephropathy. Pediatric nephrology (Berlin, Germany), 23(10), 1883–1885.

[1566] Coussement P. A. (1999). Inulin and oligofructose: safe intakes and legal status. The Journal of nutrition, 129(7 Suppl), 1412S–7S.

[1567] Crane, E. (1991). Honey from honeybees and other insects. Ethology Ecology & Evolution, 3(sup1), 100–105.

[1568] Marlowe et al (2014). Honey, Hadza, hunter-gatherers, and human evolution. Journal of human evolution, 71, 119–128.

[1569] Gheldof et al (2003). Buckwheat honey increases serum antioxidant capacity in humans. Journal of agricultural and food chemistry, 51(5), 1500–1505.

[1570] Khalil et al (2015). Cardioprotective Effects of Tualang Honey: Amelioration of Cholesterol and Cardiac Enzymes Levels. BioMed research international, 2015, 286051.

[1571] Alvarez-Suarez et al (2010). Antioxidant and antimicrobial capacity of several monofloral Cuban honeys and their correlation with color, polyphenol content and other chemical compounds. Food and chemical toxicology : an international journal published for the British Industrial Biological Research Association, 48(8-9), 2490–2499.

[1572] Beretta et al (2005). Standardization of antioxidant properties of honey by a combination of spectrophotometric/fluorimetric assays and chemometrics. Analytica Chimica Acta, 533(2), 185–191.

[1573] Asaduzzaman et al (2015). Effects of Honey Supplementation on Hepatic and Cardiovascular Disease(CVD) Marker in Streptozotocin-Induced Diabetic Rats. Journal of diabetes & metabolism, 6, 1-6.

[1574] Porcza, L. M., Simms, C., & Chopra, M. (2016). Honey and Cancer: Current Status and Future Directions. Diseases (Basel, Switzerland), 4(4), 30.

[1575] Tan et al (2009). The antibacterial properties of Malaysian tualang honey against wound and enteric microorganisms in comparison to manuka honey. BMC complementary and alternative medicine, 9, 34.

316

[1576] van den Berg et al (2008). An in vitro examination of the antioxidant and anti-inflammatory properties of buckwheat honey. Journal of wound care, 17(4), 172–178.

[1577] Weston, R.J. (2000). The contribution of catalase and other natural products to the antibacterial activity of honey: a review. Food Chemistry, 71, 235-239.

[1578] Mandal, M. D., & Mandal, S. (2011). Honey: its medicinal property and antibacterial activity. Asian Pacific journal of tropical biomedicine, 1(2), 154–160.

[1579] Erejuwa et al (2012). Hepatoprotective effect of tualang honey supplementation in streptozotocin-induced diabetic rats. International Journal of Applied Research in Natural Products, 4, 37-41.

[1580] Erejuwa et al (2010). Hypoglycemic and antioxidant effects of honey supplementation in streptozotocin-induced diabetic rats. International journal for vitamin and nutrition research. Internationale Zeitschrift fur Vitamin- und Ernahrungsforschung. Journal international de vitaminologie et de nutrition, 80(1), 74–82.

[1581] Erejuwa et al (2010). Antioxidant protective effect of glibenclamide and metformin in combination with honey in pancreas of streptozotocin-induced diabetic rats. International journal of molecular sciences, 11(5), 2056–2066.

[1582] Abdulrhman, M. A. (2016). Honey as a Sole Treatment of Type 2 Diabetes Mellitus. Endocrinology & Metabolic Syndrome, 05(02).

[1583] Ahmad et al (2008). Natural honey modulates physiological glycemic response compared to simulated honey and D-glucose. Journal of food science, 73(7), H165–H167.

[1584] Al-Waili N. S. (2004). Natural honey lowers plasma glucose, C-reactive protein, homocysteine, and blood lipids in healthy, diabetic, and hyperlipidemic subjects: comparison with dextrose and sucrose. Journal of medicinal food, 7(1), 100–107.

[1585] Agrawal et al (2007). Subjects with impaired glucose tolerance exhibit a high degree of tolerance to honey. Journal of medicinal food, 10(3), 473–478.

[1586] Abdulrhman et al (2013). Effects of honey, sucrose and glucose on blood glucose and C-peptide in patients with type 1 diabetes mellitus. Complementary therapies in clinical practice, 19(1), 15–19.

[1587] Abdulrhman et al (2011). The glycemic and peak incremental indices of honey, sucrose and glucose in patients with type 1 diabetes mellitus: effects on C-peptide level-a pilot study. Acta diabetologica, 48(2), 89–94.

[1588] Watford M. (2002). Small amounts of dietary fructose dramatically increase hepatic glucose uptake through a novel mechanism of glucokinase activation. Nutrition reviews, 60(8), 253–257.

[1589] Abdulrhman et al (2011). The glycemic and peak incremental indices of honey, sucrose and glucose in patients with type 1 diabetes mellitus: effects on C-peptide level-a pilot study. Acta diabetologica, 48(2), 89–94.

[1590] Kwon, S., Kim, Y. J., & Kim, M. K. (2008). Effect of fructose or sucrose feeding with different levels on oral glucose tolerance test in normal and type 2 diabetic rats. Nutrition research and practice, 2(4), 252–258.

[1591] Erejuwa et al (2012). Fructose might contribute to the hypoglycemic effect of honey. Molecules (Basel, Switzerland), 17(2), 1900–1915.

[1592] Yaghoobi et al (2008). Natural honey and cardiovascular risk factors; effects on blood glucose, cholesterol, triacylglycerole, CRP, and body weight compared with sucrose. TheScientificWorldJournal, 8, 463–469.

[1593] Bahrami et al (2009). Effects of natural honey consumption in diabetic patients: an 8-week randomized clinical trial. International journal of food sciences and nutrition, 60(7), 618–626.

[1594] Alvarez-Suarez et al (2016) 'Activation of AMPK/Nrf2 signalling by Manuka honey protects human dermal fibroblasts against oxidative damage by improving antioxidant response and mitochondrial function promoting wound healing', Journal of Functional Foods, Volume 25, August 2016, Pages 38-49.

[1595] Alam et al (2014). Honey: a potential therapeutic agent for managing diabetic wounds. Evidence-based complementary and alternative medicine : eCAM, 2014, 169130.

[1596] Estevinho et al (2008). Antioxidant and antimicrobial effects of phenolic compounds extracts of Northeast Portugal honey. Food and chemical toxicology : an international journal published for the British Industrial Biological Research Association, 46(12), 3774–3779.

[1597] Cooper et al (1999). Antibacterial activity of honey against strains of Staphylococcus aureus from infected wounds. Journal of the Royal Society of Medicine, 92(6), 283–285.

[1598] Mathews K. A., Binnington A. G. Wound management using honey. Compendium on Continuing Education for the Practicing Verterinarian. 2002;24(1):53–59.

[1599] Al-Waili, N. S., & Boni, N. S. (2004). Honey increased saliva, plasma, and urine content of total nitrite concentrations in normal individuals. Journal of medicinal food, 7(3), 377–380.

[1600] Lotfy et al (2006). Combined use of honey, bee propolis and myrrh in healing a deep, infected wound in a patient with diabetes mellitus. British journal of biomedical science, 63(4), 171–173.

[1601] Shukrimi et al (2008). A comparative study between honey and povidone iodine as dressing solution for Wagner type II diabetic foot ulcers. The Medical journal of Malaysia, 63(1), 44–46.

[1602] Kamaratos et al (2014). Manuka honey-impregnated dressings in the treatment of neuropathic diabetic foot ulcers. International wound journal, 11(3), 259–263.

[1603] Tanzi, M. & Gabay, M. (2002). Association between honey consumption and infant botulism. *Pharmacotherapy* 22 (11): 1479–1483. Review.

[1604] Lagacé et al (2019). Effect of the new high vacuum technology on the chemical composition of maple sap and syrup. Heliyon, 5(6), e01786.

[1605] Schroeder H. A. (1967). Cadmium, chromium, and cardiovascular disease. Circulation, 35(3), 570–582. https://doi.org/10.1161/01.cir.35.3.570

[1606] Apostolidis et al (2011). In vitro evaluation of phenolic-enriched maple syrup extracts for inhibition of carbohydrate hydrolyzing enzymes relevant to type 2 diabetes management. Journal of Functional Foods, 3(2), 100–106.

[1607] St-Pierre et al (2014). Comparative analysis of maple syrup to other natural sweeteners and evaluation of their metabolic responses in healthy rats. Journal of Functional Foods, 11, 460–471.

[1608] Nagai, N., Ito, Y., & Taga, A. (2013). Comparison of the enhancement of plasma glucose levels in type 2 diabetes Otsuka Long-Evans Tokushima Fatty rats by oral administration of sucrose or maple syrup. Journal of oleo science, 62(9), 737–743.

[1609] Toyoda, T., Kamei, A., Ishijima, T. et al. A maple syrup extract alters lipid metabolism in obese type 2 diabetic model mice. Nutr Metab (Lond) 16, 84 (2019).

[1610] DiNicolantonio (2017) 'Low-Salt Diets May Be Sensitizing Us to Addiction', VICE, Accessed Online May 6th 2022: https://www.vice.com/amp/en/article/9k5bwe/low-salt-diets-may-be-screwing-with-evolution

[1611] Clark, J. J., & Bernstein, I. L. (2006). A role for D2 but not D1 dopamine receptors in the cross-sensitization between amphetamine and salt appetite. Pharmacology Biochemistry and Behavior, 83(2), 277–284. https://doi.org/10.1016/j.pbb.2006.02.008

[1612] Roitman, M. F., Na, E., Anderson, G., Jones, T. A., & Bernstein, I. L. (2002). Induction of a salt appetite alters dendritic morphology in nucleus accumbens and sensitizes rats to amphetamine. The Journal of neuroscience : the official journal of the Society for Neuroscience, 22(11), RC225. https://doi.org/10.1523/JNEUROSCI.22-11-j0001.2002

[1613] Sakai, R. R., Fine, W. B., Epstein, A. N., & Frankmann, S. P. (1987). Salt appetite is enhanced by one prior episode of sodium depletion in the rat. Behavioral neuroscience, 101(5), 724–731. https://doi.org/10.1037//0735-7044.101.5.724

[1614] Denton, D. A., McKinley, M. J., & Weisinger, R. S. (1996). Hypothalamic integration of body fluid regulation. Proceedings of the National Academy of Sciences of the United States of America, 93(14), 7397–7404. https://doi.org/10.1073/pnas.93.14.7397

[1615] Liedtke, W. B., McKinley, M. J., Walker, L. L., Zhang, H., Pfenning, A. R., Drago, J., Hochendoner, S. J., Hilton, D. L., Lawrence, A. J., & Denton, D. A. (2011). Relation of addiction genes to hypothalamic gene changes subserving genesis and gratification of a classic instinct, sodium appetite. Proceedings of the National Academy of Sciences of the United States of America, 108(30), 12509–12514. https://doi.org/10.1073/pnas.1109199108

[1616] Robinson, T. E., & Berridge, K. C. (1993). The neural basis of drug craving: an incentive-sensitization theory of addiction. Brain research. Brain research reviews, 18(3), 247–291. https://doi.org/10.1016/0165-0173(93)90013-p

[1617] Robinson, T. E., & Kolb, B. (1997). Persistent structural modifications in nucleus accumbens and prefrontal cortex neurons produced by previous experience with amphetamine. The Journal of neuroscience : the official journal of the Society for Neuroscience, 17(21), 8491–8497. https://doi.org/10.1523/JNEUROSCI.17-21-08491.1997

[1618] Clark, J. J., & Bernstein, I. L. (2006). A role for D2 but not D1 dopamine receptors in the cross-sensitization between amphetamine and salt appetite. Pharmacology, biochemistry, and behavior, 83(2), 277–284. https://doi.org/10.1016/j.pbb.2006.02.008

[1619] Heaney R. P. (2015). Making Sense of the Science of Sodium. Nutrition today, 50(2), 63–66. https://doi.org/10.1097/NT.0000000000000084

[1620] Guinard, J. X., & Brun, P. (1998). Sensory-specific satiety: comparison of taste and texture effects. Appetite, 31(2), 141–157. https://doi.org/10.1006/appe.1998.0159

[1621] Rolls et al (1981) 'Sensory specific satiety in man', Physiology & Behavior, Volume 27, Issue 1, July 1981, Pages 137-142.

[1622] Rolls, B. J., Rowe, E. A., Rolls, E. T., Kingston, B., Megson, A., & Gunary, R. (1981). Variety in a meal enhances food intake in man. Physiology & behavior, 26(2), 215–221. https://doi.org/10.1016/0031-9384(81)90014-7

[1623] Rolls, B. J., Rolls, E. T. & Rowe, E. A. (1982b). The influence of variety on food selection and intake in man. In L. M. Barker (Ed.), Psychobiology of Human Food Selection. Pp. 101–122. Westport, CT: A.V.I. Publishing Co.

[1624] Rolls, B. J., Rowe, E. A., & Rolls, E. T. (1982). How sensory properties of foods affect human feeding behavior. Physiology & behavior, 29(3), 409–417. https://doi.org/10.1016/0031-9384(82)90259-1

[1625] DiMeglio, L. A., Evans-Molina, C., & Oram, R. A. (2018). Type 1 diabetes. Lancet (London, England), 391(10138), 2449–2462. https://doi.org/10.1016/S0140-6736(18)31320-5

[1626] Katsarou et al (2017). Type 1 diabetes mellitus. Nature reviews. Disease primers, 3, 17016.

[1627] Knip et al (2005). Environmental triggers and determinants of type 1 diabetes. Diabetes, 54 Suppl 2, S125–S136.

[1628] Butler, A. E., & Misselbrook, D. (2020). Distinguishing between type 1 and type 2 diabetes. BMJ (Clinical research ed.), 370, m2998. https://doi.org/10.1136/bmj.m2998

[1629] Diabetes Research Institute Foundation (2023) 'Living With Diabetes', Accessed Online March 6th 2023: https://diabetesresearch.org/type-1-diabetes-cure/

[1630] Diabetes Research Institute Foundation (2023) 'Curing Diabetes', Accessed Online March 6th 2023: https://diabetesresearch.org/DRI-clinical-trials/

[1631] Silverstein, A. M. (2014). Autoimmunity. The Autoimmune Diseases, 11–17. doi:10.1016/b978-0-12-384929-8.00002-2

[1632] Silverstein, A. M. (2001). Autoimmunity versus horror autotoxicus: The struggle for recognition. Nature Immunology, 2(4), 279–281. doi:10.1038/86280

[1633] Poletaev, A. B., Churilov, L. P., Stroev, Y. I., & Agapov, M. M. (2012). Immunophysiology versus immunopathology: Natural autoimmunity in human health and disease. Pathophysiology : the official journal of the International Society for Pathophysiology, 19(3), 221–231. https://doi.org/10.1016/j.pathophys.2012.07.003

[1634] Stefanová, I., Dorfman, J. R., & Germain, R. N. (2002). Self-recognition promotes the foreign antigen sensitivity of naive T lymphocytes. Nature, 420(6914), 429–434. doi:10.1038/nature01146

[1635] Blumberg, R. S., Dittel, B., Hafler, D., von Herrath, M., & Nestle, F. O. (2012). Unraveling the autoimmune translational research process layer by layer. Nature Medicine, 18(1), 35–41. doi:10.1038/nm.2632

[1636] Bluestone, J. A., Tang, Q., & Sedwick, C. E. (2008). T Regulatory Cells in Autoimmune Diabetes: Past Challenges, Future Prospects. Journal of Clinical Immunology, 28(6), 677–684. doi:10.1007/s10875-008-9242-z

[1637] Yurasov, S., Wardemann, H., Hammersen, J., Tsuiji, M., Meffre, E., Pascual, V., & Nussenzweig, M. C. (2005). Defective B cell tolerance checkpoints in systemic lupus erythematosus. Journal of Experimental Medicine, 201(5), 703–711. doi:10.1084/jem.20042251

[1638] Mohan, J. F., & Unanue, E. R. (2012). Unconventional recognition of peptides by T cells and the implications for autoimmunity. Nature Reviews Immunology, 12(10), 721–728. doi:10.1038/nri3294

[1639] Audiger, C., Rahman, M. J., Yun, T. J., Tarbell, K. V., & Lesage, S. (2017). The Importance of Dendritic Cells in Maintaining Immune Tolerance. The Journal of Immunology, 198(6), 2223–2231. doi:10.4049/jimmunol.1601629

[1640] Ganguly, D., Haak, S., Sisirak, V., & Reizis, B. (2013). The role of dendritic cells in autoimmunity. Nature Reviews Immunology, 13(8), 566–577. doi:10.1038/nri3477

[1641] Hardin, J. A. (2005). Dendritic cells: potential triggers of autoimmunity and targets for therapy. Annals of the Rheumatic Diseases, 64(suppl_4), iv86–iv90. doi:10.1136/ard.2005.044560

[1642] Litman, G. W., Cannon, J. P., & Dishaw, L. J. (2005). Reconstructing immune phylogeny: new perspectives. Nature Reviews Immunology, 5(11), 866–879. doi:10.1038/nri1712

[1643] Pancer, Z., & Cooper, M. D. (2006). THE EVOLUTION OF ADAPTIVE IMMUNITY. Annual Review of Immunology, 24(1), 497–518. doi:10.1146/annurev.immunol.24.021605.090542

[1644] Stiemsma L, Reynolds L, Turvey S, Finlay B. The hygiene hypothesis: current perspectives and future therapies. Immunotargets Ther. 2015;4:143-157

[1645] Shaw, S. Y., Blanchard, J. F., & Bernstein, C. N. (2010). Association Between the Use of Antibiotics in the First Year of Life and Pediatric Inflammatory Bowel Disease. American Journal of Gastroenterology, 105(12), 2687–2692. doi:10.1038/ajg.2010.398

[1646] Olszak, T., An, D., Zeissig, S., Vera, M. P., Richter, J., Franke, A., Glickman, J. N., Siebert, R., Baron, R. M., Kasper, D. L., & Blumberg, R. S. (2012). Microbial exposure during early life has persistent effects on natural killer T cell function. Science (New York, N.Y.), 336(6080), 489–493. https://doi.org/10.1126/science.1219328

[1647] Blustein, J., & Liu, J. (2015). Time to consider the risks of caesarean delivery for long term child health. BMJ, 350(jun09 3), h2410–h2410. doi:10.1136/bmj.h2410

[1648] Bach, J.-F., & Chatenoud, L. (2012). The Hygiene Hypothesis: An Explanation for the Increased Frequency of Insulin-Dependent Diabetes. Cold Spring Harbor Perspectives in Medicine, 2(2), a007799–a007799. doi:10.1101/cshperspect.a007799

[1649] Procaccini, C., Carbone, F., Galgani, M., La Rocca, C., De Rosa, V., Cassano, S., & Matarese, G. (2011). Obesity and susceptibility to autoimmune diseases. Expert Review of Clinical Immunology, 7(3), 287–294. doi:10.1586/eci.11.18

[1650] Rosenblum, M. D., Remedios, K. A., & Abbas, A. K. (2015). Mechanisms of human autoimmunity. Journal of Clinical Investigation, 125(6), 2228–2233. doi:10.1172/jci78088

[1651] Zenewicz, L. A., Abraham, C., Flavell, R. A., & Cho, J. H. (2010). Unraveling the Genetics of Autoimmunity. Cell, 140(6), 791–797. doi:10.1016/j.cell.2010.03.003

[1652] Criswell, L. A., Pfeiffer, K. A., Lum, R. F., Gonzales, B., Novitzke, J., Kern, M., … Gregersen, P. K. (2005). Analysis of Families in the Multiple Autoimmune Disease Genetics Consortium (MADGC) Collection: the PTPN22 620W Allele Associates with Multiple Autoimmune Phenotypes. The American Journal of Human Genetics, 76(4), 561–571. doi:10.1086/429096

[1653] Bottini, N., Musumeci, L., Alonso, A., Rahmouni, S., Nika, K., Rostamkhani, M., … Mustelin, T. (2004). A functional variant of lymphoid tyrosine phosphatase is associated with type I diabetes. Nature Genetics, 36(4), 337–338. doi:10.1038/ng1323

[1654] Kyogoku, C., Ortmann, W. A., Lee, A., Selby, S., Carlton, V. E. H., Chang, M., … Behrens, T. W. (2004). Genetic Association of the R620W Polymorphism of Protein Tyrosine Phosphatase PTPN22 with Human SLE. The American Journal of Human Genetics, 75(3), 504–507. doi:10.1086/423790

[1655] Begovich, A. B., Caillier, S. J., Alexander, H. C., Penko, J. M., Hauser, S. L., Barcellos, L. F., & Oksenberg, J. R. (2005). The R620W Polymorphism of the Protein Tyrosine Phosphatase PTPN22 Is Not Associated with Multiple Sclerosis. The American Journal of Human Genetics, 76(1), 184–187. doi:10.1086/427244

[1656] Begovich, A. B., Carlton, V. E. H., Honigberg, L. A., Schrodi, S. J., Chokkalingam, A. P., Alexander, H. C., … Gregersen, P. K. (2004). A Missense Single-Nucleotide Polymorphism in a Gene Encoding a Protein Tyrosine Phosphatase (PTPN22) Is Associated with Rheumatoid Arthritis. The American Journal of Human Genetics, 75(2), 330–337. doi:10.1086/422827

[1657] Cerosaletti, K., Schneider, A., Schwedhelm, K., Frank, I., Tatum, M., Wei, S., … Long, S. A. (2013). Multiple Autoimmune-Associated Variants Confer Decreased IL-2R Signaling in CD4+CD25hi T Cells of Type 1 Diabetic and Multiple Sclerosis Patients. PLoS ONE, 8(12), e83811. doi:10.1371/journal.pone.0083811

[1658] Klein, J., & Sato, A. (2000). The HLA System. New England Journal of Medicine, 343(11), 782–786. doi:10.1056/nejm200009143431106

[1659] Cruz-Tapias et al (2012). HLA and Sjögren's syndrome susceptibility. A meta-analysis of worldwide studies. Autoimmunity reviews, 11(4), 281–287.

[1660] Nguyen et al (2013) 'Definition of High-Risk Type 1 Diabetes HLA-DR and HLA-DQ Types Using Only Three Single Nucleotide Polymorphisms ', Diabetes 2013;62(6):2135–2140.

[1661] Noble, J. A., & Valdes, A. M. (2011). Genetics of the HLA region in the prediction of type 1 diabetes. Current diabetes reports, 11(6), 533–542.

[1662] Jaraquemada (1984) 'Association of HLA-DR4/Dw4 and DR2/Dw2 with radiologic changes in a prospective study of patients with rheumatoid arthritis', Arthritis and Rheumatism, Vol 27, No 1.

[1663] Kuhn, A., Wenzel, J., & Weyd, H. (2014). Photosensitivity, Apoptosis, and Cytokines in the Pathogenesis of Lupus Erythematosus: a Critical Review. Clinical Reviews in Allergy & Immunology, 47(2), 148–162. doi:10.1007/s12016-013-8403-x

[1664] Stojanovich, L., & Marisavljevich, D. (2008). Stress as a trigger of autoimmune disease. Autoimmunity Reviews, 7(3), 209–213. doi:10.1016/j.autrev.2007.11.007

[1665] Root-Bernstein, R., & Fairweather, D. (2013). Complexities in the Relationship Between Infection and Autoimmunity. Current Allergy and Asthma Reports, 14(1). doi:10.1007/s11882-013-0407-3

[1666] Patel, B., Schutte, R., Sporns, P., Doyle, J., Jewel, L., & Fedorak, R. N. (2002). Potato Glycoalkaloids Adversely Affect Intestinal Permeability and Aggravate Inflammatory Bowel Disease. Inflammatory Bowel Diseases, 8(5), 340–346. doi:10.1097/00054725-200209000-00005

[1667] Freed, D. L. J. (1999). Do dietary lectins cause disease? BMJ, 318(7190), 1023–1024. doi:10.1136/bmj.318.7190.1023

[1668] Sanchez, A., Reeser, J. L., Lau, H. S., Yahiku, P. Y., Willard, R. E., McMillan, P. J., … Register, U. D. (1973). Role of sugars in human neutrophilic phagocytosis. The American Journal of Clinical Nutrition, 26(11), 1180–1184. doi:10.1093/ajcn/26.11.1180

[1669] Lerner, A., Shoenfeld, Y., & Matthias, T. (2017). Adverse effects of gluten ingestion and advantages of gluten withdrawal in nonceliac autoimmune disease. Nutrition Reviews, 75(12), 1046–1058. doi:10.1093/nutrit/nux054

[1670] Vojdani, A., & Tarash, I. (2013). Cross-Reaction between Gliadin and Different Food and Tissue Antigens. Food and Nutrition Sciences, 04(01), 20–32. doi:10.4236/fns.2013.41005

[1671] Taylor, P. C., & Feldmann, M. (2009). Anti-TNF biologic agents: still the therapy of choice for rheumatoid arthritis. Nature Reviews Rheumatology, 5(10), 578–582. doi:10.1038/nrrheum.2009.181

[1672] Patel, D. D., Lee, D. M., Kolbinger, F., & Antoni, C. (2012). Effect of IL-17A blockade with secukinumab in autoimmune diseases. Annals of the Rheumatic Diseases, 72(suppl 2), iii116–iii123. doi:10.1136/annrheumdis-2012-202371

[1673] Buckner, J. H. (2010). Mechanisms of impaired regulation by CD4+CD25+FOXP3+ regulatory T cells in human autoimmune diseases. Nature Reviews Immunology, 10(12), 849–859. doi:10.1038/nri2889

[1674] Sanchez Rodriguez, R., Pauli, M. L., Neuhaus, I. M., Yu, S. S., Arron, S. T., Harris, H. W., … Rosenblum, M. D. (2014). Memory regulatory T cells reside in human skin. Journal of Clinical Investigation, 124(3), 1027–1036. doi:10.1172/jci72932

[1675] Kuehn, H. S., Ouyang, W., Lo, B., Deenick, E. K., Niemela, J. E., Avery, D. T., … Uzel, G. (2014). Immune dysregulation in human subjects with heterozygous germline mutations in CTLA4. Science, 345(6204), 1623–1627. doi:10.1126/science.1255904

[1676] Lucier, J., & Tabatabai, L. (2020). SAT-677 A Case of Opdivo Induced Type 1 Diabetes. Journal of the Endocrine Society, 4(Supplement_1).

[1677] Thayer et al (2012). Role of environmental chemicals in diabetes and obesity: a National Toxicology Program workshop review. Environmental health perspectives, 120(6), 779–789.

[1678] Repaske D. R. (2016). Medication-induced diabetes mellitus. Pediatric diabetes, 17(6), 392–397.

[1679] Nikoopour, E., Schwartz, J. A., & Singh, B. (2008). Therapeutic benefits of regulating inflammation in autoimmunity. Inflammation & allergy drug targets, 7(3), 203–210. https://doi.org/10.2174/187152808785748155

[1680] Manzel, A., Muller, D. N., Hafler, D. A., Erdman, S. E., Linker, R. A., & Kleinewietfeld, M. (2013). Role of "Western Diet" in Inflammatory Autoimmune Diseases. Current Allergy and Asthma Reports, 14(1). doi:10.1007/s11882-013-0404-6

[1681] Hedström, A. K., Lima Bomfim, I., Hillert, J., Olsson, T., & Alfredsson, L. (2014). Obesity interacts with infectious mononucleosis in risk of multiple sclerosis. European Journal of Neurology, 22(3), 578–e38. doi:10.1111/ene.12620

[1682] Van den Elsen, L. W., Poyntz, H. C., Weyrich, L. S., Young, W., & Forbes-Blom, E. E. (2017). Embracing the gut microbiota: the new frontier for inflammatory and infectious diseases. Clinical & Translational Immunology, 6(1), e125. doi:10.1038/cti.2016.91

[1683] Lazar, V., Ditu, L.-M., Pircalabioru, G. G., Gheorghe, I., Curutiu, C., Holban, A. M., … Chifiriuc, M. C. (2018). Aspects of Gut Microbiota and Immune System Interactions in Infectious Diseases, Immunopathology, and Cancer. Frontiers in Immunology, 9. doi:10.3389/fimmu.2018.01830

[1684] Thaiss, C. A., Zmora, N., Levy, M., & Elinav, E. (2016). The microbiome and innate immunity. Nature, 535(7610), 65–74. doi:10.1038/nature18847

[1685] Zhou, X., Du, L., Shi, R., Chen, Z., Zhou, Y., & Li, Z. (2018). Early-life food nutrition, microbiota maturation and immune development shape life-long health. Critical Reviews in Food Science and Nutrition, 59(sup1), S30–S38. doi:10.1080/10408398.2018.1485628

[1686] Scher, J. U., Sczesnak, A., Longman, R. S., Segata, N., Ubeda, C., Bielski, C., … Littman, D. R. (2013). Expansion of intestinal Prevotella copri correlates with enhanced susceptibility to arthritis. eLife, 2. doi:10.7554/elife.01202

[1687] Khan, M. T., Duncan, S. H., Stams, A. J. M., van Dijl, J. M., Flint, H. J., & Harmsen, H. J. M. (2012). The gut anaerobe Faecalibacterium prausnitzii uses an extracellular electron shuttle to grow at oxic–anoxic interphases. The ISME Journal, 6(8), 1578–1585. doi:10.1038/ismej.2012.5

[1688] M'koma, A. E. (2013). Inflammatory Bowel Disease: An Expanding Global Health Problem. Clinical Medicine Insights: Gastroenterology, 6, CGast.S12731. doi:10.4137/cgast.s12731

[1689] Zhou et al (2020). Evaluating the Causal Role of Gut Microbiota in Type 1 Diabetes and Its Possible Pathogenic Mechanisms. Frontiers in Endocrinology, 11.

[1690] Vatanen, T., Franzosa, E.A., Schwager, R. et al. The human gut microbiome in early-onset type 1 diabetes from the TEDDY study. Nature 562, 589–594 (2018).

[1691] Alkanani, A. K., Hara, N., Gottlieb, P. A., Ir, D., Robertson, C. E., Wagner, B. D., … Zipris, D. (2015). Alterations in Intestinal Microbiota Correlate With Susceptibility to Type 1 Diabetes. Diabetes, 64(10), 3510–3520. doi:10.2337/db14-1847

[1692] Jamshidi, P., Hasanzadeh, S., Tahvildari, A. et al. Is there any association between gut microbiota and type 1 diabetes? A systematic review. Gut Pathog 11, 49 (2019).

[1693] Maffeis, C., Martina, A., Corradi, M., Quarella, S., Nori, N., Torriani, S., … Felis, G. E. (2016). Association between intestinal permeability and faecal microbiota composition in Italian children with beta cell autoimmunity at risk for type 1 diabetes. Diabetes/Metabolism Research and Reviews, 32(7), 700–709. doi:10.1002/dmrr.2790

[1694] De Goffau, M. C., Luopajarvi, K., Knip, M., Ilonen, J., Ruohtula, T., Harkonen, T., … Vaarala, O. (2012). Fecal Microbiota Composition Differs Between Children With -Cell Autoimmunity and Those Without. Diabetes, 62(4), 1238–1244. doi:10.2337/db12-0526

[1695] Van den Elsen, L. W., Poyntz, H. C., Weyrich, L. S., Young, W., & Forbes-Blom, E. E. (2017). Embracing the gut microbiota: the new frontier for inflammatory and infectious diseases. Clinical & Translational Immunology, 6(1), e125. doi:10.1038/cti.2016.91

[1696] Matsuguchi, T., Takagi, A., Matsuzaki, T., Nagaoka, M., Ishikawa, K., Yokokura, T., & Yoshikai, Y. (2003). Lipoteichoic Acids from Lactobacillus Strains Elicit Strong Tumor Necrosis Factor Alpha-Inducing Activities in Macrophages through Toll-Like Receptor 2. Clinical Diagnostic Laboratory Immunology, 10(2), 259–266. doi:10.1128/cdli.10.2.259-266.2003

[1697] Ventura et al (2006). Intestinal permeability in patients with adverse reactions to food. Digestive and liver disease : official journal of the Italian Society of Gastroenterology and the Italian Association for the Study of the Liver, 38(10), 732–736.

[1698] Arrieta, M. C., Bistritz, L., & Meddings, J. B. (2006). Alterations in intestinal permeability. Gut, 55(10), 1512–1520. https://doi.org/10.1136/gut.2005.085373

[1699] Vaarala O. (2008). Leaking gut in type 1 diabetes. Current opinion in gastroenterology, 24(6), 701–706.

[1700] de Kort, S., Keszthelyi, D., & Masclee, A. A. (2011). Leaky gut and diabetes mellitus: what is the link?. Obesity reviews : an official journal of the International Association for the Study of Obesity, 12(6), 449–458.

[1701] Visser et al (2009). Tight junctions, intestinal permeability, and autoimmunity: celiac disease and type 1 diabetes paradigms. Annals of the New York Academy of Sciences, 1165, 195–205.

[1702] Meddings et al (1999). Increased gastrointestinal permeability is an early lesion in the spontaneously diabetic BB rat. The American journal of physiology, 276(4), G951–G957.

[1703] Bischoff et al (2014). Intestinal permeability--a new target for disease prevention and therapy. BMC gastroenterology, 14, 189.

[1704] Hietbrink et al (2009). Systemic inflammation increases intestinal permeability during experimental human endotoxemia. Shock (Augusta, Ga.), 32(4), 374–378.

[1705] Konturek et al (2011). Stress and the gut: pathophysiology, clinical consequences, diagnostic approach and treatment options. Journal of physiology and pharmacology : an official journal of the Polish Physiological Society, 62(6), 591–599.

[1706] Ferrier et al (2006). Impairment of the intestinal barrier by ethanol involves enteric microflora and mast cell activation in rodents. The American journal of pathology, 168(4), 1148–1154.

[1707] Spruss, A., & Bergheim, I. (2009). Dietary fructose and intestinal barrier: potential risk factor in the pathogenesis of nonalcoholic fatty liver disease. The Journal of nutritional biochemistry, 20(9), 657–662.

[1708] Bjarnason, I., & Takeuchi, K. (2009). Intestinal permeability in the pathogenesis of NSAID-induced enteropathy. Journal of gastroenterology, 44 Suppl 19, 23–29.

[1709] Fasano, A. (2011). Zonulin and Its Regulation of Intestinal Barrier Function: The Biological Door to Inflammation, Autoimmunity, and Cancer. Physiological Reviews, 91(1), 151–175.

[1710] Fasano A. (2012). Intestinal permeability and its regulation by zonulin: diagnostic and therapeutic implications. Clinical gastroenterology and hepatology : the official clinical practice journal of the American Gastroenterological Association, 10(10), 1096–1100.

[1711] Sapone et al (2006). Zonulin upregulation is associated with increased gut permeability in subjects with type 1 diabetes and their relatives. Diabetes, 55(5), 1443–1449.

[1712] Suzuki, T., & Hara, H. (2011). Role of flavonoids in intestinal tight junction regulation. The Journal of Nutritional Biochemistry, 22(5), 401–408. doi:10.1016/j.jnutbio.2010.08.001

[1713] Illescas-Montes R, Melguizo-Rodríguez L, Ruiz C, Costela-Ruiz VJ. Vitamin D and autoimmune diseases. Life Sci. 2019;233:116744. doi:10.1016/j.lfs.2019.116744

[1714] Yang, C.-Y., Leung, P. S. C., Adamopoulos, I. E., & Gershwin, M. E. (2013). The Implication of Vitamin D and Autoimmunity: a Comprehensive Review. Clinical Reviews in Allergy & Immunology, 45(2), 217–226. doi:10.1007/s12016-013-8361-3

[1715] Holick, M. F. (2004). Sunlight and vitamin D for bone health and prevention of autoimmune diseases, cancers, and cardiovascular disease. The American Journal of Clinical Nutrition, 80(6), 1678S–1688S. doi:10.1093/ajcn/80.6.1678s

[1716] Lopez, E. R., Regulla, K., Pani, M. A., Krause, M., Usadel, K.-H., & Badenhoop, K. (2004). CYP27B1 polymorphisms variants are associated with type 1 diabetes mellitus in Germans. The Journal of Steroid Biochemistry and Molecular Biology, 89-90, 155–157. doi:10.1016/j.jsbmb.2004.03.095

[1717] Fichna, M., Żurawek, M., Januszkiewicz-Lewandowska, D., Gryczyñska, M., Fichna, P., Sowiñski, J., & Nowak, J. (2009). Association of the CYP27B1 C(−1260)A Polymorphism with Autoimmune Addison's Disease. Experimental and Clinical Endocrinology & Diabetes, 118(08), 544–549. doi:10.1055/s-0029-1241206

[1718] Lopez, E., Zwermann, O., Segni, M., Meyer, G., Reincke, M., Seissler, J., … Badenhoop, K. (2004). A promoter polymorphism of the CYP27B1 gene is associated with Addison's disease, Hashimoto's thyroiditis, Graves' disease and type 1 diabetes mellitus in Germans. European Journal of Endocrinology, 193–197. doi:10.1530/eje.0.1510193

[1719] Acheson, E. D., Bachrach, C. A., & Wright, F. M. (1960). SOME COMMENTS ON THE RELATIONSHIP OF THE DISTRIBUTION OF MULTIPLE SCLEROSIS TO LATITUDE, SOLAR RADIATION, AND OTHER VARIABLES. Acta Psychiatrica Scandinavica, 35(S147), 132–147. doi:10.1111/j.1600-0447.1960.tb08674.x

[1720] Meier, D. S., Balashov, K. E., Healy, B., Weiner, H. L., & Guttmann, C. R. G. (2010). Seasonal prevalence of MS disease activity. Neurology, 75(9), 799–806. doi:10.1212/wnl.0b013e3181f0734c

[1721] Embry, A. F., Snowdon, L. R., & Vieth, R. (2000). Vitamin D and seasonal fluctuations of gadolinium-enhancing magnetic resonance imaging lesions in multiple sclerosis. Annals of neurology, 48(2), 271–272.

[1722] Simpson, S., Blizzard, L., Otahal, P., Van der Mei, I., & Taylor, B. (2011). Latitude is significantly associated with the prevalence of multiple sclerosis: a meta-analysis. Journal of Neurology, Neurosurgery & Psychiatry, 82(10), 1132–1141. doi:10.1136/jnnp.2011.240432

[1723] McDowell, T.-Y., Amr, S., Culpepper, W. J., Langenberg, P., Royal, W., Bever, C., & Bradham, D. D. (2011). Sun Exposure, Vitamin D and Age at Disease Onset in Relapsing Multiple Sclerosis. Neuroepidemiology, 36(1), 39–45. doi:10.1159/000322512

[1724] Van der Mei, I. A. F. (2003). Past exposure to sun, skin phenotype, and risk of multiple sclerosis: case-control study. BMJ, 327(7410), 316–0. doi:10.1136/bmj.327.7410.316

[1725] Hayes, C. E., Hubler, S. L., Moore, J. R., Barta, L. E., Praska, C. E., & Nashold, F. E. (2015). Vitamin D Actions on CD4+ T Cells in Autoimmune Disease. Frontiers in Immunology, 6. doi:10.3389/fimmu.2015.00100

[1726] Moltchanova, E. V., Schreier, N., Lammi, N., & Karvonen, M. (2009). Seasonal variation of diagnosis of Type 1 diabetes mellitus in children worldwide. Diabetic Medicine, 26(7), 673–678. doi:10.1111/j.1464-5491.2009.02743.x

[1727] Hyppönen, E., Läärä, E., Reunanen, A., Järvelin, M.-R., & Virtanen, S. M. (2001). Intake of vitamin D and risk of type 1 diabetes: a birth-cohort study. The Lancet, 358(9292), 1500–1503. doi:10.1016/s0140-6736(01)06580-1

[1728] Boitard, C. (2013). T-lymphocyte recognition of beta cells in type 1 diabetes: Clinical perspectives. Diabetes & Metabolism, 39(6), 459–466. doi:10.1016/j.diabet.2013.08.001

[1729] Severson, C., & Hafler, D. A. (2009). T-Cells in Multiple Sclerosis. Molecular Basis of Multiple Sclerosis, 75–98. doi:10.1007/400_2009_9012

[1730] Yang, C.-Y., Leung, P. S. C., Adamopoulos, I. E., & Gershwin, M. E. (2013). The Implication of Vitamin D and Autoimmunity: a Comprehensive Review. Clinical Reviews in Allergy & Immunology, 45(2), 217–226. doi:10.1007/s12016-013-8361-3

[1731] Aspray, T. J., Bowring, C., Fraser, W., Gittoes, N., Javaid, M. K., Macdonald, H., … Francis, R. M. (2014). National Osteoporosis Society Vitamin D Guideline Summary. Age and Ageing, 43(5), 592–595. doi:10.1093/ageing/afu093

[1732] Raftery, T., Martineau, A. R., Greiller, C. L., Ghosh, S., McNamara, D., Bennett, K., … O'Sullivan, M. (2015). Effects of vitamin D supplementation on intestinal permeability, cathelicidin and disease markers in Crohn's disease: Results from a randomised double-blind placebo-controlled study. United European Gastroenterology Journal, 3(3), 294–302. doi:10.1177/2050640615572176

[1733] Wortsman J, Matsuoka LY, Chen TC, Lu Z, Holick MF. Decreased bioavailability of vitamin D in obesity [published correction appears in Am J Clin Nutr. 2003 May;77(5):1342]. Am J Clin Nutr. 2000;72(3):690-693. doi:10.1093/ajcn/72.3.690

[1734] Simopoulos A. P. (2002). Omega-3 fatty acids in inflammation and autoimmune diseases. Journal of the American College of Nutrition, 21(6), 495–505. https://doi.org/10.1080/07315724.2002.10719248

[1735] Hathcock, J. N., Shao, A., Vieth, R., & Heaney, R. (2007). Risk assessment for vitamin D. The American journal of clinical nutrition, 85(1), 6–18. https://doi.org/10.1093/ajcn/85.1.6

[1736] Masterjohn C. (2007). Vitamin D toxicity redefined: vitamin K and the molecular mechanism. Medical hypotheses, 68(5), 1026–1034. https://doi.org/10.1016/j.mehy.2006.09.051

[1737] Camargo, A., Ruano, J., Fernandez, J. M., Parnell, L. D., Jimenez, A., Santos-Gonzalez, M., … Perez-Jimenez, F. (2010). Gene expression changes in mononuclear cells in patients with metabolic syndrome after acute intake of phenol-rich virgin olive oil. BMC Genomics, 11(1), 253. doi:10.1186/1471-2164-11-253

[1738] Wessels, I., Maywald, M., & Rink, L. (2017). Zinc as a Gatekeeper of Immune Function. Nutrients, 9(12), 1286. https://doi.org/10.3390/nu9121286

[1739] Foster, M., & Samman, S. (2012). Zinc and Regulation of Inflammatory Cytokines: Implications for Cardiometabolic Disease. Nutrients, 4(7), 676–694. doi:10.3390/nu4070676

[1740] Sanna, A., Firinu, D., Zavattari, P., & Valera, P. (2018). Zinc Status and Autoimmunity: A Systematic Review and Meta-Analysis. Nutrients, 10(1), 68. doi:10.3390/nu10010068

[1741] Prasad, A. S. (2000). Effects of Zinc Deficiency on Th1 and Th2 Cytokine Shifts. The Journal of Infectious Diseases, 182(s1), S62–S68. doi:10.1086/315916

[1742] Rosenkranz, E., Metz, C. H. D., Maywald, M., Hilgers, R.-D., Weßels, I., Senff, T., … Rink, L. (2015). Zinc supplementation induces regulatory T cells by inhibition of Sirt-1 deacetylase in mixed lymphocyte cultures. Molecular Nutrition & Food Research, 60(3), 661–671. doi:10.1002/mnfr.201500524

[1743] Uusitalo, L., Kenward, M. G., Virtanen, S. M., Uusitalo, U., Nevalainen, J., Niinistö, S., … Knip, M. (2008). Intake of antioxidant vitamins and trace elements during pregnancy and risk of advanced β cell autoimmunity in the child. The American Journal of Clinical Nutrition, 88(2), 458–464. doi:10.1093/ajcn/88.2.458

[1744] Zamora-Ros, R., Rabassa, M., Cherubini, A., Urpí-Sardà, M., Bandinelli, S., Ferrucci, L., & Andres-Lacueva, C. (2013). High Concentrations of a Urinary Biomarker of Polyphenol Intake Are Associated with Decreased Mortality in Older Adults. The Journal of Nutrition, 143(9), 1445–1450. doi:10.3945/jn.113.177121

[1745] Pérez-Jiménez, J., Neveu, V., Vos, F., & Scalbert, A. (2010). Identification of the 100 richest dietary sources of polyphenols: an application of the Phenol-Explorer database. European Journal of Clinical Nutrition, 64(S3), S112–S120. doi:10.1038/ejcn.2010.221

[1746] Aryaeian, N., Shahram, F., Mahmoudi, M., Tavakoli, H., Yousefi, B., Arablou, T., & Jafari Karegar, S. (2019). The effect of ginger supplementation on some immunity and inflammation intermediate genes expression in patients with active Rheumatoid Arthritis. Gene, 698, 179–185. doi:10.1016/j.gene.2019.01.048

[1747] Niu, X., Wu, C., Li, M., Zhao, Q., Meydani, S. N., Wang, J., & Wu, D. (2018). Naringenin is an inhibitor of T cell effector functions. The Journal of Nutritional Biochemistry, 58, 71–79. doi:10.1016/j.jnutbio.2018.04.008

[1748] Wang, J., Qi, Y., Niu, X., Tang, H., Meydani, S. N., & Wu, D. (2018). Dietary naringenin supplementation attenuates experimental autoimmune encephalomyelitis by modulating autoimmune inflammatory responses in mice. The Journal of Nutritional Biochemistry, 54, 130–139. doi:10.1016/j.jnutbio.2017.12.004

[1749] Wong, C. P., Nguyen, L. P., Noh, S. K., Bray, T. M., Bruno, R. S., & Ho, E. (2011). Induction of regulatory T cells by green tea polyphenol EGCG. Immunology Letters, 139(1-2), 7–13. doi:10.1016/j.imlet.2011.04.009

[1750] Bright, J. J. (n.d.). CURCUMIN AND AUTOIMMUNE DISEASE. The Molecular Targets and Therapeutic Uses of Curcumin in Health and Disease, 425–451. doi:10.1007/978-0-387-46401-5_19

[1751] Klune et al (2008). HMGB1: endogenous danger signaling. Molecular medicine (Cambridge, Mass.), 14(7-8), 476–484.

[1752] Ferrari, S., Finelli, P., Rocchi, M., & Bianchi, M. E. (1996). The active gene that encodes human high mobility group 1 protein (HMG1) contains introns and maps to chromosome 13. Genomics, 35(2), 367–371.

[1753] Zhang, J., Zhang, L., Zhang, S., Yu, Q., Xiong, F., Huang, K., Wang, C. Y., & Yang, P. (2017). HMGB1, an innate alarmin, plays a critical role in chronic inflammation of adipose tissue in obesity. Molecular and cellular endocrinology, 454, 103–111. https://doi.org/10.1016/j.mce.2017.06.012

[1754] Biscetti, F.; Rando, M.M.; Nardella, E.; Cecchini, A.L.; Pecorini, G.; Landolfi, R.; Flex, A. High Mobility Group Box-1 and Diabetes Mellitus Complications: State of the Art and Future Perspectives. Int. J. Mol. Sci. 2019, 20, 6258.

[1755] Cai, J., Yuan, H., Wang, Q., Yang, H., Al-Abed, Y., Hua, Z., Wang, J., Chen, D., Wu, J., Lu, B., Pribis, J. P., Jiang, W., Yang, K., Hackam, D. J., Tracey, K. J., Billiar, T. R., & Chen, A. F. (2015). HMGB1-Driven Inflammation and Intimal Hyperplasia After Arterial Injury Involves Cell-Specific Actions Mediated by TLR4. Arteriosclerosis, thrombosis, and vascular biology, 35(12), 2579–2593. https://doi.org/10.1161/ATVBAHA.115.305789

[1756] Cirillo, F., Catellani, C., Sartori, C., Lazzeroni, P., Morini, D., Nicoli, A., Giorgi-Rossi, P., Amarri, S., La Sala, G. B., & Street, M. E. (2019). CFTR and FOXO1 gene expression are reduced and high mobility group box 1 (HMGB1) is increased in the ovaries and serum of women with polycystic ovarian syndrome. Gynecological endocrinology : the official journal of the International Society of Gynecological Endocrinology, 35(10), 842–846. https://doi.org/10.1080/09513590.2019.1599349

[1757] Zhang et al (2020). Extracellular HMGB1 exacerbates autoimmune progression and recurrence of type 1 diabetes by impairing regulatory T cell stability. Diabetologia, 63(5), 987–1001.

[1758] Chen et al (2015). HMGB1 is activated in type 2 diabetes mellitus patients and in mesangial cells in response to high glucose. International journal of clinical and experimental pathology, 8(6), 6683–6691.

[1759] Biscetti et al (2019). High Mobility Group Box-1 and Diabetes Mellitus Complications: State of the Art and Future Perspectives. International journal of molecular sciences, 20(24), 6258.

[1760] Ishibashi (2010) 'Serum HMGB1 Level in Patients with Type 2 Diabetes', American Diabetes Association, Accessed Online March 8th 2023: https://professional.diabetes.org/abstract/serum-hmgb1-level-patients-type-2-diabetes

[1761] Wang et al (2015). Plasma HMGB-1 Levels in Subjects with Obesity and Type 2 Diabetes: A Cross-Sectional Study in China. PloS one, 10(8), e0136564.

[1762] Zhang et al (2009). HMGB1, an innate alarmin, in the pathogenesis of type 1 diabetes. International journal of clinical and experimental pathology, 3(1), 24–38.

[1763] Han et al (2008). Extracellular high-mobility group box 1 acts as an innate immune mediator to enhance autoimmune progression and diabetes onset in NOD mice. Diabetes, 57(8), 2118–2127.

[1764] Chen et al (2018) Blockade of HMGB1 Attenuates Diabetic Nephropathy in Mice. Sci Rep 8, 8319.

[1765] Itoh et al (2015). HMGB1-Mediated Early Loss of Transplanted Islets Is Prevented by Anti-IL-6R Antibody in Mice. Pancreas, 44(1), 166–171.

[1766] Matsuoka et al (2010). High-mobility group box 1 is involved in the initial events of early loss of transplanted islets in mice. The Journal of clinical investigation, 120(3), 735–743.

[1767] Itoh et al (2014). Elevation of high-mobility group box 1 after clinical autologous islet transplantation and its inverse correlation with outcomes. Cell transplantation, 23(2), 153–165.

[1768] Rauvala, H., & Rouhiainen, A. (2007). RAGE as a receptor of HMGB1 (Amphoterin): roles in health and disease. Current molecular medicine, 7(8), 725–734. https://doi.org/10.2174/156652407783220750

[1769] Yang, H., Hreggvidsdottir, H. S., Palmblad, K., Wang, H., Ochani, M., Li, J., … Tracey, K. J. (2010). A critical cysteine is required for HMGB1 binding to Toll-like receptor 4 and activation of macrophage cytokine release. Proceedings of the National Academy of Sciences, 107(26), 11942–11947. doi:10.1073/pnas.1003893107

[1770] Bierhaus et al (2001). Diabetes-Associated Sustained Activation of the Transcription Factor Nuclear Factor-κB. Diabetes, 50(12), 2792–2808.

[1771] Luevano-Contreras, C., & Chapman-Novakofski, K. (2010). Dietary advanced glycation end products and aging. Nutrients, 2(12), 1247–1265.

[1772] Uribarri et al (2007). Circulating glycotoxins and dietary advanced glycation endproducts: two links to inflammatory response, oxidative stress, and aging. The journals of gerontology. Series A, Biological sciences and medical sciences, 62(4), 427–433.

[1773] Gasparotto et al (2019). Systemic Inflammation Changes the Site of RAGE Expression from Endothelial Cells to Neurons in Different Brain Areas. Molecular neurobiology, 56(5), 3079–3089.

[1774] Gasparotto, J., Girardi, C. S., Somensi, N., Ribeiro, C. T., Moreira, J., Michels, M., Sonai, B., Rocha, M., Steckert, A. V., Barichello, T., Quevedo, J., Dal-Pizzol, F., & Gelain, D. P. (2018). Receptor for advanced glycation end products mediates sepsis-triggered amyloid-β accumulation, Tau phosphorylation, and cognitive impairment. The Journal of biological chemistry, 293(1), 226–244. https://doi.org/10.1074/jbc.M117.786756

[1775] Yammani R. R. (2012). S100 proteins in cartilage: role in arthritis. Biochimica et biophysica acta, 1822(4), 600–606.

[1776] Jandeleit-Dahm, K., & Cooper, M. E. (2008). The role of AGEs in cardiovascular disease. Current pharmaceutical design, 14(10), 979–986.

[1777] Srikanth et al (2011). Advanced glycation endproducts and their receptor RAGE in Alzheimer's disease. Neurobiology of aging, 32(5), 763–777.

[1778] Simm et al (2007). Advanced glycation endproducts: a biomarker for age as an outcome predictor after cardiac surgery?. Experimental gerontology, 42(7), 668–675.

[1779] Gugliucci, A., & Bendayan, M. (1996). Renal fate of circulating advanced glycated end products (AGE): evidence for reabsorption and catabolism of AGE-peptides by renal proximal tubular cells. Diabetologia, 39(2), 149–160.

[1780] Zimmerman et al (1995). Neurotoxicity of advanced glycation endproducts during focal stroke and neuroprotective effects of aminoguanidine. Proceedings of the National Academy of Sciences of the United States of America, 92(9), 3744–3748.

[1781] Goh, S.-Y., & Cooper, M. E. (2008). The Role of Advanced Glycation End Products in Progression and Complications of Diabetes. The Journal of Clinical Endocrinology & Metabolism, 93(4), 1143–1152.

[1782] Prasad, A., Bekker, P., & Tsimikas, S. (2012). Advanced glycation end products and diabetic cardiovascular disease. Cardiology in review, 20(4), 177–183.

322

[1783] Di Marco et al (2013). Diabetes alters activation and repression of pro- and anti-inflammatory signaling pathways in the vasculature. Frontiers in endocrinology, 4, 68.

[1784] Sabbatinelli, J., Castiglione, S., Macrì, F. et al. Circulating levels of AGEs and soluble RAGE isoforms are associated with all-cause mortality and development of cardiovascular complications in type 2 diabetes: a retrospective cohort study. Cardiovasc Diabetol 21, 95 (2022).

[1785] Uribarri et al (2010). Advanced glycation end products in foods and a practical guide to their reduction in the diet. Journal of the American Dietetic Association, 110(6), 911–16.e12.

[1786] Sebeková et al (2001). Plasma levels of advanced glycation end products in healthy, long-term vegetarians and subjects on a western mixed diet. European journal of nutrition, 40(6), 275–281.

[1787] Ahmed, N., & Furth, A. J. (1992). Failure of common glycation assays to detect glycation by fructose. Clinical chemistry, 38(7), 1301–1303.

[1788] Uribarri et al (2010). Advanced glycation end products in foods and a practical guide to their reduction in the diet. Journal of the American Dietetic Association, 110(6), 911–16.e12.

[1789] Mark et al (2014). Consumption of a diet low in advanced glycation end products for 4 weeks improves insulin sensitivity in overweight women. Diabetes care, 37(1), 88–95.

[1790] de Courten et al (2016). Diet low in advanced glycation end products increases insulin sensitivity in healthy overweight individuals: a double-blind, randomized, crossover trial. The American journal of clinical nutrition, 103(6), 1426–1433.

[1791] Baye, E., Kiriakova, V., Uribarri, J. et al. Consumption of diets with low advanced glycation end products improves cardiometabolic parameters: meta-analysis of randomised controlled trials. Sci Rep 7, 2266 (2017).

[1792] Ottum, M. S., & Mistry, A. M. (2015). Advanced glycation end-products: modifiable environmental factors profoundly mediate insulin resistance. Journal of clinical biochemistry and nutrition, 57(1), 1–12.

[1793] Reiser K. M. (1994). Influence of age and long-term dietary restriction on enzymatically mediated crosslinks and nonenzymatic glycation of collagen in mice. Journal of gerontology, 49(2), B71–B79.

[1794] Sell, D. R., Kleinman, N. R., & Monnier, V. M. (2000). Longitudinal determination of skin collagen glycation and glycoxidation rates predicts early death in C57BL/6NNIA mice. FASEB journal : official publication of the Federation of American Societies for Experimental Biology, 14(1), 145–156.

[1795] Cefalu et al (1995). Caloric restriction decreases age-dependent accumulation of the glycoxidation products, N epsilon-(carboxymethyl)lysine and pentosidine, in rat skin collagen. The journals of gerontology. Series A, Biological sciences and medical sciences, 50(6), B337–B341.

[1796] Flanagan et al (2020). Calorie Restriction and Aging in Humans. Annual review of nutrition, 40, 105–133.

[1797] Waziry et al (2023) 'Effect of long-term caloric restriction on DNA methylation measures of biological aging in healthy adults from the CALERIE trial', Nat Aging 3, 248–257 (2023). https://doi.org/10.1038/s43587-022-00357-y

[1798] Mune, M., Meydani, M., Jahngen-Hodge, J. et al. Effect of calorie restriction on liver and kidney glutathione in aging emory mice. AGE 18, 43–49 (1995). https://doi.org/10.1007/BF02432518

[1799] Nowotny, K., Jung, T., Höhn, A., Weber, D., & Grune, T. (2015). Advanced glycation end products and oxidative stress in type 2 diabetes mellitus. Biomolecules, 5(1), 194–222.

[1800] Deuther-Conrad et al (2001). Advanced glycation endproducts change glutathione redox status in SH-SY5Y human neuroblastoma cells by a hydrogen peroxide dependent mechanism. Neuroscience letters, 312(1), 29–32.

[1801] Handayani et al (2020) 'The role of reduced glutathione on oxidative stress, reticulum endoplasmic stress and glycation in human lens epithelial cell culture', Journal of Pharmacy & Pharmacognosy Research 9(2):175-181.

[1802] Pusterla et al (2013). Receptor for advanced glycation endproducts (RAGE) is a key regulator of oval cell activation and inflammation-associated liver carcinogenesis in mice. Hepatology (Baltimore, Md.), 58(1), 363–373. https://doi.org/10.1002/hep.26395

[1803] Venereau, E., De Leo, F., Mezzapelle, R., Careccia, G., Musco, G., & Bianchi, M. E. (2016). HMGB1 as biomarker and drug target. Pharmacological research, 111, 534–544. https://doi.org/10.1016/j.phrs.2016.06.031

[1804] Rietschel ET, Kirikae T, Schade FU, Mamat U, Schmidt G, Loppnow H, Ulmer AJ, Zähringer U, Seydel U, Di Padova F (1994). "Bacterial endotoxin: molecular relationships of structure to activity and function". FASEB J. 8 (2): 217–25.

[1805] Beutler, B., & Cerami, A. (1988). Tumor Necrosis, Cachexia, Shock, and Inflammation: A Common Mediator. Annual Review of Biochemistry, 57(1), 505–518. doi:10.1146/annurev.bi.57.070188.002445

[1806] Rietschel, E. T., Kirikae, T., Schade, F. U., Mamat, U., Schmidt, G., Loppnow, H., … Brade, H. (1994). Bacterial endotoxin: molecular relationships of structure to activity and function. The FASEB Journal, 8(2), 217–225. doi:10.1096/fasebj.8.2.8119492

[1807] Epstein, F. H., & Parrillo, J. E. (1993). Pathogenetic Mechanisms of Septic Shock. New England Journal of Medicine, 328(20), 1471–1477. doi:10.1056/nejm199305203282008

[1808] Bernard, G. R., Vincent, J.-L., Laterre, P.-F., LaRosa, S. P., Dhainaut, J.-F., Lopez-Rodriguez, A., … Fisher, C. J. (2001). Efficacy and Safety of Recombinant Human Activated Protein C for Severe Sepsis. New England Journal of Medicine, 344(10), 699–709. doi:10.1056/nejm200103083441001

[1809] Parlesak, A., Schäfer, C., Schütz, T., Bode, J. C., & Bode, C. (2000). Increased intestinal permeability to macromolecules and endotoxemia in patients with chronic alcohol abuse in different stages of alcohol-induced liver disease. Journal of Hepatology, 32(5), 742–747. doi:10.1016/s0168-8278(00)80242-1

[1810] Moreno-Navarrete JM, Ortega F, Serino M, Luche E, Waget A, Pardo G, Salvador J, Ricart W, Frühbeck G, Burcelin R, Fernández-Real JM (2012). "Circulating lipopolysaccharide-binding protein (LBP) as a marker of obesity-related insulin resistance". Int J Obes (Lond). 36 (11): 1442–9.

[1811] Cani PD, Amar J, Iglesias MA, Poggi M, Knauf C, Bastelica D, Neyrinck AM, Fava F, Tuohy KM, Chabo C, Waget A, Delmée E, Cousin B, Sulpice T, Chamontin B, Ferrières J, Tanti JF, Gibson GR, Casteilla L, Delzenne NM, Alessi MC, Burcelin R (2007). "Metabolic endotoxemia initiates obesity and insulin resistance". Diabetes. 56 (7): 1761–72.

[1812] Rietschel, E. T., Kirikae, T., Schade, F. U., Mamat, U., Schmidt, G., Loppnow, H., … Brade, H. (1994). Bacterial endotoxin: molecular relationships of structure to activity and function. The FASEB Journal, 8(2), 217–225. doi:10.1096/fasebj.8.2.8119492

[1813] Rahiman, F., & Pool, E. J. (2013). THE IN VITRO EFFECTS OF ARTIFICIAL AND NATURAL SWEETENERS ON THE IMMUNE SYSTEM USING WHOLE BLOOD CULTURE ASSAYS. Journal of Immunoassay and Immunochemistry, 35(1), 26–36. doi:10.1080/15321819.2013.784197

[1814] https://www.ncbi.nlm.nih.gov/pmc/articles/PMC291248/

[1815] Babic, I., Nguyen-the, C., Amiot, M. J., & Aubert, S. (1994). Antimicrobial activity of shredded carrot extracts on food-borne bacteria and yeast. Journal of Applied Bacteriology, 76(2), 135–141. doi:10.1111/j.1365-2672.1994.tb01608.x

323

[1816] Liu, Z., Chang, Y., Zhang, J., Huang, X., Jiang, J., Li, S., & Wang, Z. (2013). Magnesium deficiency promotes secretion of high-mobility group box 1 protein from lipopolysaccharide-activated macrophages in vitro. Journal of Surgical Research, 180(2), 310–316. doi:10.1016/j.jss.2012.04.045

[1817] Voziyan, P. A., & Hudson, B. G. (2005). Pyridoxamine: the many virtues of a maillard reaction inhibitor. Annals of the New York Academy of Sciences, 1043, 807–816.

[1818] Vasan, S., Foiles, P., & Founds, H. (2003). Therapeutic potential of breakers of advanced glycation end product-protein crosslinks. Archives of biochemistry and biophysics, 419(1), 89–96.

[1819] Dearlove et al (2008). Inhibition of protein glycation by extracts of culinary herbs and spices. Journal of medicinal food, 11(2), 275–281.

[1820] Jin, S., & Cho, K. H. (2011). Water extracts of cinnamon and clove exhibits potent inhibition of protein glycation and anti-atherosclerotic activity in vitro and in vivo hypolipidemic activity in zebrafish. Food and chemical toxicology : an international journal published for the British Industrial Biological Research Association, 49(7), 1521–1529.

[1821] Gkogkolou, P., & Böhm, M. (2012). Advanced glycation end products: Key players in skin aging?. Dermato-endocrinology, 4(3), 259–270.

[1822] Ou et al (2018) 'Protective effect of rosmarinic acid and carnosic acid against streptozotocin-induced oxidation, glycation, inflammation and microbiota imbalance in diabetic rats', Food & Function 9(2).

[1823] Wu, C. H., & Yen, G. C. (2005). Inhibitory effect of naturally occurring flavonoids on the formation of advanced glycation endproducts. Journal of agricultural and food chemistry, 53(8), 3167–3173.

[1824] Draelos et al (2009). An evaluation of the effect of a topical product containing C-xyloside and blueberry extract on the appearance of type II diabetic skin. Journal of cosmetic dermatology, 8(2), 147–151.

[1825] Adeva-Andany et al (2018). Insulin resistance and glycine metabolism in humans. Amino acids, 50(1), 11–27. https://doi.org/10.1007/s00726-017-2508-0

[1826] Wang et al (2019). Glycine Suppresses AGE/RAGE Signaling Pathway and Subsequent Oxidative Stress by Restoring Glo1 Function in the Aorta of Diabetic Rats and in HUVECs. Oxidative medicine and cellular longevity, 2019, 4628962. https://doi.org/10.1155/2019/4628962

[1827] Sekhar (2022) 'GlyNAC (Glycine and N-Acetylcysteine) Supplementation Improves Impaired Mitochondrial Fuel Oxidation and Lowers Insulin Resistance in Patients with Type 2 Diabetes: Results of a Pilot Study', Antioxidants 11(1):154.

[1828] Reddy, V. P., Garrett, M. R., Perry, G., & Smith, M. A. (2005). Carnosine: a versatile antioxidant and antiglycating agent. Science of aging knowledge environment : SAGE KE, 2005(18), pe12.

[1829] Ghodsi, R., & Kheirouri, S. (2018). Carnosine and advanced glycation end products: a systematic review. Amino acids, 50(9), 1177–1186.

[1830] Houjeghani et al (2018). l-Carnosine supplementation attenuated fasting glucose, triglycerides, advanced glycation end products, and tumor necrosis factor-α levels in patients with type 2 diabetes: a double-blind placebo-controlled randomized clinical trial. Nutrition research (New York, N.Y.), 49, 96–106.

[1831] Freund et al (2018). The Inhibition of Advanced Glycation End Products by Carnosine and Other Natural Dipeptides to Reduce Diabetic and Age-Related Complications. Comprehensive reviews in food science and food safety, 17(5), 1367–1378.

[1832] Freund, M. A., Chen, B., & Decker, E. A. (2018). The Inhibition of Advanced Glycation End Products by Carnosine and Other Natural Dipeptides to Reduce Diabetic and Age-Related Complications. Comprehensive reviews in food science and food safety, 17(5), 1367–1378.

[1833] Ghelani, H., Razmovski-Naumovski, V., Pragada, R.R. et al. (R)-α-Lipoic acid inhibits fructose-induced myoglobin fructation and the formation of advanced glycation end products (AGEs) in vitro. BMC Complement Altern Med 18, 13 (2018).

[1834] Muellenbach et al (2008). Interactions of the advanced glycation end product inhibitor pyridoxamine and the antioxidant alpha-lipoic acid on insulin resistance in the obese Zucker rat. Metabolism: clinical and experimental, 57(10), 1465–1472.

[1835] Reyad-ul-Ferdous et al (2022) 'Glycyrrhizin (Glycyrrhizic Acid) HMGB1 (high mobility group box 1) inhibitor upregulate mitochondrial function in adipocyte, cell viability and in-silico study', Journal of Saudi Chemical Society, Volume 26, Issue 3, May 2022, 101454.

[1836] Li, C., Peng, S., Liu, X., Han, C., Wang, X., Jin, T., … Teng, W. (2017). Glycyrrhizin, a Direct HMGB1 Antagonist, Ameliorates Inflammatory Infiltration in a Model of Autoimmune Thyroiditis via Inhibition of TLR2-HMGB1 Signaling. Thyroid, 27(5), 722–731. doi:10.1089/thy.2016.0432

[1837] Fu et al (2014). Glycyrrhizin inhibits lipopolysaccharide-induced inflammatory response by reducing TLR4 recruitment into lipid rafts in RAW264.7 cells. Biochimica et biophysica acta, 1840(6), 1755–1764.

[1838] Liu et al (2014). Zhongguo Zhong yao za zhi = Zhongguo zhongyao zazhi = China journal of Chinese materia medica, 39(19), 3841–3845.

[1839] Lee et al (2019). Effects of glycyrrhizin on lipopolysaccharide-induced acute lung injury in a mouse model. Journal of thoracic disease, 11(4), 1287–1302.

[1840] Wang et al (2017). Glycyrrhizin inhibits LPS-induced inflammatory mediator production in endometrial epithelial cells. Microbial pathogenesis, 109, 110–113.

[1841] Liu et al (2021). Ferulic acid inhibits LPS-induced apoptosis in bovine mammary epithelial cells by regulating the NF-κB and Nrf2 signalling pathways to restore mitochondrial dynamics and ROS generation. Veterinary research, 52(1), 104.

[1842] Huang et al (2016) 'Ferulic acid prevents LPS-induced up-regulation of PDE4B and stimulates the cAMP/CREB signaling pathway in PC12 cells'. Acta Pharmacol Sin 37, 1543–1554 (2016).

[1843] Shao, S., Gao, Y., Liu, J., Tian, M., Gou, Q., & Su, X. (2018). Ferulic Acid Mitigates Radiation Injury in Human Umbilical Vein Endothelial Cells In Vitro via the Thrombomodulin Pathway. Radiation research, 190(3), 298–308. https://doi.org/10.1667/RR14696.1

[1844] Mir et al (2018). Ferulic acid protects lipopolysaccharide-induced acute kidney injury by suppressing inflammatory events and upregulating antioxidant defenses in Balb/c mice. Biomedicine & pharmacotherapy = Biomedecine & pharmacotherapie, 100, 304–315.

[1845] Sompong et al (2015). Protective Effects of Ferulic Acid on High Glucose-Induced Protein Glycation, Lipid Peroxidation, and Membrane Ion Pump Activity in Human Erythrocytes. PLOS ONE, 10(6), e0129495.

[1846] Quinde-Axtell, Z., & Baik, B. K. (2006). Phenolic compounds of barley grain and their implication in food product discoloration. Journal of agricultural and food chemistry, 54(26), 9978–9984. https://doi.org/10.1021/jf060974w

[1847] Beejmohun, V., Fliniaux, O., Grand, É., Lamblin, F., Bensaddek, L., Christen, P., … Mesnard, F. (2007). Microwave-assisted extraction of the main phenolic compounds in flaxseed. Phytochemical Analysis, 18(4), 275–282. doi:10.1002/pca.973

[1848] Pietrofesa, R. A., Velalopoulou, A., Arguiri, E., Menges, C. W., Testa, J. R., Hwang, W.-T., … Christofidou-Solomidou, M. (2015). Flaxseed lignans enriched in secoisolariciresinol diglucoside prevent acute asbestos-induced peritoneal inflammation in mice. Carcinogenesis, 37(2), 177–187. doi:10.1093/carcin/bgv174

[1849] Lee, W., Cho, S.-H., Kim, J.-E., Lee, C., Lee, J.-H., Baek, M.-C., ... Bae, J.-S. (2019). Suppressive Effects of Ginsenoside Rh1 on HMGB1-Mediated Septic Responses. The American Journal of Chinese Medicine, 47(01), 119–133. doi:10.1142/s0192415x1950006x

[1850] Wang, H., Li, W., Li, J., Rendon-Mitchell, B., Ochani, M., Ashok, M., Yang, L., Yang, H., Tracey, K. J., Wang, P., & Sama, A. E. (2006). The aqueous extract of a popular herbal nutrient supplement, Angelica sinensis, protects mice against lethal endotoxemia and sepsis. The Journal of nutrition, 136(2), 360–365. https://doi.org/10.1093/jn/136.2.360

[1851] Lim, D. S., Bae, K. G., Jung, I. S., Kim, C. H., Yun, Y. S., & Song, J. Y. (2002). Anti-Septicaemic Effect of Polysaccharide from Panax ginseng by Macrophage Activation. Journal of Infection, 45(1), 32–38. doi:10.1053/jinf.2002.1007

[1852] MAEKAWA, L. E., VALERA, M. C., OLIVEIRA, L. D. de, CARVALHO, C. A. T., CAMARGO, C. H. R., & JORGE, A. O. C. (2013). Effect of Zingiber officinale and propolis on microorganisms and endotoxins in root canals. Journal of Applied Oral Science, 21(1), 25–31. doi:10.1590/1678-7757201302129

[1853] Chen, X., Li, W., & Wang, H. (2006). More tea for septic patients? – Green tea may reduce endotoxin-induced release of high mobility group box 1 and other pro-inflammatory cytokines. Medical Hypotheses, 66(3), 660–663. doi:10.1016/j.mehy.2005.09.025

[1854] Saiwichai, T., Sangalangkarn, V., Kawahara, K., Oyama, Y., Chaichalotornkul, S., Narkpinit, S., Harnyuttanakorn, P., Singhasivanon, P., Maruyama, I., & Tancharoen, S. (2010). Green tea extract supplement inhibition of HMGB1 release in rats exposed to cigarette smoke. The Southeast Asian journal of tropical medicine and public health, 41(1), 250–258.

[1855] Li, Y., Chen, L., Guo, F., Cao, Y., Hu, W., Shi, Y., ... Guo, Y. (2019). Effects of epigallocatechin-3-gallate on the HMGB1/RAGE pathway in PM2.5-exposed asthmatic rats. Biochemical and Biophysical Research Communications, 513(4), 898–903. doi:10.1016/j.bbrc.2019.03.165

[1856] Li, W., Zhu, S., Li, J., Assa, A., Jundoria, A., Xu, J., ... Wang, H. (2011). EGCG stimulates autophagy and reduces cytoplasmic HMGB1 levels in endotoxin-stimulated macrophages. Biochemical Pharmacology, 81(9), 1152–1163. doi:10.1016/j.bcp.2011.02.015

[1857] dos Santos Danziger Silvério et al (2021) 'Coffee intake (Coffea arabica L.) reduces advanced glycation end product (AGEs) formation and platelet aggregation in diabetic rats', Revista de Ciencias Farmaceuticas Basica e Aplicada 42:e711.

[1858] Fernandez-Gomez, B., Nitride, C., Ullate, M. et al. Inhibitors of advanced glycation end products from coffee bean roasting by-product. Eur Food Res Technol 244, 1101–1110 (2018). https://doi.org/10.1007/s00217-017-3023-y

[1859] Takeuchi et al (2015). Assessment of the concentrations of various advanced glycation end-products in beverages and foods that are commonly consumed in Japan. PloS one, 10(3), e0118652.

[1860] Mortaz, E., Adcock, I. M., Ricciardolo, F. L., Varahram, M., Jamaati, H., Velayati, A. A., Folkerts, G., & Garssen, J. (2015). Anti-Inflammatory Effects of Lactobacillus Rahmnosus and Bifidobacterium Breve on Cigarette Smoke Activated Human Macrophages. PloS one, 10(8), e0136455. https://doi.org/10.1371/journal.pone.0136455

[1861] Ali, M., Heyob, K., & Rogers, L. K. (2016). DHA Suppresses Primary Macrophage Inflammatory Responses via Notch 1/ Jagged 1 Signaling. Scientific reports, 6, 22276. https://doi.org/10.1038/srep22276

[1862] Choi et al (2014). DHA suppresses Prevotella intermedia lipopolysaccharide-induced production of proinflammatory mediators in murine macrophages. The British journal of nutrition, 111(7), 1221–1230.

[1863] Cao, S., Ren, J., Sun, L., Gu, G., Yuan, Y., & Li, J. (2011). Fish oil-supplemented parenteral nutrition prolongs survival while beneficially altering phospholipids' Fatty Acid composition and modulating immune function in rat sepsis. Shock (Augusta, Ga.), 36(2), 184–190. https://doi.org/10.1097/SHK.0b013e31821e4f8b

[1864] Kim, K., Jung, N., Lee, K., Choi, J., Kim, S., Jun, J., Kim, E., & Kim, D. (2013). Dietary omega-3 polyunsaturated fatty acids attenuate hepatic ischemia/reperfusion injury in rats by modulating toll-like receptor recruitment into lipid rafts. Clinical nutrition (Edinburgh, Scotland), 32(5), 855–862. https://doi.org/10.1016/j.clnu.2012.11.026

[1865] Schierbeck, H., Wähämaa, H., Andersson, U., & Harris, H. E. (2010). Immunomodulatory drugs regulate HMGB1 release from activated human monocytes. Molecular medicine (Cambridge, Mass.), 16(9-10), 343–351. https://doi.org/10.2119/molmed.2010.00031

[1866] Yang, M., Cao, L., Xie, M., Yu, Y., Kang, R., Yang, L., ... Tang, D. (2013). Chloroquine inhibits HMGB1 inflammatory signaling and protects mice from lethal sepsis. Biochemical Pharmacology, 86(3), 410–418. doi:10.1016/j.bcp.2013.05.013

[1867] Tang, D., Kang, R., Xiao, W., Zhang, H., Lotze, M. T., Wang, H., & Xiao, X. (2009). Quercetin Prevents LPS-Induced High-Mobility Group Box 1 Release and Proinflammatory Function. American Journal of Respiratory Cell and Molecular Biology, 41(6), 651–660. doi:10.1165/rcmb.2008-0119oc

[1868] Li, X., Jin, Q., Yao, Q., Xu, B., Li, Z., & Tu, C. (2016). Quercetin attenuates the activation of hepatic stellate cells and liver fibrosis in mice through modulation of HMGB1-TLR2/4-NF-κB signaling pathways. Toxicology Letters, 261, 1–12. doi:10.1016/j.toxlet.2016.09.002

[1869] Satish, M., Gunasekar, P., Asensio, J. A., & Agrawal, D. K. (2020). Vitamin D attenuates HMGB1-mediated neointimal hyperplasia after percutaneous coronary intervention in swine. Molecular and cellular biochemistry, 10.1007/s11010-020-03847-y. Advance online publication. https://doi.org/10.1007/s11010-020-03847-y

[1870] Qiao et al (2017). Zhongguo dang dai er ke za zhi = Chinese journal of contemporary pediatrics, 19(1), 95–103.

[1871] Gmiat et al (2017). Changes in pro-inflammatory markers and leucine concentrations in response to Nordic Walking training combined with vitamin D supplementation in elderly women. Biogerontology, 18(4), 535–548.

[1872] Ge (2019) et al. Vitamin D/VDR signaling inhibits LPS-induced IFNγ and IL-1β in Oral epithelia by regulating hypoxia-inducible factor-1α signaling pathway. Cell Commun Signal 17, 18.

[1873] Mazur-Bialy, A. I., Pochec, E., & Plytycz, B. (2015). Immunomodulatory effect of riboflavin deficiency and enrichment - reversible pathological response versus silencing of inflammatory activation. Journal of physiology and pharmacology : an official journal of the Polish Physiological Society, 66(6), 793–802.

[1874] Goh, J., Hofmann, P., Aw, N. H., Tan, P. L., Tschakert, G., Mueller, A., ... Gan, L. S. H. (2020). Concurrent high-intensity aerobic and resistance exercise modulates systemic release of alarmins (HMGB1, S100A8/A9, HSP70) and inflammatory biomarkers in healthy young men: a pilot study. Translational Medicine Communications, 5(1). doi:10.1186/s41231-020-00056-z

[1875] Izuishi, K., Tsung, A., Jeyabalan, G., Critchlow, N. D., Li, J., Tracey, K. J., ... Billiar, T. R. (2006). Cutting Edge: High-Mobility Group Box 1 Preconditioning Protects against Liver Ischemia-Reperfusion Injury. The Journal of Immunology, 176(12), 7154–7158. doi:10.4049/jimmunol.176.12.7154

[1876] Palumbo, R., Sampaolesi, M., De Marchis, F., Tonlorenzi, R., Colombetti, S., Mondino, A., Cossu, G., & Bianchi, M. E. (2004). Extracellular HMGB1, a signal of tissue damage, induces mesoangioblast migration and proliferation. The Journal of cell biology, 164(3), 441–449. https://doi.org/10.1083/jcb.200304135

[1877] Aneja, R., Odoms, K., Dunsmore, K., Shanley, T. P., & Wong, H. R. (2006). Extracellular Heat Shock Protein-70 Induces Endotoxin Tolerance in THP-1 Cells. The Journal of Immunology, 177(10), 7184–7192. doi:10.4049/jimmunol.177.10.7184

[1878] Tang, D., Kang, R., Xiao, W., Wang, H., Calderwood, S. K., & Xiao, X. (2007). The Anti-inflammatory Effects of Heat Shock Protein 72 Involve Inhibition of High-Mobility-Group Box 1 Release and Proinflammatory Function in Macrophages. The Journal of Immunology, 179(2), 1236–1244. doi:10.4049/jimmunol.179.2.1236

325

[1879] Tang, D., Kang, R., Xiao, W., Jiang, L., Liu, M., Shi, Y., ... Xiao, X. (2007). Nuclear Heat Shock Protein 72 as a Negative Regulator of Oxidative Stress (Hydrogen Peroxide)-Induced HMGB1 Cytoplasmic Translocation and Release. The Journal of Immunology, 178(11), 7376–7384. doi:10.4049/jimmunol.178.11.7376

[1880] Bi, X., Xu, M., Li, J., Huang, T., Jiang, B., Shen, L., ... Yin, Z. (2019). Heat shock protein 27 inhibits HMGB1 translocation by regulating CBP acetyltransferase activity and ubiquitination. Molecular Immunology, 108, 45–55. doi:10.1016/j.molimm.2019.02.008

[1881] Wolf, M., Lossdörfer, S., Römer, P., Kirschneck, C., Küpper, K., Deschner, J., & Jäger, A. (2015). Short-term heat pre-treatment modulates the release of HMGB1 and pro-inflammatory cytokines in hPDL cells following mechanical loading and affects monocyte behavior. Clinical Oral Investigations, 20(5), 923–931. doi:10.1007/s00784-015-1580-7

[1882] Edgar et al (2012). Peroxiredoxins are conserved markers of circadian rhythms. Nature, 485(7399), 459–464.

[1883] Nagoshi E et al (2004) 'Circadian Gene Expression in Individual Fibroblasts', Cell, VOLUME 119, ISSUE 5, P693-705.

[1884] Farha, R.A. and Alefishat, E. (2018), 'Shift Work and the Risk of Cardiovascular Diseases and Metabolic Syndrome Among Jordanian Employees', Oman Med J. 2018 May; 33(3): 235–242.

[1885] Vetter, C et al (2016) 'Association between rotating night shift work and risk of coronary heart disease among women', JAMA. 2016 Apr 26; 315(16): 1726–1734.

[1886] Garcia-Saenz, A. et al (2018) 'Evaluating the Association between Artificial Light-at-Night Exposure and Breast and Prostate Cancer Risk in Spain (MCC-Spain Study)', Environmental Health Perspectives, 126 (04).

[1887] Erren et al (2010). Shift work and cancer: the evidence and the challenge. Deutsches Arzteblatt international, 107(38), 657–662.

[1888] Vetter et al (2018). Night Shift Work, Genetic Risk, and Type 2 Diabetes in the UK Biobank. Diabetes care, 41(4), 762–769.

[1889] Young et al (2012). Control of type 1 diabetes mellitus and shift work. Occupational Medicine, 63(1), 70–72.

[1890] Manodpitipong et al (2017). Night-shift work is associated with poorer glycaemic control in patients with type 2 diabetes. Journal of sleep research, 26(6), 764–772.

[1891] Kondratov R. V. (2007). A role of the circadian system and circadian proteins in aging. Ageing research reviews, 6(1), 12–27. https://doi.org/10.1016/j.arr.2007.02.003

[1892] Kondratova, A. A., & Kondratov, R. V. (2012). The circadian clock and pathology of the ageing brain. Nature reviews. Neuroscience, 13(5), 325–335. https://doi.org/10.1038/nrn3208

[1893] Orozco-Solis, R., & Sassone-Corsi, P. (2014). Circadian clock: linking epigenetics to aging. Current opinion in genetics & development, 26, 66–72. https://doi.org/10.1016/j.gde.2014.06.003

[1894] Halberg, F. (1959). "Physiologic 24-hour periodicity: general and procedural considerations with reference to the adrenal cycle". Zeitschrift für Vitamin- Hormone- und Fermentforschung. 10: 225–296.

[1895] Halberg et al (1977). "[Glossary of chronobiology (author's transl)]". Chronobiologia. 4 Suppl 1: 1–189.

[1896] Duffy, J. F., & Wright, K. P. (2005). Entrainment of the Human Circadian System by Light. Journal of Biological Rhythms, 20(4), 326–338.

[1897] Cromie, William (1999). "Human Biological Clock Set Back an Hour". Harvard Gazette.

[1898] King (2005). Lange Q&A USMLE Step 1 (6th ed.). New York: McGraw-Hill Medical. p. 82. ISBN 978-0-07-144578-8.

[1899] Piroli, G. G., Grillo, C. A., Reznikov, L. R., Adams, S., McEwen, B. S., Charron, M. J., & Reagan, L. P. (2007). Corticosterone impairs insulin-stimulated translocation of GLUT4 in the rat hippocampus. Neuroendocrinology, 85(2), 71–80. https://doi.org/10.1159/000101694

[1900] Adam et al (2017). Diurnal cortisol slopes and mental and physical health outcomes: A systematic review and meta-analysis. Psychoneuroendocrinology, 83, 25–41.

[1901] Joseph, J. J., & Golden, S. H. (2017). Cortisol dysregulation: the bidirectional link between stress, depression, and type 2 diabetes mellitus. Annals of the New York Academy of Sciences, 1391(1), 20–34. https://doi.org/10.1111/nyas.13217

[1902] Debono et al (2009). Modified-release hydrocortisone to provide circadian cortisol profiles. The Journal of clinical endocrinology and metabolism, 94(5), 1548–1554.

[1903] Benloucif et al (2005). Stability of melatonin and temperature as circadian phase markers and their relation to sleep times in humans. Journal of biological rhythms, 20(2), 178–188.

[1904] Ferracioli-Oda et al (2013). Meta-analysis: melatonin for the treatment of primary sleep disorders. PloS one, 8(5), e63773.

[1905] Ramis, MR. et al (2015) 'Caloric restriction, resveratrol and melatonin: Role of SIRT1 and implications for aging and related-diseases', Mechanisms of Ageing and Development, 146-148:28-41.

[1906] Liu, J., Huang, F., & He, H.-W. (2013). Melatonin Effects on Hard Tissues: Bone and Tooth. International Journal of Molecular Sciences, 14(5), 10063–10074.

[1907] Boga et al (2018). Therapeutic potential of melatonin related to its role as an autophagy regulator: A review. Journal of Pineal Research, 66(1), e12534. doi:10.1111/jpi.12534

[1908] Yi et al (2005). Effects of melatonin in age-related macular degeneration. Annals of the New York Academy of Sciences, 1057, 384–392.

[1909] Claustrat, B., & Leston, J. (2015). Melatonin: Physiological effects in humans. Neuro-Chirurgie, 61(2-3), 77–84. https://doi.org/10.1016/j.neuchi.2015.03.002

[1910] Rodella et al (2013). Vascular endothelial cells and dysfunctions: role of melatonin. Frontiers in bioscience (Elite edition), 5, 119–129.

[1911] Radogna et al (2010). Melatonin: a pleiotropic molecule regulating inflammation. Biochemical pharmacology, 80(12), 1844–1852.

[1912] Kurdi, M. S., & Muthukalai, S. P. (2016). The Efficacy of Oral Melatonin in Improving Sleep in Cancer Patients with Insomnia: A Randomized Double-Blind Placebo-Controlled Study. Indian journal of palliative care, 22(3), 295–300.

[1913] Quera Salva et al (2011). Circadian rhythms, melatonin and depression. Current pharmaceutical design, 17(15), 1459–1470.

[1914] Reiter et al (2012). Obesity and metabolic syndrome: association with chronodisruption, sleep deprivation, and melatonin suppression. Annals of medicine, 44(6), 564–577.

[1915] Davis, S., & Mirick, D. K. (2006). Circadian disruption, shift work and the risk of cancer: a summary of the evidence and studies in Seattle. Cancer causes & control : CCC, 17(4), 539–545.

[1916] Dominguez-Rodriguez et al (2010). Melatonin and circadian biology in human cardiovascular disease. Journal of Pineal Research, no–no.

[1917] Grivas, T. B., & Savvidou, O. D. (2007). Melatonin the "light of night" in human biology and adolescent idiopathic scoliosis. Scoliosis, 2, 6. https://doi.org/10.1186/1748-7161-2-6

[1918] Jarrett, R. J., & Keen, H. (1970). Further observations on the diurnal variation in oral glucose tolerance. British medical journal, 4(5731), 334–337.

[1919] Grabner et al (1975). Untersuchungen zur circadianen Rhythmik der Glucosetoleranz [Diurnal variation of glucose tolerance and insulin secretion in man (author's transl)]. Klinische Wochenschrift, 53(16), 773–778.

[1920] Carroll, K. F., & Nestel, P. J. (1973). Diurnal variation in glucose tolerance and in insulin secretion in man. Diabetes, 22(5), 333–348.

[1921] Mayer et al (1976). Epidemiologic findings on the relationship of time of day and time since last meal to glucose tolerance. Diabetes, 25(10), 936–943.

[1922] Bowen, A. J., & Reeves, R. L. (1967). Diurnal variation in glucose tolerance. Archives of internal medicine, 119(3), 261–264.

[1923] Jarrett, R. J., & Keen, H. (1969). Diurnal variation of oral glucose tolerance: a possible pointer to the evolution of diabetes mellitus. British medical journal, 2(5653), 341–344.

[1924] Jarrett et al (1972). Diurnal variation in oral glucose tolerance: blood sugar and plasma insulin levels morning, afternoon, and evening. British medical journal, 1(5794), 199–201.

[1925] Basse et al (2018). Skeletal Muscle Insulin Sensitivity Show Circadian Rhythmicity Which Is Independent of Exercise Training Status. Frontiers in Physiology, 9.

[1926] Sonnier et al (2014). Glycemic control is impaired in the evening in prediabetes through multiple diurnal rhythms. Journal of diabetes and its complications, 28(6), 836–843.

[1927] Hulmán et al (2013). Effect of time of day and fasting duration on measures of glycaemia: analysis from the Whitehall II Study. Diabetologia, 56(2), 294–297.

[1928] Sonnier et al (2014). Glycemic control is impaired in the evening in prediabetes through multiple diurnal rhythms. Journal of diabetes and its complications, 28(6), 836–843.

[1929] Whichelow et al (1974). Diurnal variation in response to intravenous glucose. British medical journal, 1(5906), 488–491.

[1930] Morris et al (2015). Endogenous circadian system and circadian misalignment impact glucose tolerance via separate mechanisms in humans. Proceedings of the National Academy of Sciences of the United States of America, 112(17), E2225–E2234.

[1931] Lee et al (1992). Diurnal variation in glucose tolerance. Cyclic suppression of insulin action and insulin secretion in normal-weight, but not obese, subjects. Diabetes, 41(6), 750–759.

[1932] Calles-Escandon et al (1989). Postprandial oscillatory patterns of blood glucose and insulin in NIDDM. Abnormal diurnal insulin secretion patterns and glucose homeostasis independent of obesity. Diabetes care, 12(10), 709–714.

[1933] Boden, G., Ruiz, J., Urbain, J. L., & Chen, X. (1996). Evidence for a circadian rhythm of insulin secretion. The American journal of physiology, 271(2 Pt 1), E246–E252.

[1934] Poggiogalle et al (2018). Circadian regulation of glucose, lipid, and energy metabolism in humans. Metabolism: clinical and experimental, 84, 11–27.

[1935] Lee et al (1992). Diurnal variation in glucose tolerance. Cyclic suppression of insulin action and insulin secretion in normal-weight, but not obese, subjects. Diabetes, 41(6), 750–759.

[1936] Zimmet et al (1974). Diurnal variation in glucose tolerance: associated changes in plasma insulin, growth hormone, and non-esterified fatty acids. British medical journal, 1(5906), 485–488.

[1937] Plat et al (1999). Metabolic effects of short-term elevations of plasma cortisol are more pronounced in the evening than in the morning. The Journal of clinical endocrinology and metabolism, 84(9), 3082–3092.

[1938] Plat et al (1996). Effects of morning cortisol elevation on insulin secretion and glucose regulation in humans. The American journal of physiology, 270(1 Pt 1), E36–E42.

[1939] Møller et al (1991). Effects of growth hormone on glucose metabolism. Hormone research, 36 Suppl 1, 32–35.

[1940] Van Cauter et al (1991). Modulation of glucose regulation and insulin secretion by circadian rhythmicity and sleep. The Journal of clinical investigation, 88(3), 934–942.

[1941] Yoshino et al (2014). Diurnal variation in insulin sensitivity of glucose metabolism is associated with diurnal variations in whole-body and cellular fatty acid metabolism in metabolically normal women. The Journal of clinical endocrinology and metabolism, 99(9), E1666–E1670.

[1942] Pisu et al (1980). Diurnal variations in insulin secretion and insulin sensitivity in aged subjects. Acta diabetologica latina, 17(2), 153–160.

[1943] Pinkhasov et al (2016). Circadian Rhythms of Carbohydrate Metabolism in Women with Different Types of Obesity. Bulletin of experimental biology and medicine, 161(3), 323–326.

[1944] Walsh CH, Wright ADDiurnal patterns of oral glucose tolerance in diabeticsPostgraduate Medical Journal 1975;51:169-172.

[1945] Boden et al (1996). Evidence for a circadian rhythm of insulin sensitivity in patients with NIDDM caused by cyclic changes in hepatic glucose production. Diabetes, 45(8), 1044–1050.

[1946] Radziuk, J., & Pye, S. (2006). Diurnal rhythm in endogenous glucose production is a major contributor to fasting hyperglycaemia in type 2 diabetes. Suprachiasmatic deficit or limit cycle behaviour?. Diabetologia, 49(7), 1619–1628.

[1947] Macauley et al (2015). Diurnal variation in skeletal muscle and liver glycogen in humans with normal health and Type 2 diabetes. Clinical science (London, England : 1979), 128(10), 707–713.

[1948] Poggiogalle et al (2018). Circadian regulation of glucose, lipid, and energy metabolism in humans. Metabolism: clinical and experimental, 84, 11–27.

[1949] Carrasco-Benso et al (2016). Human adipose tissue expresses intrinsic circadian rhythm in insulin sensitivity. FASEB journal : official publication of the Federation of American Societies for Experimental Biology, 30(9), 3117–3123.

[1950] McGinnis, G. R., & Young, M. E. (2016). Circadian regulation of metabolic homeostasis: causes and consequences. Nature and science of sleep, 8, 163–180.

[1951] Reinke, H., & Asher, G. (2016). Circadian Clock Control of Liver Metabolic Functions. Gastroenterology, 150(3), 574–580.

[1952] Ma, D., Li, S., Molusky, M. M., & Lin, J. D. (2012). Circadian autophagy rhythm: a link between clock and metabolism?. Trends in endocrinology and metabolism: TEM, 23(7), 319–325. https://doi.org/10.1016/j.tem.2012.03.004

[1953] Cella, L. K., Van Cauter, E., & Schoeller, D. A. (1995). Diurnal rhythmicity of human cholesterol synthesis: normal pattern and adaptation to simulated "jet lag". The American journal of physiology, 269(3 Pt 1), E489–E498.

[1954] Cella, L. K., Van Cauter, E., & Schoeller, D. A. (1995). Effect of meal timing on diurnal rhythm of human cholesterol synthesis. The American journal of physiology, 269(5 Pt 1), E878–E883.

[1955] Romon et al (1997). Circadian variation of postprandial lipemia. The American journal of clinical nutrition, 65(4), 934–940.

[1956] van Kerkhof et al (2015). Diurnal Variation of Hormonal and Lipid Biomarkers in a Molecular Epidemiology-Like Setting. PloS one, 10(8), e0135652.

[1957] Sennels et al (2015). Diurnal changes of biochemical metabolic markers in healthy young males - the Bispebjerg study of diurnal variations. Scandinavian journal of clinical and laboratory investigation, 75(8), 686–692.

[1958] Singh et al (2016). Circadian Time Structure of Circulating Plasma Lipid Components in Healthy Indians of Different Age Groups. Indian journal of clinical biochemistry : IJCB, 31(2), 215–223.

[1959] Rivera-Coll et al (1994). Circadian rhythmic variations in serum concentrations of clinically important lipids. Clinical chemistry, 40(8), 1549–1553.

327

[1960] Demacker et al (1982). Intra-individual variation of serum cholesterol, triglycerides and high density lipoprotein cholesterol in normal humans. Atherosclerosis, 45(3), 259–266.

[1961] Halkes et al (2001). Gender differences in diurnal triglyceridemia in lean and overweight subjects. International journal of obesity and related metabolic disorders : journal of the International Association for the Study of Obesity, 25(12), 1767–1774.

[1962] Tahara, Y., Aoyama, S. & Shibata, S. The mammalian circadian clock and its entrainment by stress and exercise. J Physiol Sci 67, 1–10 (2017). https://doi.org/10.1007/s12576-016-0450-7

[1963] Touitou, Y., Selmaoui, B., Lambrozo, J., & Auzeby, A. (2002). Evaluation de l'effet des champs magnétiques (50 Hz) sur la sécrétion de mélatonine chez l'homme et le rat. Etude circadienne [Evaluation of the effect of magnetic fields on the secretion of melatonin in humans and rats. Circadian study]. Bulletin de l'Academie nationale de medecine, 186(9), 1625–1641.

[1964] Buhr, E. D., Yoo, S.-H., & Takahashi, J. S. (2010). Temperature as a Universal Resetting Cue for Mammalian Circadian Oscillators. Science, 330(6002), 379–385. doi:10.1126/science.1195262

[1965] Johnston J. D. (2014). Physiological responses to food intake throughout the day. Nutrition research reviews, 27(1), 107–118. https://doi.org/10.1017/S0954422414000055

[1966] Cheung IN et al (2016) 'Morning and Evening Blue-Enriched Light Exposure Alters Metabolic Function in Normal Weight Adults', PLoS One. 2016 May 18;11(5):e0155601.

[1967] Utiger (1992) 'Melatonin--the hormone of darkness', N Engl J Med. 1992 Nov 5;327(19):1377-9.

[1968] Park, S. J., & Tokura, H. (1999). Bright light exposure during the daytime affects circadian rhythms of urinary melatonin and salivary immunoglobulin A. Chronobiology international, 16(3), 359–371.

[1969] Mishima et al (2001). Diminished melatonin secretion in the elderly caused by insufficient environmental illumination. The Journal of clinical endocrinology and metabolism, 86(1), 129–134.

[1970] Wurtman (2000) 'Age-Related Decreases in Melatonin Secretion—Clinical Consequences', The Journal of Clinical Endocrinology & Metabolism, Volume 85, Issue 6, 1 June 2000, Pages 2135–2136, https://doi.org/10.1210/jcem.85.6.6660.

[1971] Carrier, J., Monk, T. H., Buysse, D. J., & Kupfer, D. J. (1997). Sleep and morningness-eveningness in the 'middle' years of life (20-59 y). Journal of sleep research, 6(4), 230–237. https://doi.org/10.1111/j.1365-2869.1997.00230.x

[1972] Duffy et al (2002). Peak of circadian melatonin rhythm occurs later within the sleep of older subjects. American journal of physiology. Endocrinology and metabolism, 282(2), E297–E303. https://doi.org/10.1152/ajpendo.00268.2001

[1973] Dijk, D. J., Duffy, J. F., & Czeisler, C. A. (2000). Contribution of circadian physiology and sleep homeostasis to age-related changes in human sleep. Chronobiology international, 17(3), 285–311. https://doi.org/10.1081/cbi-100101049

[1974] Turner, P. L., & Mainster, M. A. (2008). Circadian photoreception: ageing and the eye's important role in systemic health. British Journal of Ophthalmology, 92(11), 1439–1444. doi:10.1136/bjo.2008.141747

[1975] Obayashi, K., Saeki, K., Iwamoto, J., Ikada, Y., & Kurumatani, N. (2014). Independent associations of exposure to evening light and nocturnal urinary melatonin excretion with diabetes in the elderly. Chronobiology international, 31(3), 394–400. https://doi.org/10.3109/07420528.2013.864299

[1976] Obayashi, K., Saeki, K., Iwamoto, J., Okamoto, N., Tomioka, K., Nezu, S., Ikada, Y., & Kurumatani, N. (2013). Exposure to light at night, nocturnal urinary melatonin excretion, and obesity/dyslipidemia in the elderly: a cross-sectional analysis of the HEIJO-KYO study. The Journal of clinical endocrinology and metabolism, 98(1), 337–344. https://doi.org/10.1210/jc.2012-2874

[1977] Obayashi et al (2014). Independent associations of exposure to evening light and nocturnal urinary melatonin excretion with diabetes in the elderly. Chronobiology international, 31(3), 394–400.

[1978] Albreiki et al (2017). A single night light exposure acutely alters hormonal and metabolic responses in healthy participants. Endocrine connections, 6(2), 100–110.

[1979] Gil-Lozano et al (2016). Short-term sleep deprivation with nocturnal light exposure alters time-dependent glucagon-like peptide-1 and insulin secretion in male volunteers. American journal of physiology. Endocrinology and metabolism, 310(1), E41–E50.

[1980] Afroz-Hossain et al (2019) 'Sleep and Environmental Factors Affecting Glycemic Control in People with Type 2 Diabetes Mellitus'. Curr Diab Rep 19, 40.

[1981] Obayashi, K., Saeki, K., & Kurumatani, N. (2016). Ambient Light Exposure and Changes in Obesity Parameters: A Longitudinal Study of the HEIJO-KYO Cohort. The Journal of clinical endocrinology and metabolism, 101(9), 3539–3547.

[1982] Obayashi et al (2013). Exposure to light at night, nocturnal urinary melatonin excretion, and obesity/dyslipidemia in the elderly: a cross-sectional analysis of the HEIJO-KYO study. The Journal of clinical endocrinology and metabolism, 98(1), 337–344.

[1983] Hysing et al (2014) 'Sleep and use of electronic devices in adolescence: results from a large population-based study BMJ Open 2015;5:e006748. doi: 10.1136/bmjopen-2014-006748.

[1984] Gooley et al (2011) 'Exposure to Room Light before Bedtime Suppresses Melatonin Onset and Shortens Melatonin Duration in Humans', J Clin Endocrinol Metab. 2011 Mar; 96(3): E463–E472.

[1985] Falchi et al (2011) 'Limiting the impact of light pollution on human health, environment and stellar visibility', J Environ Manage. 2011 Oct;92(10):2714-22. doi: 10.1016/j.jenvman.2011.06.029. Epub 2011 Jul 13.

[1986] Zhao et al (2012). Red light and the sleep quality and endurance performance of Chinese female basketball players. Journal of athletic training, 47(6), 673–678. https://doi.org/10.4085/1062-6050-47.6.08

[1987] Bennett et al (2009). Use of modified spectacles and light bulbs to block blue light at night may prevent postpartum depression. Medical hypotheses, 73(2), 251–253.

[1988] Hester et al (2021). Evening wear of blue-blocking glasses for sleep and mood disorders: a systematic review. Chronobiology international, 38(10), 1375–1383.

[1989] Shechter et al (2018). Blocking nocturnal blue light for insomnia: A randomized controlled trial. Journal of psychiatric research, 96, 196–202.

[1990] Skobowiat and Slominski (2015) 'Ultraviolet B (UVB) activates hypothalamic-pituitary-adrenal (HPA) axis in C57BL/6 mice', J Invest Dermatol. 2015 Jun; 135(6): 1638–1648.

[1991] Cui et al (2007) 'Central role of p53 in the suntan response and pathologic hyperpigmentation.' Cell. 2007 Mar 9;128(5):853-64.

[1992] Bathina, S., & Das, U. N. (2015). Brain-derived neurotrophic factor and its clinical implications. Archives of medical science : AMS, 11(6), 1164–1178. https://doi.org/10.5114/aoms.2015.56342

[1993] Molendijk et al (2012). Serum BDNF concentrations show strong seasonal variation and correlations with the amount of ambient sunlight. PloS one, 7(11), e48046. https://doi.org/10.1371/journal.pone.0048046

[1994] Allen et al (1992). Insulin sensitivity after phototherapy for seasonal affective disorder. Lancet (London, England), 339(8800), 1065–1066.

[1995] Nieuwenhuis, R. F., Spooren, P. F., & Tilanus, J. J. (2009). Verminderde insulinebehoefte; een verrassend effect van lichttherapie bij insulineafhankelijke diabetes mellitus [Less need for insulin, a surprising effect of phototherapy in insulin-dependent diabetes mellitus]. Tijdschrift voor psychiatrie, 51(9), 693–697.

[1996] Dunai et al (2007). Moderate exercise and bright light treatment in overweight and obese individuals. Obesity (Silver Spring, Md.), 15(7), 1749–1757.

[1997] Danilenko et al (2013). Bright light for weight loss: results of a controlled crossover trial. Obesity facts, 6(1), 28–38.

[1998] Albreiki et al (2015) 'Are leptin responses influenced by bright light treatment in healthy young individuals', Proceedings of The Nutrition Society 74(OCE4).

[1999] Figueiro et al (2012). Light modulates leptin and ghrelin in sleep-restricted adults. International journal of endocrinology, 2012, 530726.

[2000] Buhr, E. D., Yoo, S.-H., & Takahashi, J. S. (2010). Temperature as a Universal Resetting Cue for Mammalian Circadian Oscillators. Science, 330(6002), 379–385. doi:10.1126/science.1195262

[2001] Obradovich et al (2017) 'Nighttime temperature and human sleep loss in a changing climate', Science Advances, 26 May 2017: Vol. 3, no. 5, e1601555, DOI: 10.1126/sciadv.1601555.

[2002] Mizuno (2012) 'Effects of thermal environment on sleep and circadian rhythm', J Physiol Anthropol. 2012; 31(1): 14.

[2003] Lack et al (2008) 'The relationship between insomnia and body temperatures', Sleep Medicine Reviews, Volume 12, Issue 4, August 2008, Pages 307-317.

[2004] National Sleep Foundation 'The Ideal Temperature for Sleep', Accessed Online: https://www.sleep.org/articles/temperature-for-sleep/

[2005] Mindell, J. A., Li, A. M., Sadeh, A., Kwon, R., & Goh, D. Y. (2015). Bedtime routines for young children: a dose-dependent association with sleep outcomes. Sleep, 38(5), 717–722. https://doi.org/10.5665/sleep.4662

[2006] Bailey, B. W., Allen, M. D., LeCheminant, J. D., Tucker, L. A., Errico, W. K., Christensen, W. F., & Hill, M. D. (2014). Objectively Measured Sleep Patterns in Young Adult Women and the Relationship to Adiposity. American Journal of Health Promotion, 29(1), 46–54. doi:10.4278/ajhp.121012-quan-500

[2007] Dworak et al (2017). Creatine supplementation reduces sleep need and homeostatic sleep pressure in rats. Journal of sleep research, 26(3), 377–385.

[2008] McMorris et al (2007). Creatine supplementation, sleep deprivation, cortisol, melatonin and behavior. Physiology & behavior, 90(1), 21–28.

[2009] McMorris et al (2006). Effect of creatine supplementation and sleep deprivation, with mild exercise, on cognitive and psychomotor performance, mood state, and plasma concentrations of catecholamines and cortisol. Psychopharmacology, 185(1), 93–103.

[2010] Irwin et al (2020). Effects of acute caffeine consumption following sleep loss on cognitive, physical, occupational and driving performance: A systematic review and meta-analysis. Neuroscience and biobehavioral reviews, 108, 877–888.

[2011] Cook et al (2011). Skill execution and sleep deprivation: effects of acute caffeine or creatine supplementation - a randomized placebo-controlled trial. Journal of the International Society of Sports Nutrition, 8, 2.

[2012] Costello et al (2014). The effectiveness of melatonin for promoting healthy sleep: a rapid evidence assessment of the literature. Nutrition journal, 13, 106.

[2013] Kurdi, M. S., & Muthukalai, S. P. (2016). The Efficacy of Oral Melatonin in Improving Sleep in Cancer Patients with Insomnia: A Randomized Double-Blind Placebo-Controlled Study. Indian journal of palliative care, 22(3), 295–300.

[2014] Statland, B. E., & Demas, T. J. (1980). Serum caffeine half-lives. Healthy subjects vs. patients having alcoholic hepatic disease. American journal of clinical pathology, 73(3), 390–393.

[2015] Ferracioli-Oda et al (2013). Meta-analysis: melatonin for the treatment of primary sleep disorders. PloS one, 8(5), e63773.

[2016] Dollins et al (1994). Effect of inducing nocturnal serum melatonin concentrations in daytime on sleep, mood, body temperature, and performance. Proceedings of the National Academy of Sciences of the United States of America, 91(5), 1824–1828.

[2017] Reid et al (1996). Day-time melatonin administration: effects on core temperature and sleep onset latency. Journal of sleep research, 5(3), 150–154.

[2018] Andersen, L.P.H., Gögenur, I., Rosenberg, J. et al. The Safety of Melatonin in Humans. Clin Drug Investig 36, 169–175 (2016).

[2019] Dasgupta (2020) 'All you need to know about melatonin', Medical News Today, Accessed Online March 14th 2023: https://www.medicalnewstoday.com/articles/232138

[2020] Tordjman et al (2017). Melatonin: Pharmacology, Functions and Therapeutic Benefits. Current neuropharmacology, 15(3), 434–443.

[2021] Karasek, M., & Winczyk, K. (2006). Melatonin in humans. Journal of physiology and pharmacology : an official journal of the Polish Physiological Society, 57 Suppl 5, 19–39.

[2022] Hack et al (2003). The effects of low-dose 0.5-mg melatonin on the free-running circadian rhythms of blind subjects. Journal of biological rhythms, 18(5), 420–429.

[2023] Matsumoto et al (1997). The amplitude of endogenous melatonin production is not affected by melatonin treatment in humans. Journal of pineal research, 22(1), 42–44.

[2024] Silman R. E. (1993). Melatonin: a contraceptive for the nineties. European journal of obstetrics, gynecology, and reproductive biology, 49(1-2), 3–9.

[2025] Presl J. (1993). Melatonin a orální kontracepce [Melatonin and oral contraception]. Ceskoslovenska gynekologie, 58(3), 141–142.

[2026] Nogueira LM, Sampson JN, Chu LW, Yu K, Andriole G, Church T, et al. (2013) Individual Variations in Serum Melatonin Levels through Time: Implications for Epidemiologic Studies. PLoS ONE 8(12): e83208.

[2027] Behram Kandemir et al (2018). Melatonin protects against streptozotocin-induced diabetic cardiomyopathy by the phosphorylation of vascular endothelial growth factor-A (VEGF-A). Cellular and Molecular Biology, 64(14), 47–52.

[2028] Doosti-Irani et al (2018). The Effects of Melatonin Supplementation on Glycemic Control: A Systematic Review and Meta-Analysis of Randomized Controlled Trials. Hormone and Metabolic Research, 50(11), 783–790.

[2029] Rezvanfar et al (2016). Effect of bedtime melatonin consumption on diabetes control and lipid profile. International Journal of Diabetes in Developing Countries, 37(1), 74–77.

[2030] Kadhim et al (2006). Effects of melatonin and zinc on lipid profile and renal function in type 2 diabetic patients poorly controlled with metformin. Journal of pineal research, 41(2), 189–193.

[2031] Doron Garfinkel et al (2011) Efficacy and safety of prolonged-release melatonin in insomnia patients with diabetes: a randomized, double-blind, crossover study, Diabetes, Metabolic Syndrome and Obesity, 4:, 307-313, DOI: 10.2147/DMSO.S23904

[2032] Mohammadi-Sartang et al (2018). Effects of melatonin supplementation on blood lipid concentrations: A systematic review and meta-analysis of randomized controlled trials. Clinical nutrition (Edinburgh, Scotland), 37(6 Pt A), 1943–1954.

[2033] Sun et al (2018). Melatonin Treatment Improves Insulin Resistance and Pigmentation in Obese Patients with Acanthosis Nigricans. International journal of endocrinology, 2018, 2304746.

[2034] Pourhanifeh et al (2020). Melatonin: new insights on its therapeutic properties in diabetic complications. Diabetology & Metabolic Syndrome, 12(1).

[2035] Meryem Ergenc et al (2022) Melatonin reverses depressive and anxiety like-behaviours induced by diabetes: involvement of oxidative stress, age, rage and S100B levels in the hippocampus and prefrontal cortex of rats, Archives of Physiology and Biochemistry, 128:2, 402-410.

[2036] Espino et al (2019). Melatonin and Oxidative Stress in the Diabetic State: Clinical Implications and Potential Therapeutic Applications. Current medicinal chemistry, 26(22), 4178–4190.

2037 Fernstrom and Wurtman (1971) 'Brain serotonin content: physiological dependence on plasma tryptophan levels', Science. 1971 Jul 9;173(3992):149-52.

[2038] van Hall et al (1995). Ingestion of branched-chain amino acids and tryptophan during sustained exercise in man: failure to affect performance. The Journal of physiology, 486 (Pt 3)(Pt 3), 789–794.

2039 Halson (2014) 'Sleep in Elite Athletes and Nutritional Interventions to Enhance Sleep', Sports Med. 2014; 44(Suppl 1): 13–23.

[2040] Meng et al (2017) 'Dietary Sources and Bioactivities of Melatonin', Nutrients. 2017 Apr; 9(4): 367.

2041 Oba et al (2008) 'Consumption of vegetables alters morning urinary 6-sulfatoxymelatonin concentration', J Pineal Res. 2008 Aug;45(1):17-23. doi: 10.1111/j.1600-079X.2007.00549.x. Epub 2008 Jan 15.

2042 Howatson et al (2012) 'Effect of tart cherry juice (Prunus cerasus) on melatonin levels and enhanced sleep quality', Eur J Nutr. 2012 Dec;51(8):909-16. doi: 10.1007/s00394-011-0263-7. Epub 2011 Oct 30.

[2043] Oladi E et al (2014) 'Spectrofluorimetric determination of melatonin in kernels of four different Pistacia varieties after ultrasound-assisted solid-liquid extraction', Spectrochim Acta A Mol Biomol Spectrosc. 2014 Nov 11;132:326-9. doi: 10.1016/j.saa.2014.05.010. Epub 2014 May 16.

[2044] Tan et al (2014) 'Melatonin identified in meats and other food stuffs: potentially nutritional impact', J Pineal Res. 2014 Sep;57(2):213-8. doi: 10.1111/jpi.12152. Epub 2014 Jul 8.

[2045] Karunanithi et al (2014) 'Quantitative determination of melatonin in milk by LC-MS/MS', J Food Sci Technol. 2014 Apr;51(4):805-12. doi: 10.1007/s13197-013-1221-6. Epub 2013 Dec 1.

[2046] Wang et al (2016) 'Effect of Cultivar, Temperature, and Environmental Conditions on the Dynamic Change of Melatonin in Mulberry Fruit Development and Wine Fermentation', J Food Sci. 2016 Apr;81(4):M958-67. doi: 10.1111/1750-3841.13263. Epub 2016 Mar 8.

[2047] Mrowicka et al (2022). Lutein and Zeaxanthin and Their Roles in Age-Related Macular Degeneration-Neurodegenerative Disease. Nutrients, 14(4), 827.

[2048] Wilson et al (2021). The Effect of Lutein/Zeaxanthin Intake on Human Macular Pigment Optical Density: A Systematic Review and Meta-Analysis. Advances in nutrition (Bethesda, Md.), 12(6), 2244–2254.

[2049] Kukula-Koch et al (2021). Is Phytomelatonin Complex Better Than Synthetic Melatonin? The Assessment of the Antiradical and Anti-Inflammatory Properties. Molecules (Basel, Switzerland), 26(19), 6087.

2050 Lin et al (2011) 'Effect of kiwifruit consumption on sleep quality in adults with sleep problems', Asia Pac J Clin Nutr. 2011;20(2):169-74.

[2051] Halson (2014) 'Sleep in Elite Athletes and Nutritional Interventions to Enhance Sleep', Sports Med. 2014; 44(Suppl 1): 13–23.

[2052] Fourtillan et al (2000) 'Bioavailability of melatonin in humans after day-time administration of D(7) melatonin', Biopharm Drug Dispos. 2000 Jan;21(1):15-22.

[2053] DeMuro et al (2000) 'The absolute bioavailability of oral melatonin', J Clin Pharmacol. 2000 Jul;40(7):781-4.

[2054] Tahara, Y., & Shibata, S. (2016). Circadian rhythms of liver physiology and disease: experimental and clinical evidence. Nature Reviews Gastroenterology & Hepatology, 13(4), 217–226. doi:10.1038/nrgastro.2016.8

[2055] Longo, V. D., & Panda, S. (2016). Fasting, Circadian Rhythms, and Time-Restricted Feeding in Healthy Lifespan. Cell metabolism, 23(6), 1048-1059.

[2056] Alirezaei et al (2010). Short-term fasting induces profound neuronal autophagy. Autophagy, 6(6), 702–710.

[2057] Liu et al (2009). Hepatic autophagy is suppressed in the presence of insulin resistance and hyperinsulinemia: inhibition of FoxO1-dependent expression of key autophagy genes by insulin. The Journal of biological chemistry, 284(45), 31484–31492.

[2058] Gupta, N. J., Kumar, V., & Panda, S. (2017). A camera-phone based study reveals erratic eating pattern and disrupted daily eating-fasting cycle among adults in India. PloS one, 12(3), e0172852.

[2059] Gill, S., & Panda, S. (2015). A Smartphone App Reveals Erratic Diurnal Eating Patterns in Humans that Can Be Modulated for Health Benefits. Cell metabolism, 22(5), 789-98.

[2060] Jiang, P., & Turek, F. W. (2017). Timing of meals: when is as critical as what and how much. American journal of physiology. Endocrinology and metabolism, 312(5), E369–E380.

[2061] Damiola et al (2001) 'Restricted feeding uncouples circadian oscillators in peripheral tissues from the central pacemaker in the suprachiasmatic nucleus', Genes & Development 14(23):2950-61

[2062] Davidson, A. J., Poole, A. S., Yamazaki, S., & Menaker, M. (2003). Is the food-entrainable circadian oscillator in the digestive system? Genes, Brain and Behavior, 2(1), 32–39. doi:10.1034/j.1601-183x.2003.00005.x

[2063] Shimizu et al (2018). Delayed first active-phase meal, a breakfast-skipping model, led to increased body weight and shifted the circadian oscillation of the hepatic clock and lipid metabolism-related genes in rats fed a high-fat diet. PloS one, 13(10), e0206669.

[2064] Kolbe, I., Leinweber, B., Brandenburger, M., & Oster, H. (2019). Circadian clock network desynchrony promotes weight gain and alters glucose homeostasis in mice. Molecular metabolism, 30, 140–151.

[2065] Nováková, M., Polidarová, L., Sládek, M., & Sumová, A. (2011). Restricted feeding regime affects clock gene expression profiles in the suprachiasmatic nucleus of rats exposed to constant light. Neuroscience, 197, 65–71.

[2066] Hamaguchi, Y., Tahara, Y., Hitosugi, M., & Shibata, S. (2015). Impairment of Circadian Rhythms in Peripheral Clocks by Constant Light Is Partially Reversed by Scheduled Feeding or Exercise. Journal of biological rhythms, 30(6), 533–542.

[2067] Wang et al (2017). Time-Restricted Feeding Shifts the Skin Circadian Clock and Alters UVB-Induced DNA Damage. Cell reports, 20(5), 1061–1072.

[2068] Woodie et al (2018). Restricted feeding for 9h in the active period partially abrogates the detrimental metabolic effects of a Western diet with liquid sugar consumption in mice. Metabolism: clinical and experimental, 82, 1–13.

[2069] Delahaye et al (2018). Time-restricted feeding of a high-fat diet in male C57BL/6 mice reduces adiposity but does not protect against increased systemic inflammation. Applied physiology, nutrition, and metabolism = Physiologie appliquee, nutrition et metabolisme, 43(10), 1033–1042.

[2070] Olsen et al (2017). Time-restricted feeding on weekdays restricts weight gain: A study using rat models of high-fat diet-induced obesity. Physiology & behavior, 173, 298–304.

[2071] Villanueva et al (2019). Time-restricted feeding restores muscle function in Drosophila models of obesity and circadian-rhythm disruption. Nature communications, 10(1), 2700.

[2072] Hatori et al (2012). Time-restricted feeding without reducing caloric intake prevents metabolic diseases in mice fed a high-fat diet. Cell metabolism, 15(6), 848–860.

[2073] Chaix, A., Zarrinpar, A., Miu, P., & Panda, S. (2014). Time-restricted feeding is a preventative and therapeutic intervention against diverse nutritional challenges. Cell metabolism, 20(6), 991–1005.

[2074] Hatori, M., Vollmers, C., Zarrinpar, A., DiTacchio, L., Bushong, E. A., Gill, S., … Panda, S. (2012). Time-Restricted Feeding without Reducing Caloric Intake Prevents Metabolic Diseases in Mice Fed a High-Fat Diet. Cell Metabolism, 15(6), 848–860. doi:10.1016/j.cmet.2012.04.019

[2075] Moro, T., Tinsley, G., Bianco, A. et al. Effects of eight weeks of time-restricted feeding (16/8) on basal metabolism, maximal strength, body composition, inflammation, and cardiovascular risk factors in resistance-trained males. J Transl Med 14, 290 (2016). https://doi.org/10.1186/s12967-016-1044-0

[2076] Zare, A., Hajhashemi, M., Hassan, Z. M., Zarrin, S., Pourpak, Z., Moin, M., Salarilak, S., Masudi, S., & Shahabi, S. (2011). Effect of Ramadan fasting on serum heat shock protein 70 and serum lipid profile. Singapore medical journal, 52(7), 491–495.

[2077] Rothschild, J., Hoddy, K. K., Jambazian, P., & Varady, K. A. (2014). Time-restricted feeding and risk of metabolic disease: a review of human and animal studies. Nutrition reviews, 72(5), 308–318. https://doi.org/10.1111/nure.12104

[2078] Jamshed, H., Beyl, R. A., Della Manna, D. L., Yang, E. S., Ravussin, E., & Peterson, C. M. (2019). Early Time-Restricted Feeding Improves 24-Hour Glucose Levels and Affects Markers of the Circadian Clock, Aging, and Autophagy in Humans. Nutrients, 11(6), 1234. https://doi.org/10.3390/nu11061234

[2079] Sutton et al (2018) 'Early Time-Restricted Feeding Improves Insulin Sensitivity, Blood Pressure, and Oxidative Stress Even without Weight Loss in Men with Prediabetes', CLINICAL AND TRANSLATIONAL REPORT| VOLUME 27, ISSUE 6, P1212-1221.E3, JUNE 05, 2018

[2080] Stote et al (2007). A controlled trial of reduced meal frequency without caloric restriction in healthy, normal-weight, middle-aged adults. The American journal of clinical nutrition, 85(4), 981–988.

[2081] Chow et al (2020). Time-Restricted Eating Effects on Body Composition and Metabolic Measures in Humans who are Overweight: A Feasibility Study. Obesity (Silver Spring, Md.), 28(5), 860–869.

[2082] Anton et al (2019). The Effects of Time Restricted Feeding on Overweight, Older Adults: A Pilot Study. Nutrients, 11(7), 1500.

[2083] Moro et al (2016). Effects of eight weeks of time-restricted feeding (16/8) on basal metabolism, maximal strength, body composition, inflammation, and cardiovascular risk factors in resistance-trained males. Journal of translational medicine, 14(1), 290.

[2084] Gabel et al (2020). Effect of time restricted feeding on the gut microbiome in adults with obesity: A pilot study. Nutrition and Health, 26(2), 79–85. doi:10.1177/0260106020910907

[2085] LeCheminant et al (2013). Restricting night-time eating reduces daily energy intake in healthy young men: a short-term cross-over study. The British journal of nutrition, 110(11), 2108–2113. https://doi.org/10.1017/S0007114513001359

[2086] Gill, S., & Panda, S. (2015). A Smartphone App Reveals Erratic Diurnal Eating Patterns in Humans that Can Be Modulated for Health Benefits. Cell metabolism, 22(5), 789-98.

[2087] Sutton, E. F., Beyl, R., Early, K. S., Cefalu, W. T., Ravussin, E., & Peterson, C. M. (2018). Early Time-Restricted Feeding Improves Insulin Sensitivity, Blood Pressure, and Oxidative Stress Even without Weight Loss in Men with Prediabetes. Cell metabolism, 27(6), 1212–1221.e3.

[2088] Jamshed et al (2019). Early Time-Restricted Feeding Improves 24-Hour Glucose Levels and Affects Markers of the Circadian Clock, Aging, and Autophagy in Humans. Nutrients, 11(6), 1234.

[2089] Ravussin et al (2019). Early Time-Restricted Feeding Reduces Appetite and Increases Fat Oxidation But Does Not Affect Energy Expenditure in Humans. Obesity (Silver Spring, Md.), 27(8), 1244–1254.

[2090] Moro et al (2016) 'Effects of eight weeks of time-restricted feeding (16/8) on basal metabolism, maximal strength, body composition, inflammation, and cardiovascular risk factors in resistance-trained males', J Transl Med. 2016 Oct 13;14(1):290.

[2091] Panda S. (2016). Circadian physiology of metabolism. Science (New York, N.Y.), 354(6315), 1008–1015. https://doi.org/10.1126/science.aah4967

[2092] de Cabo et al (2018) 'A time to fast', Science, Vol. 362, Issue 6416, pp. 770-775.

[2093] Longo, V. D., & Mattson, M. P. (2014). Fasting: Molecular Mechanisms and Clinical Applications. Cell Metabolism, 19(2), 181–192. doi:10.1016/j.cmet.2013.12.008

[2094] Hayashida, S., Arimoto, A., Kuramoto, Y., Kozako, T., Honda, S., Shimeno, H., & Soeda, S. (2010). Fasting promotes the expression of SIRT1, an NAD+-dependent protein deacetylase, via activation of PPARα in mice. Molecular and Cellular Biochemistry, 339(1-2), 285–292. doi:10.1007/s11010-010-0391-z

[2095] Bi et al (2015). Breakfast skipping and the risk of type 2 diabetes: A meta-analysis of observational studies. Public Health Nutrition, 18(16), 3013-3019.

[2096] Nakajima, K., & Suwa, K. (2015). Association of hyperglycemia in a general Japanese population with late-night-dinner eating alone, but not breakfast skipping alone. Journal of Diabetes & Metabolic Disorders, 14(1). doi:10.1186/s40200-015-0147-0

[2097] Okada et al (2019). The Association of Having a Late Dinner or Bedtime Snack and Skipping Breakfast with Overweight in Japanese Women. Journal of Obesity, 2019, 1–5. doi:10.1155/2019/2439571

[2098] Azami et al (2018). Long working hours and skipping breakfast concomitant with late evening meals are associated with suboptimal glycemic control among young male Japanese patients with type 2 diabetes. Journal of Diabetes Investigation, 10(1), 73–83. doi:10.1111/jdi.12852

[2099] Kahleova et al (2014). Eating two larger meals a day (breakfast and lunch) is more effective than six smaller meals in a reduced-energy regimen for patients with type 2 diabetes: a randomised crossover study. Diabetologia, 57(8), 1552–1560. doi:10.1007/s00125-014-3253-5

[2100] Rudic et al (2004). BMAL1 and CLOCK, two essential components of the circadian clock, are involved in glucose homeostasis. PLoS biology, 2(11), e377.

[2101] Sonnier, T., Rood, J., Gimble, J. M., & Peterson, C. M. (2014). Glycemic control is impaired in the evening in prediabetes through multiple diurnal rhythms. Journal of diabetes and its complications, 28(6), 836–843. https://doi.org/10.1016/j.jdiacomp.2014.04.001

[2102] Basse et al (2018). Skeletal Muscle Insulin Sensitivity Show Circadian Rhythmicity Which Is Independent of Exercise Training Status. Frontiers in physiology, 9, 1198.

[2103] Jamshed et al (2019) 'Early Time-Restricted Feeding Improves 24-Hour Glucose Levels and Affects Markers of the Circadian Clock, Aging, and Autophagy in Humans', Nutrients. 2019 May 30;11(6). pii: E1234. doi: 10.3390/nu11061234.

[2104] Gabel et al (2018) 'Effects of 8-hour time restricted feeding on body weight and metabolic disease risk factors in obese adults: A pilot study', Nutr Healthy Aging. 2018; 4(4): 345–353.

[2105] Loboda et al (2009). Diurnal variation of the human adipose transcriptome and the link to metabolic disease. BMC medical genomics, 2, 7.

[2106] Tinsley et al (2019). Time-restricted feeding plus resistance training in active females: a randomized trial. The American journal of clinical nutrition, 110(3), 628–640.

[2107] Carlson et al (2007). Impact of reduced meal frequency without caloric restriction on glucose regulation in healthy, normal-weight middle-aged men and women. Metabolism: clinical and experimental, 56(12), 1729–1734.

[2108] Shimizu et al (2018). Delayed first active-phase meal, a breakfast-skipping model, led to increased body weight and shifted the circadian oscillation of the hepatic clock and lipid metabolism-related genes in rats fed a high-fat diet. PloS one, 13(10), e0206669.

[2109] Hutchinson et al (2019) 'Time-Restricted Feeding Improves Glucose Tolerance in Men at Risk for Type 2 Diabetes: A Randomized Crossover Trial', Obesity, Volume 27, Issue 5, Pages 724-732.

[2110] Meessen et al (2022) 'Differential Effects of One Meal per Day in the Evening on Metabolic Health and Physical Performance in Lean Individuals', Front. Physiol., 11 January 2022 |

[2111] Stote et al (2007). A controlled trial of reduced meal frequency without caloric restriction in healthy, normal-weight, middle-aged adults. The American journal of clinical nutrition, 85(4), 981–988.

[2112] Dunbar, R. I. M. (2017). Breaking Bread: the Functions of Social Eating. Adaptive Human Behavior and Physiology, 3(3), 198–211. doi:10.1007/s40750-017-0061-4

[2113] Holten et al (2004) 'Strength training increases insulin-mediated glucose uptake, GLUT4 content, and insulin signaling in skeletal muscle in patients with type 2 diabetes', Diabetes. 2004 Feb;53(2):294-305.

[2114] Intensive blood-glucose control with sulphonylureas or insulin compared with conventional treatment and risk of complications in patients with type 2 diabetes (UKPDS 33). UK Prospective Diabetes Study (UKPDS) Group. Lancet. 1998 Sep 12;352(9131):837-53. Erratum in: Lancet 1999 Aug 14;354(9178):602. PMID: 9742976.

[2115] Nathan, D. M., & DCCT/EDIC Research Group (2014). The diabetes control and complications trial/epidemiology of diabetes interventions and complications study at 30 years: overview. Diabetes care, 37(1), 9–16. https://doi.org/10.2337/dc13-2112

[2116] Adler et al (2000). Association of systolic blood pressure with macrovascular and microvascular complications of type 2 diabetes (UKPDS 36): prospective observational study. BMJ (Clinical research ed.), 321(7258), 412–419. https://doi.org/10.1136/bmj.321.7258.412

[2117] Nathan DM, Cleary PA, Backlund JY, Genuth SM, Lachin JM, Orchard TJ, Raskin P, Zinman B; Diabetes Control and Complications Trial/Epidemiology of Diabetes Interventions and Complications (DCCT/EDIC) Study Research Group. Intensive diabetes treatment and cardiovascular disease in patients with type 1 diabetes. N Engl J Med. 2005 Dec 22;353(25):2643-53. doi: 10.1056/NEJMoa052187. PMID: 16371630; PMCID: PMC2637991.

[2118] Matthews, D.R., Hosker, J.P., Rudenski, A.S. et al. Homeostasis model assessment: insulin resistance and β-cell function from fasting plasma glucose and insulin concentrations in man. Diabetologia 28, 412–419 (1985). https://doi.org/10.1007/BF00280883

[2119] Baek et al (2018). Insulin Resistance and the Risk of Diabetes and Dysglycemia in Korean General Adult Population. Diabetes & Metabolism Journal, 42(4), 296.

[2120] Lee et al (2016). Optimal Cut-Offs of Homeostasis Model Assessment of Insulin Resistance (HOMA-IR) to Identify Dysglycemia and Type 2 Diabetes Mellitus: A 15-Year Prospective Study in Chinese. PLOS ONE, 11(9), e0163424.

[2121] Salgado et al (2010). Insulin resistance index (HOMA-IR) in the differentiation of patients with non-alcoholic fatty liver disease and healthy individuals. Arquivos de gastroenterologia, 47(2), 165–169.

[2122] Abdesselam et al (2021). Estimate of the HOMA-IR Cut-off Value for Identifying Subjects at Risk of Insulin Resistance Using a Machine Learning Approach. Sultan Qaboos University medical journal, 21(4), 604–612.

[2123] Horáková et al (2019). Optimal Homeostasis Model Assessment of Insulin Resistance (HOMA-IR) Cut-Offs: A Cross-Sectional Study in the Czech Population. Medicina, 55(5), 158.

[2124] Davidson LE, Hudson R, Kilpatrick K, et al. Effects of Exercise Modality on Insulin Resistance and Functional Limitation in Older Adults: A Randomized Controlled Trial. Arch Intern Med. 2009;169(2):122–131.

[2125] Manson et al (1992). A prospective study of exercise and incidence of diabetes among US male physicians. JAMA, 268(1), 63–67.

[2126] Knowler et al (2002). Reduction in the incidence of type 2 diabetes with lifestyle intervention or metformin. The New England journal of medicine, 346(6), 393–403.

[2127] Manson et al (1991). Physical activity and incidence of non-insulin-dependent diabetes mellitus in women. Lancet (London, England), 338(8770), 774–778.

[2128] Pan et al (1997). Effects of Diet and Exercise in Preventing NIDDM in People With Impaired Glucose Tolerance: The Da Qing IGT and Diabetes Study. Diabetes Care, 20(4), 537–544.

[2129] Roberts et al (2013). Metabolic syndrome and insulin resistance: underlying causes and modification by exercise training. Comprehensive Physiology, 3(1), 1–58.

[2130] Magkos et al (2008). Improved insulin sensitivity after a single bout of exercise is curvilinearly related to exercise energy expenditure. Clinical science (London, England : 1979), 114(1), 59–64.

[2131] Newsom et al (2013). A single session of low-intensity exercise is sufficient to enhance insulin sensitivity into the next day in obese adults. Diabetes care, 36(9), 2516–2522.

[2132] Sheri R. Colberg, Ronald J. Sigal, Jane E. Yardley, Michael C. Riddell, David W. Dunstan, Paddy C. Dempsey, Edward S. Horton, Kristin Castorino, Deborah F. Tate; Physical Activity/Exercise and Diabetes: A Position Statement of the American Diabetes Association. Diabetes Care 1 November 2016; 39 (11): 2065–2079.

[2133] Little et al (2011). Low-volume high-intensity interval training reduces hyperglycemia and increases muscle mitochondrial capacity in patients with type 2 diabetes. Journal of applied physiology (Bethesda, Md. : 1985), 111(6), 1554–1560.

[2134] Jelleyman et al (2015). The effects of high-intensity interval training on glucose regulation and insulin resistance: a meta-analysis. Obesity reviews : an official journal of the International Association for the Study of Obesity, 16(11), 942–961.

[2135] Yardley et al (2013). Resistance versus aerobic exercise: acute effects on glycemia in type 1 diabetes. Diabetes care, 36(3), 537–542.

[2136] Tonoli et al (2012). Effects of different types of acute and chronic (training) exercise on glycaemic control in type 1 diabetes mellitus: a meta-analysis. Sports medicine (Auckland, N.Z.), 42(12), 1059–1080.

[2137] Dubé et al (2013). Glucose or intermittent high-intensity exercise in glargine/glulisine users with T1DM. Medicine and science in sports and exercise, 45(1), 3–7.

2138 Hejnová, J., Majerčík, M., Polák, J., Richterová, B., Crampes, F., deGlisezinski, I., & Stich, V. (2004). Vliv silove-dynamického tréninku na inzulínovou senzitivitu u inzulínorezistentních mužů [Effect of dynamic strength training on insulin sensitivity in men with insulin resistance]. Casopis lekaru ceskych, 143(11), 762–765.

2139 Burns, R. D., Fu, Y., & Zhang, P. (2019). Resistance Training and Insulin Sensitivity in Youth: A Meta-analysis. American journal of health behavior, 43(2), 228–242. https://doi.org/10.5993/AJHB.43.2.1

2140 Hansen, E., Landstad, B. J., Gundersen, K. T., Torjesen, P. A., & Svebak, S. (2012). Insulin sensitivity after maximal and endurance resistance training. Journal of strength and conditioning research, 26(2), 327–334. https://doi.org/10.1519/JSC.0b013e318220e70f

2141 Shaibi, G. Q., Cruz, M. L., Ball, G. D., Weigensberg, M. J., Salem, G. J., Crespo, N. C., & Goran, M. I. (2006). Effects of resistance training on insulin sensitivity in overweight Latino adolescent males. Medicine and science in sports and exercise, 38(7), 1208–1215. https://doi.org/10.1249/01.mss.0000227304.88406.0f

2142 Heilbronn, L., Smith, S. R., & Ravussin, E. (2004). Failure of fat cell proliferation, mitochondrial function and fat oxidation results in ectopic fat storage, insulin resistance and type II diabetes mellitus. International Journal of Obesity, 28(S4), S12–S21. doi:10.1038/sj.ijo.0802853

2143 Kullmann, S., Valenta, V., Wagner, R., Tschritter, O., Machann, J., Häring, H.-U., … Heni, M. (2020). Brain insulin sensitivity is linked to adiposity and body fat distribution. Nature Communications, 11(1). doi:10.1038/s41467-020-15686-y

2144 Caro, J. F., Dohm, L. G., Pories, W. J., & Sinha, M. K. (1989). Cellular alterations in liver, skeletal muscle, and adipose tissue responsible for insulin resistance in obesity and type II diabetes. Diabetes/metabolism reviews, 5(8), 665–689. https://doi.org/10.1002/dmr.5610050804

2145 Holten, M. K., Zacho, M., Gaster, M., Juel, C., Wojtaszewski, J. F. P., & Dela, F. (2004). Strength Training Increases Insulin-Mediated Glucose Uptake, GLUT4 Content, and Insulin Signaling in Skeletal Muscle in Patients With Type 2 Diabetes. Diabetes, 53(2), 294–305. doi:10.2337/diabetes.53.2.294

[2146] Gordon et al (2009). Resistance training improves metabolic health in type 2 diabetes: a systematic review. Diabetes research and clinical practice, 83(2), 157–175.

[2147] Dimeo et al (2012) 'Aerobic Exercise Reduces Blood Pressure in Resistant Hypertension', Hypertension, Vol. 60, No. 3.

[2148] Nishitani et al (2011). Impact of diabetes on muscle mass, muscle strength, and exercise tolerance in patients after coronary artery bypass grafting. Journal of cardiology, 58(2), 173–180.

[2149] Leenders et al (2013). Patients with type 2 diabetes show a greater decline in muscle mass, muscle strength, and functional capacity with aging. Journal of the American Medical Directors Association, 14(8), 585–592.

[2150] Anton et al (2013). Obesity and diabetes as accelerators of functional decline: can lifestyle interventions maintain functional status in high risk older adults?. Experimental gerontology, 48(9), 888–897.

[2151] Mesinovic et al (2019). Sarcopenia and type 2 diabetes mellitus: a bidirectional relationship. Diabetes, metabolic syndrome and obesity : targets and therapy, 12, 1057–1072.

[2152] Perry et al (2016). Muscle atrophy in patients with Type 2 Diabetes Mellitus: roles of inflammatory pathways, physical activity and exercise. Exercise immunology review, 22, 94–109.

[2153] Lecker et al (2006). Protein degradation by the ubiquitin-proteasome pathway in normal and disease states. Journal of the American Society of Nephrology : JASN, 17(7), 1807–1819.

[2154] Pickup et al (1997). NIDDM as a disease of the innate immune system: association of acute-phase reactants and interleukin-6 with metabolic syndrome X. Diabetologia, 40(11), 1286–1292.

[2155] Spranger et al (2003). Inflammatory cytokines and the risk to develop type 2 diabetes: results of the prospective population-based European Prospective Investigation into Cancer and Nutrition (EPIC)-Potsdam Study. Diabetes, 52(3), 812–817.

[2156] Herder et al (2006). Chemokines as risk factors for type 2 diabetes: results from the MONICA/KORA Augsburg study, 1984-2002. Diabetologia, 49(5), 921–929.

[2157] de Boer et al (2007). The temporal responses of protein synthesis, gene expression and cell signalling in human quadriceps muscle and patellar tendon to disuse. The Journal of physiology, 585(Pt 1), 241–251.

[2158] Bassil et al (2013). Muscle protein anabolism in type 2 diabetes. Current opinion in clinical nutrition and metabolic care, 16(1), 83–88.

[2159] Siew et al (2007). Insulin resistance is associated with skeletal muscle protein breakdown in non-diabetic chronic hemodialysis patients. Kidney international, 71(2), 146–152.

[2160] Wang et al 2006). Insulin resistance accelerates muscle protein degradation: Activation of the ubiquitin-proteasome pathway by defects in muscle cell signaling. Endocrinology, 147(9), 4160–4168.

[2161] Sriwijitkamol et al (2006). Reduced skeletal muscle inhibitor of kappaB beta content is associated with insulin resistance in subjects with type 2 diabetes: reversal by exercise training. Diabetes, 55(3), 760–767.

[2162] You et al (2006). Chronic inflammation: role of adipose tissue and modulation by weight loss. Current diabetes reviews, 2(1), 29–37.

[2163] Hayashino et al (2014). Effects of exercise on C-reactive protein, inflammatory cytokine and adipokine in patients with type 2 diabetes: a meta-analysis of randomized controlled trials. Metabolism: clinical and experimental, 63(3), 431–440.

[2164] Kadoglou et al (2007). The anti-inflammatory effects of exercise training in patients with type 2 diabetes mellitus. European journal of cardiovascular prevention and rehabilitation : official journal of the European Society of Cardiology, Working Groups on Epidemiology & Prevention and Cardiac Rehabilitation and Exercise Physiology, 14(6), 837–843.

[2165] Balducci et al (2010). Anti-inflammatory effect of exercise training in subjects with type 2 diabetes and the metabolic syndrome is dependent on exercise modalities and independent of weight loss. Nutrition, metabolism, and cardiovascular diseases : NMCD, 20(8), 608–617.

[2166] Watson et al (2015). Progressive Resistance Exercise Training in CKD: A Feasibility Study. American journal of kidney diseases : the official journal of the National Kidney Foundation, 66(2), 249–257.

[2167] Chen et al (2021). Effects of resistance training in healthy older people with sarcopenia: a systematic review and meta-analysis of randomized controlled trials. European Review of Aging and Physical Activity, 18(1).

[2168] Alkner, B. A., & Tesch, P. A. (2004). Knee extensor and plantar flexor muscle size and function following 90 days of bed rest with or without resistance exercise. European journal of applied physiology, 93(3), 294–305.

[2169] Holten et al (2004). Strength training increases insulin-mediated glucose uptake, GLUT4 content, and insulin signaling in skeletal muscle in patients with type 2 diabetes. Diabetes, 53(2), 294–305.

[2170] Jorge et al (2011). The effects of aerobic, resistance, and combined exercise on metabolic control, inflammatory markers, adipocytokines, and muscle insulin signaling in patients with type 2 diabetes mellitus. Metabolism: clinical and experimental, 60(9), 1244–1252.

[2171] Geirsdottir et al (2012). Effect of 12-week resistance exercise program on body composition, muscle strength, physical function, and glucose metabolism in healthy, insulin-resistant, and diabetic elderly Icelanders. The journals of gerontology. Series A, Biological sciences and medical sciences, 67(11), 1259–1265.

[2172] Brooks et al (2006). Strength training improves muscle quality and insulin sensitivity in Hispanic older adults with type 2 diabetes. International journal of medical sciences, 4(1), 19–27.

[2173] Gonzalez et al (2015). Association between myosin heavy chain protein isoforms and intramuscular anabolic signaling following resistance exercise in trained men. Physiological reports, 3(1), e12268.

[2174] Figueiredo et al (2015). Ribosome biogenesis adaptation in resistance training-induced human skeletal muscle hypertrophy. American journal of physiology. Endocrinology and metabolism, 309(1), E72–E83.

333

[2175] Apró et al (2015). Resistance exercise-induced S6K1 kinase activity is not inhibited in human skeletal muscle despite prior activation of AMPK by high-intensity interval cycling. American journal of physiology. Endocrinology and metabolism, 308(6), E470–E481.

[2176] Goodman C. A. (2014). The role of mTORC1 in regulating protein synthesis and skeletal muscle mass in response to various mechanical stimuli. Reviews of physiology, biochemistry and pharmacology, 166, 43–95.

[2177] Watson, K., & Baar, K. (2014). mTOR and the health benefits of exercise. Seminars in cell & developmental biology, 36, 130–139.

[2178] Jacobs et al (2013). Eccentric contractions increase the phosphorylation of tuberous sclerosis complex-2 (TSC2) and alter the targeting of TSC2 and the mechanistic target of rapamycin to the lysosome. The Journal of physiology, 591(18), 4611–4620.

2179 Garber et al (2011). Quantity and Quality of Exercise for Developing and Maintaining Cardiorespiratory, Musculoskeletal, and Neuromotor Fitness in Apparently Healthy Adults. Medicine & Science in Sports & Exercise, 43(7), 1334–1359. doi:10.1249/mss.0b013e318213fefb

2180 Slysz et al (2016) 'The efficacy of blood flow restricted exercise: A systematic review & meta-analysis', Journal of Science and Medicine in Sports, Volume 19, Issue 8, Pages 669–675. DOI: https://doi.org/10.1016/j.jsams.2015.09.005

2181 Schoenfeld BJ et al (2016) 'Effects of Resistance Training Frequency on Measures of Muscle Hypertrophy: A Systematic Review and Meta-Analysis', Sports Med, Vol 46(11), p 1689-1697.

2182 Schoenfeld, B. J. (2010). The Mechanisms of Muscle Hypertrophy and Their Application to Resistance Training. Journal of Strength and Conditioning Research, 24(10), 2857–2872. doi:10.1519/jsc.0b013e3181e840f3

[2183] Hu et al (2020). Evaluation of walking exercise on glycemic control in patients with type 2 diabetes mellitus: A protocol for systematic review and meta-analysis of randomized cross-over controlled trials. Medicine, 99(47), e22735.

[2184] Moghetti et al (2020) 'Walking for subjects with type 2 diabetes: A systematic review and joint AMD/SID/SISMES evidence-based practical guideline', Nutrition, Metabolism and Cardiovascular Diseases, Volume 30, Issue 11, 30 October 2020, Pages 1882-1898.

[2185] Jesus del Pozo-Cruz, Francisco Alvarez-Barbosa, Daniel Gallardo-Gomez, Borja del Pozo Cruz; Optimal Number of Steps per Day to Prevent All-Cause Mortality in People With Prediabetes and Diabetes. Diabetes Care 1 September 2022; 45 (9): 2156–2158.

[2186] Iwasaki et al (2021). Fast walking is a preventive factor against new-onset diabetes mellitus in a large cohort from a Japanese general population. Scientific Reports, 11(1).

[2187] White et al (2013). Trajectories of gait speed predict mortality in well-functioning older adults: the Health, Aging and Body Composition study. The journals of gerontology. Series A, Biological sciences and medical sciences, 68(4), 456–464.

[2188] Buffey, A.J., Herring, M.P., Langley, C.K. et al. The Acute Effects of Interrupting Prolonged Sitting Time in Adults with Standing and Light-Intensity Walking on Biomarkers of Cardiometabolic Health in Adults: A Systematic Review and Meta-analysis. Sports Med 52, 1765–1787 (2022).

[2189] Dunstan et al (2007). Association of television viewing with fasting and 2-h postchallenge plasma glucose levels in adults without diagnosed diabetes. Diabetes care, 30(3), 516–522.

[2190] Fritschi et al (2016). Association Between Daily Time Spent in Sedentary Behavior and Duration of Hyperglycemia in Type 2 Diabetes. Biological research for nursing, 18(2), 160–166.

[2191] Alternating Bouts of Sitting and Standing Attenuate Postprandial Glucose Responses-Corrigendum. (2020). Medicine and science in sports and exercise, 52(9), 2058–2059.

[2192] Buckley et al (2014). Standing-based office work shows encouraging signs of attenuating post-prandial glycaemic excursion. Occupational and environmental medicine, 71(2), 109–111.

[2193] David W. Dunstan, Bronwyn A. Kingwell, Robyn Larsen, Genevieve N. Healy, Ester Cerin, Marc T. Hamilton, Jonathan E. Shaw, David A. Bertovic, Paul Z. Zimmet, Jo Salmon, Neville Owen; Breaking Up Prolonged Sitting Reduces Postprandial Glucose and Insulin Responses. Diabetes Care 1 May 2012; 35 (5): 976–983.

[2194] Larsen et al (2015). Breaking up of prolonged sitting over three days sustains, but does not enhance, lowering of postprandial plasma glucose and insulin in overweight and obese adults. Clinical science (London, England : 1979), 129(2), 117–127.

[2195] Henson et al (2016). Breaking Up Prolonged Sitting With Standing or Walking Attenuates the Postprandial Metabolic Response in Postmenopausal Women: A Randomized Acute Study. Diabetes care, 39(1), 130–138.

[2196] van Dijk et al (2013). Effect of moderate-intensity exercise versus activities of daily living on 24-hour blood glucose homeostasis in male patients with type 2 diabetes. Diabetes care, 36(11), 3448–3453.

[2197] Colberg et al (2009). Postprandial walking is better for lowering the glycemic effect of dinner than pre-dinner exercise in type 2 diabetic individuals. Journal of the American Medical Directors Association, 10(6), 394–397.

[2198] Cinti S. (2005). The adipose organ. Prostaglandins, leukotrienes, and essential fatty acids, 73(1), 9–15. https://doi.org/10.1016/j.plefa.2005.04.010

[2199] Enerbäck S. (2009). The origins of brown adipose tissue. The New England journal of medicine, 360(19), 2021–2023. https://doi.org/10.1056/NEJMcibr0809610

[2200] Kozak, L. P. (2010). Brown Fat and the Myth of Diet-Induced Thermogenesis. Cell Metabolism, 11(4), 263–267. https://doi.org/10.1016/j.cmet.2010.03.009

[2201] Gesta, S., Tseng, Y. H., & Kahn, C. R. (2007). Developmental origin of fat: tracking obesity to its source. Cell, 131(2), 242–256. https://doi.org/10.1016/j.cell.2007.10.004

[2202] Saito, M., Okamatsu-Ogura, Y., Matsushita, M., Watanabe, K., Yoneshiro, T., Nio-Kobayashi, J., Iwanaga, T., Miyagawa, M., Kameya, T., Nakada, K., Kawai, Y., & Tsujisaki, M. (2009). High incidence of metabolically active brown adipose tissue in healthy adult humans: effects of cold exposure and adiposity. Diabetes, 58(7), 1526–1531. https://doi.org/10.2337/db09-0530

[2203] Nedergaard, J., Bengtsson, T., & Cannon, B. (2007). Unexpected evidence for active brown adipose tissue in adult humans. American journal of physiology. Endocrinology and metabolism, 293(2), E444–E452. https://doi.org/10.1152/ajpendo.00691.2006

[2204] Samuelson, I., & Vidal-Puig, A. (2020). Studying Brown Adipose Tissue in a Human in vitro Context. Frontiers in Endocrinology, 11. https://doi.org/10.3389/fendo.2020.00629

[2205] Carrière, A., Jeanson, Y., Cousin, B., Arnaud, E., & Casteilla, L. (2013). Le recrutement et l'activation d'adipocytes bruns et/ou BRITE. Médecine/Sciences, 29(8–9), 729–735. https://doi.org/10.1051/medsci/2013298011

[2206] Cypess, A. M., & Kahn, C. R. (2010). Brown fat as a therapy for obesity and diabetes. Current opinion in endocrinology, diabetes, and obesity, 17(2), 143–149.

[2207] Liu, X., Zheng, Z., Zhu, X., Meng, M., Li, L., Shen, Y., Chi, Q., Wang, D., Zhang, Z., Li, C., Li, Y., Xue, Y., Speakman, J. R., & Jin, W. (2013). Brown adipose tissue transplantation improves whole-body energy metabolism. Cell research, 23(6), 851–854. https://doi.org/10.1038/cr.2013.64

[2208] Stanford, K. I., Middelbeek, R. J., Townsend, K. L., An, D., Nygaard, E. B., Hitchcox, K. M., Markan, K. R., Nakano, K., Hirshman, M. F., Tseng, Y. H., & Goodyear, L. J. (2013). Brown adipose tissue regulates glucose homeostasis and insulin sensitivity. The Journal of clinical investigation, 123(1), 215–223. https://doi.org/10.1172/JCI62308

[2209] Berbée, J. F., Boon, M. R., Khedoe, P. P., Bartelt, A., Schlein, C., Worthmann, A., Kooijman, S., Hoeke, G., Mol, I. M., John, C., Jung, C., Vazirpanah, N., Brouwers, L. P., Gordts, P. L., Esko, J. D., Hiemstra, P. S., Havekes, L. M., Scheja, L., Heeren, J., & Rensen, P. C. (2015). Brown fat activation reduces hypercholesterolaemia and protects from atherosclerosis development. Nature communications, 6, 6356. https://doi.org/10.1038/ncomms7356

[2210] Bartelt, A., Bruns, O. T., Reimer, R., Hohenberg, H., Ittrich, H., Peldschus, K., Kaul, M. G., Tromsdorf, U. I., Weller, H., Waurisch, C., Eychmüller, A., Gordts, P. L., Rinninger, F., Bruegelmann, K., Freund, B., Nielsen, P., Merkel, M., & Heeren, J. (2011). Brown adipose tissue activity controls triglyceride clearance. Nature medicine, 17(2), 200–205. https://doi.org/10.1038/nm.2297

[2211] Cypess, A. M., Lehman, S., Williams, G., Tal, I., Rodman, D., Goldfine, A. B., Kuo, F. C., Palmer, E. L., Tseng, Y. H., Doria, A., Kolodny, G. M., & Kahn, C. R. (2009). Identification and importance of brown adipose tissue in adult humans. The New England journal of medicine, 360(15), 1509–1517. https://doi.org/10.1056/NEJMoa0810780

[2212] Graja, A., & Schulz, T. J. (2014). Mechanisms of Aging-Related Impairment of Brown Adipocyte Development and Function. Gerontology, 61(3), 211–217. Portico. https://doi.org/10.1159/000366557

[2213] Romere, C., Duerrschmid, C., Bournat, J., Constable, P., Jain, M., Xia, F., Saha, P. K., Del Solar, M., Zhu, B., York, B., Sarkar, P., Rendon, D. A., Gaber, M. W., LeMaire, S. A., Coselli, J. S., Milewicz, D. M., Sutton, V. R., Butte, N. F., Moore, D. D., & Chopra, A. R. (2016). Asprosin, a Fasting-Induced Glucogenic Protein Hormone. Cell, 165(3), 566–579. https://doi.org/10.1016/j.cell.2016.02.063

[2214] Martínez-Sánchez N. (2020). There and Back Again: Leptin Actions in White Adipose Tissue. International journal of molecular sciences, 21(17), 6039. https://doi.org/10.3390/ijms21176039

[2215] Alan, M., Gurlek, B., Yilmaz, A., Aksit, M., Aslanipour, B., Gulhan, I., Mehmet, C., & Taner, C. E. (2019). Asprosin: a novel peptide hormone related to insulin resistance in women with polycystic ovary syndrome. Gynecological endocrinology : the official journal of the International Society of Gynecological Endocrinology, 35(3), 220–223. https://doi.org/10.1080/09513590.2018.1512967

[2216] Yuan, M., Li, W., Zhu, Y., Yu, B., & Wu, J. (2020). Asprosin: A Novel Player in Metabolic Diseases. Frontiers in endocrinology, 11, 64. https://doi.org/10.3389/fendo.2020.00064

[2217] Wang, C. Y., Lin, T. A., Liu, K. H., Liao, C. H., Liu, Y. Y., Wu, V. C., Wen, M. S., & Yeh, T. S. (2019). Serum asprosin levels and bariatric surgery outcomes in obese adults. International journal of obesity (2005), 43(5), 1019–1025. https://doi.org/10.1038/s41366-018-0248-1

[2218] Wu, J., Boström, P., Sparks, L. M., Ye, L., Choi, J. H., Giang, A.-H., Khandekar, M., Virtanen, K. A., Nuutila, P., Schaart, G., Huang, K., Tu, H., van Marken Lichtenbelt, W. D., Hoeks, J., Enerbäck, S., Schrauwen, P., & Spiegelman, B. M. (2012). Beige Adipocytes Are a Distinct Type of Thermogenic Fat Cell in Mouse and Human. Cell, 150(2), 366–376. https://doi.org/10.1016/j.cell.2012.05.016

[2219] Miao, Y., Qin, H., Zhong, Y., Huang, K., & Rao, C. (2021). Novel adipokine asprosin modulates browning and adipogenesis in white adipose tissue. The Journal of endocrinology, 249(2), 83–93. https://doi.org/10.1530/JOE-20-0503

[2220] Cedikova, M., Kripnerová, M., Dvorakova, J., Pitule, P., Grundmanova, M., Babuska, V., Mullerova, D., & Kuncova, J. (2016). Mitochondria in White, Brown, and Beige Adipocytes. Stem cells international, 2016, 6067349. https://doi.org/10.1155/2016/6067349

[2221] Lidell, M. E., Betz, M. J., & Enerbäck, S. (2014). Two types of brown adipose tissue in humans. Adipocyte, 3(1), 63–66. https://doi.org/10.4161/adip.26896

[2222] Heaton J. M. (1972). The distribution of brown adipose tissue in the human. Journal of anatomy, 112(Pt 1), 35–39.

[2223] Dempersmier et al (2015). Cold-Inducible Zfp516 Activates UCP1 Transcription to Promote Browning of White Fat and Development of Brown Fat. Molecular Cell, 57(2), 235–246. doi:10.1016/j.molcel.2014.12.005

[2224] Van Marken Lichtenbelt et al (2009). Cold-Activated Brown Adipose Tissue in Healthy Men. New England Journal of Medicine, 360(15), 1500–1508. doi:10.1056/nejmoa0808718

[2225] Saito, M. (2013). Brown Adipose Tissue as a Regulator of Energy Expenditure and Body Fat in Humans. Diabetes & Metabolism Journal, 37(1), 22. doi:10.4093/dmj.2013.37.1.22

[2226] Nie et al (2015) 'Cold exposure stimulates lipid metabolism, induces inflammatory response in the adipose tissue of mice and promotes the osteogenic differentiation of BMMSCs via the p38 MAPK pathway in vitro', Int J Clin Exp Pathol. 2015; 8(9): 10875–10886.

[2227] Claire Chevalier, Ozren Stojanović, Didier J. Colin, Nicolas Suarez-Zamorano, Valentina Tarallo, Christelle Veyrat-Durebex, Dorothée Rigo, Salvatore Fabbiano, Ana Stevanović, Stefanie Hagemann, Xavier Montet, Yann Seimbille, Nicola Zamboni, Siegfried Hapfelmeier, Mirko Trajkovski. Gut Microbiota Orchestrates Energy Homeostasis during Cold. Cell, 2015; 163 (6): 1360 DOI: 10.1016/j.cell.2015.11.004

[2228] Kulterer et al (2020). The Presence of Active Brown Adipose Tissue Determines Cold-Induced Energy Expenditure and Oxylipin Profiles in Humans. The Journal of Clinical Endocrinology & Metabolism, 105(7), 2203–2216.

[2229] Imbeault, P., Dépault, I., & Haman, F. (2009). Cold exposure increases adiponectin levels in men. Metabolism: clinical and experimental, 58(4), 552–559. https://doi.org/10.1016/j.metabol.2008.11.017

[2230] Schrauwen, P., & van Marken Lichtenbelt, W. D. (2016). Combatting type 2 diabetes by turning up the heat. Diabetologia, 59(11), 2269–2279. doi:10.1007/s00125-016-4068-3

[2231] Luo et al (2016) 'Cold-Induced Browning Dynamically Alters the Expression Profiles of Inflammatory Adipokines with Tissue Specificity in Mice', International Journal of Molecular Sciences 17(5):795.

[2232] Sugimoto et al (2022). Brown adipose tissue-derived MaR2 contributes to cold-induced resolution of inflammation. Nature Metabolism, 4(6), 775–790.

[2233] Srámek et al (2000). Human physiological responses to immersion into water of different temperatures. European journal of applied physiology, 81(5), 436–442. https://doi.org/10.1007/s004210050065

[2234] VANOOIJEN et al (2004). Seasonal changes in metabolic and temperature responses to cold air in humans. Physiology & Behavior, 82(2–3), 545–553.

[2235] Yoneshiro et al (2013). Recruited brown adipose tissue as an antiobesity agent in humans. The Journal of clinical investigation, 123(8), 3404–3408.

[2236] Hanssen et al (2015). Short-term Cold Acclimation Recruits Brown Adipose Tissue in Obese Humans. Diabetes, 65(5), 1179–1189. doi:10.2337/db15-1372

[2237] Acosta et al (2018). Physiological responses to acute cold exposure in young lean men. PLOS ONE, 13(5), e0196543. doi:10.1371/journal.pone.0196543

[2238] Langeveld et al (2016). Mild cold effects on hunger, food intake, satiety and skin temperature in humans. Endocrine connections, 5(2), 65–73.

[2239] Garritson, J. D., & Boudina, S. (2021). The Effects of Exercise on White and Brown Adipose Tissue Cellularity, Metabolic Activity and Remodeling. Frontiers in physiology, 12, 772894. https://doi.org/10.3389/fphys.2021.772894

[2240] Xu, X., Ying, Z., Cai, M., Xu, Z., Li, Y., Jiang, S. Y., Tzan, K., Wang, A., Parthasarathy, S., He, G., Rajagopalan, S., & Sun, Q. (2011). Exercise ameliorates high-fat diet-induced metabolic and vascular dysfunction, and increases adipocyte progenitor cell population in brown adipose tissue. American journal of physiology. Regulatory, integrative and comparative physiology, 300(5), R1115–R1125. https://doi.org/10.1152/ajpregu.00806.2010

[2241] Fu, P., Zhu, R., Jia, J., Hu, Y., Wu, C., Cieszczyk, P., Holmberg, H. C., & Gong, L. (2021). Aerobic exercise promotes the functions of brown adipose tissue in obese mice via a mechanism involving COX2 in the VEGF signaling pathway. Nutrition & metabolism, 18(1), 56. https://doi.org/10.1186/s12986-021-00581-0

[2242] Loustau, T., Coudiere, E., Karkeni, E., Landrier, J. F., Jover, B., & Riva, C. (2020). Murine double minute-2 mediates exercise-induced angiogenesis in adipose tissue of diet-induced obese mice. Microvascular research, 130, 104003. https://doi.org/10.1016/j.mvr.2020.104003

[2243] Ye J. (2009). Emerging role of adipose tissue hypoxia in obesity and insulin resistance. International journal of obesity (2005), 33(1), 54–66. https://doi.org/10.1038/ijo.2008.229

[2244] Kolahdouzi, S., Talebi-Garakani, E., Hamidian, G., & Safarzade, A. (2019). Exercise training prevents high-fat diet-induced adipose tissue remodeling by promoting capillary density and macrophage polarization. Life sciences, 220, 32–43. https://doi.org/10.1016/j.lfs.2019.01.037

[2245] Stanford et al (2018). 12,13-diHOME: An Exercise-Induced Lipokine that Increases Skeletal Muscle Fatty Acid Uptake. Cell Metabolism, 27(5), 1111-1120.e3.

[2246] Lee et al (2014). Irisin and FGF21 Are Cold-Induced Endocrine Activators of Brown Fat Function in Humans. Cell Metabolism, 19(2), 302–309.

[2247] Boström et al (2012). A PGC1-α-dependent myokine that drives brown-fat-like development of white fat and thermogenesis. Nature, 481(7382), 463–468.

[2248] Jiménez-Aranda et al (2013). Melatonin induces browning of inguinal white adipose tissue in Zucker diabetic fatty rats. Journal of pineal research, 55(4), 416–423.

[2249] Figueiro et al (2012). Light Modulates Leptin and Ghrelin in Sleep-Restricted Adults. International Journal of Endocrinology, 2012, 1–6.

[2250] Omisade, A., Buxton, O. M., & Rusak, B. (2010). Impact of acute sleep restriction on cortisol and leptin levels in young women. Physiology & behavior, 99(5), 651–656.

[2251] Spiegel et al (2004). Brief communication: Sleep curtailment in healthy young men is associated with decreased leptin levels, elevated ghrelin levels, and increased hunger and appetite. Annals of internal medicine, 141(11), 846–850.

[2252] Mullington et al (2003). Sleep loss reduces diurnal rhythm amplitude of leptin in healthy men. Journal of neuroendocrinology, 15(9), 851–854.

[2253] Sun et al (2020). Chronic Timed Sleep Restriction Attenuates LepRb-Mediated Signaling Pathways and Circadian Clock Gene Expression in the Rat Hypothalamus. Frontiers in Neuroscience, 14.

[2254] Ondrusova, K., Fatehi, M., Barr, A. et al. Subcutaneous white adipocytes express a light sensitive signaling pathway mediated via a melanopsin/TRPC channel axis. Sci Rep 7, 16332 (2017).

[2255] Figueiro, M. G., Plitnick, B., & Rea, M. S. (2012). Light modulates leptin and ghrelin in sleep-restricted adults. International journal of endocrinology, 2012, 530726.

[2256] O'Keefe and Bell (2007) 'Postprandial Hyperglycemia/Hyperlipidemia (Postprandial Dysmetabolism) Is a Cardiovascular Risk Factor', The American Journal of Cardiology, Volume 100, Issue 5, 1 September 2007, Pages 899-904.

[2257] Kosiborod, M. (2018). Hyperglycemia in Acute Coronary Syndromes. Endocrinology and Metabolism Clinics of North America, 47(1), 185–202.

[2258] Bonora et al (2006). Prevalence and correlates of post-prandial hyperglycaemia in a large sample of patients with type 2 diabetes mellitus. Diabetologia, 49(5), 846–854.

[2259] Catherine C. Cowie, Keith F. Rust, Danita D. Byrd-Holt, Mark S. Eberhardt, Katherine M. Flegal, Michael M. Engelgau, Sharon H. Saydah, Desmond E. Williams, Linda S. Geiss, Edward W. Gregg; Prevalence of Diabetes and Impaired Fasting Glucose in Adults in the U.S. Population: National Health and Nutrition Examination Survey 1999–2002. Diabetes Care 1 June 2006; 29 (6): 1263–1268.

[2260] Conaway et al (2005). Frequency of Undiagnosed Diabetes Mellitus in Patients With Acute Coronary Syndrome. The American Journal of Cardiology, 96(3), 363–365.

[2261] Weissman et al (2006). Power Spectral Analysis of Heart Rate Variability During the 100-g Oral Glucose Tolerance Test in Pregnant Women. Diabetes Care, 29(3), 571–574.

[2262] Cavalot et al (2006). Postprandial Blood Glucose Is a Stronger Predictor of Cardiovascular Events Than Fasting Blood Glucose in Type 2 Diabetes Mellitus, Particularly in Women: Lessons from the San Luigi Gonzaga Diabetes Study. The Journal of Clinical Endocrinology & Metabolism, 91(3), 813–819.

[2263] Mellen et al (2006) 'Diabetes, the Metabolic Syndrome, and Angiographic Progression of Coronary Arterial Disease in Postmenopausal Women', Arteriosclerosis, Thrombosis, and Vascular Biology. 2006;26:189–193.

[2264] Sasso FC, Carbonara O, Nasti R, et al. Glucose Metabolism and Coronary Heart Disease in Patients With Normal Glucose Tolerance. JAMA. 2004;291(15):1857–1863. doi:10.1001/jama.291.15.1857

[2265] Buysschaert et al (2022) '1-h post-load plasma glucose for detecting early stages of prediabetes', Diabetes & Metabolism, Volume 48, Issue 6, November 2022, 101395.

[2266] Eyth E, Basit H, Swift CJ. Glucose Tolerance Test. [Updated 2022 Oct 24]. In: StatPearls [Internet]. Treasure Island (FL): StatPearls Publishing; 2023 Jan-. Available from: https://www.ncbi.nlm.nih.gov/books/NBK532915/

[2267] Beulens et al (2007) 'High Dietary Glycemic Load and Glycemic Index Increase Risk of Cardiovascular Disease Among Middle-Aged Women: A Population-Based Follow-Up Study', Journal of the American College of Cardiology, Volume 50, Issue 1, 3 July 2007, Pages 14-21.

[2268] Teymoori, F., Farhadnejad, H., Mirmiran, P. et al. The association between dietary glycemic and insulin indices with incidence of cardiovascular disease: Tehran lipid and glucose study. BMC Public Health 20, 1496 (2020).

[2269] Greenwood et al (2013). Glycemic Index, Glycemic Load, Carbohydrates, and Type 2 Diabetes. Diabetes Care, 36(12), 4166–4171.

[2270] Jenkins, D., Kendall, C., Faulkner, D. et al. Long-term effects of a plant-based dietary portfolio of cholesterol-lowering foods on blood pressure. Eur J Clin Nutr 62, 781–788 (2008).

[2271] Bayard, V., Chamorro, F., Motta, J., Hollenberg, N.K. (2007). Does Flavanol Intake Influence Mortality from Nitric Oxide-Dependent Processes? Ischemic Heart Disease, Stroke, Diabetes Mellitus, and Cancer in Panama. International Journal of Medical Sciences, 4(1), 53-58. https://doi.org/10.7150/ijms.4.53.

[2272] Shukla et al (2017). Carbohydrate-last meal pattern lowers postprandial glucose and insulin excursions in type 2 diabetes. BMJ Open Diabetes Research & Care, 5(1), e000440.

[2273] Törrönen, R., Sarkkinen, E., Tapola, N., Hautaniemi, E., Kilpi, K., & Niskanen, L. (2010). Berries modify the postprandial plasma glucose response to sucrose in healthy subjects. The British journal of nutrition, 103(8), 1094–1097.

[2274] Törrönen, R., Kolehmainen, M., Sarkkinen, E., Poutanen, K., Mykkänen, H., & Niskanen, L. (2013). Berries reduce postprandial insulin responses to wheat and rye breads in healthy women. The Journal of nutrition, 143(4), 430–436.

[2275] Törrönen et al (2012). Postprandial glucose, insulin, and free fatty acid responses to sucrose consumed with blackcurrants and lingonberries in healthy women. The American journal of clinical nutrition, 96(3), 527–533.

[2276] Törrönen et al (2012). Postprandial glucose, insulin and glucagon-like peptide 1 responses to sucrose ingested with berries in healthy subjects. The British journal of nutrition, 107(10), 1445–1451.

[2277] Castro-Acosta, M. L., Lenihan-Geels, G. N., Corpe, C. P., & Hall, W. L. (2016). Berries and anthocyanins: promising functional food ingredients with postprandial glycaemia-lowering effects. The Proceedings of the Nutrition Society, 75(3), 342–355.

[2278] Arora, S.K., McFarlane, S.I. The case for low carbohydrate diets in diabetes management. Nutr Metab (Lond) 2, 16 (2005). https://doi.org/10.1186/1743-7075-2-16

[2279] Claudia et al (2009) Effects of a Plant-Based High-Carbohydrate/High-Fiber Diet Versus High–Monounsaturated Fat/Low-Carbohydrate Diet on Postprandial Lipids in Type 2 Diabetic Patients. Diabetes Care 1 December 2009; 32 (12): 2168–2173.

[2280] Ma et al (2006). Association between dietary fiber and serum C-reactive protein. The American journal of clinical nutrition, 83(4), 760–766.

[2281] Hall et al (2021). Effect of a plant-based, low-fat diet versus an animal-based, ketogenic diet on ad libitum energy intake. Nature Medicine, 27(2), 344–353.

[2282] Galgani, J., Aguirre, C. & Díaz, E. Acute effect of meal glycemic index and glycemic load on blood glucose and insulin responses in humans. Nutr J 5, 22 (2006).

[2283] Ceriello et al (2005) 'Effect of Atorvastatin and Irbesartan, Alone and in Combination, on Postprandial Endothelial Dysfunction, Oxidative Stress, and Inflammation in Type 2 Diabetic Patients', Circulation, Vol 111, No 19.

[2284] O'Keefe et al (2008) 'Dietary Strategies for Improving Post-Prandial Glucose, Lipids, Inflammation, and Cardiovascular Health', Journal of the American College of Cardiology, Volume 51, Issue 3, 22 January 2008, Pages 249-255.

[2285] Shuldiner et al (2004). Genes and pathophysiology of type 2 diabetes: more than just the Randle cycle all over again. The Journal of clinical investigation, 114(10), 1414–1417.

[2286] Monnier et al (2006). Activation of Oxidative Stress by Acute Glucose Fluctuations Compared With Sustained Chronic Hyperglycemia in Patients With Type 2 Diabetes. JAMA, 295(14), 1681.

[2287] Brownlee et al (2006). Glycemic Variability: A Hemoglobin A1c–Independent Risk Factor for Diabetic Complications. JAMA, 295(14), 1707.

[2288] Lichtenstein et al (2006). Diet and Lifestyle Recommendations Revision 2006. Circulation, 114(1), 82–96.

[2289] Hlebowicz et al (2007). Effect of cinnamon on postprandial blood glucose, gastric emptying, and satiety in healthy subjects. The American Journal of Clinical Nutrition, 85(6), 1552–1556.

[2290] Allen et al (2013). Cinnamon use in type 2 diabetes: an updated systematic review and meta-analysis. Annals of family medicine, 11(5), 452–459.

[2291] Iwata et al (2016). The Relation between Hepatotoxicity and the Total Coumarin Intake from Traditional Japanese Medicines Containing Cinnamon Bark. Frontiers in pharmacology, 7, 174.

[2292] Magistrelli, A., & Chezem, J. C. (2012). Effect of ground cinnamon on postprandial blood glucose concentration in normal-weight and obese adults. Journal of the Academy of Nutrition and Dietetics, 112(11), 1806–1809.

[2293] Bernardo et al (2015). Effect of Cinnamon Tea on Postprandial Glucose Concentration. Journal of diabetes research, 2015, 913651.

[2294] Kizilaslan, N., & Erdem, N. Z. (2019). The Effect of Different Amounts of Cinnamon Consumption on Blood Glucose in Healthy Adult Individuals. International journal of food science, 2019, 4138534.

[2295] Solomon, T. P. J., & Blannin, A. K. (2007). Effects of short-term cinnamon ingestion on in vivo glucose tolerance. Diabetes, Obesity and Metabolism, 9(6), 895–901.

[2296] Solomon, T. P., & Blannin, A. K. (2009). Changes in glucose tolerance and insulin sensitivity following 2 weeks of daily cinnamon ingestion in healthy humans. European journal of applied physiology, 105(6), 969–976.

[2297] Lim et al (2016). Vinegar as a functional ingredient to improve postprandial glycemic control-human intervention findings and molecular mechanisms. Molecular nutrition & food research, 60(8), 1837–1849.

[2298] Shishehbor et al (2017). Vinegar consumption can attenuate postprandial glucose and insulin responses; a systematic review and meta-analysis of clinical trials. Diabetes research and clinical practice, 127, 1–9.

[2299] Hlebowicz et al (2007). Effect of apple cider vinegar on delayed gastric emptying in patients with type 1 diabetes mellitus: a pilot study. BMC gastroenterology, 7, 46.

[2300] Siddiqui et al (2018). Diabetes Control: Is Vinegar a Promising Candidate to Help Achieve Targets?. Journal of evidence-based integrative medicine, 23, 2156587217753004.

[2301] Cheng et al (2020). A systematic review and meta-analysis: Vinegar consumption on glycaemic control in adults with type 2 diabetes mellitus. Journal of advanced nursing, 76(2), 459–474.

[2302] Budak et al (2014). Functional Properties of Vinegar. Journal of Food Science, 79(5), R757–R764.

[2303] Johnston et al (2004). Vinegar Improves Insulin Sensitivity to a High-Carbohydrate Meal in Subjects With Insulin Resistance or Type 2 Diabetes. Diabetes Care, 27(1), 281–282.

[2304] Johnston, C. S., & Buller, A. J. (2005). Vinegar and peanut products as complementary foods to reduce postprandial glycemia. Journal of the American Dietetic Association, 105(12), 1939–1942.

[2305] Östman, E., Granfeldt, Y., Persson, L. et al. Vinegar supplementation lowers glucose and insulin responses and increases satiety after a bread meal in healthy subjects. Eur J Clin Nutr 59, 983–988 (2005).

[2306] Brighenti et al (1995). Effect of neutralized and native vinegar on blood glucose and acetate responses to a mixed meal in healthy subjects. European journal of clinical nutrition, 49(4), 242–247.

[2307] Östman et al (2005). Vinegar supplementation lowers glucose and insulin responses and increases satiety after a bread meal in healthy subjects. European Journal of Clinical Nutrition, 59(9), 983–988.

[2308] Johnston, C. S., & Buller, A. J. (2005). Vinegar and peanut products as complementary foods to reduce postprandial glycemia. Journal of the American Dietetic Association, 105(12), 1939–1942

[2309] KONDO et al (2009). Vinegar Intake Reduces Body Weight, Body Fat Mass, and Serum Triglyceride Levels in Obese Japanese Subjects. Bioscience, Biotechnology, and Biochemistry, 73(8), 1837–1843.

[2310] Yagnik, D., Serafin, V., & J Shah, A. (2018). Antimicrobial activity of apple cider vinegar against Escherichia coli, Staphylococcus aureus and Candida albicans; downregulating cytokine and microbial protein expression. Scientific reports, 8(1), 1732.

[2311] Park et al (2016). Antimicrobial effects of vinegar against norovirus and Escherichia coli in the traditional Korean vinegared green laver (Enteromorpha intestinalis) salad during refrigerated storage. International journal of food microbiology, 238, 208–214.

[2312] Entani et al (1998). Antibacterial action of vinegar against food-borne pathogenic bacteria including Escherichia coli O157:H7. Journal of food protection, 61(8), 953–959.

[2313] Harsch, I. A., & Konturek, P. C. (2018). The Role of Gut Microbiota in Obesity and Type 2 and Type 1 Diabetes Mellitus: New Insights into "Old" Diseases. Medical sciences (Basel, Switzerland), 6(2), 32.

[2314] Warwick (2023) '7 Side Effects of Too Much Apple Cider Vinegar', Healthline, Accessed Online March 29th 2023: https://www.healthline.com/nutrition/apple-cider-vinegar-side-effects

[2315] Willershausen et al (2014). In vitro study on dental erosion caused by different vinegar varieties using an electron microprobe. Clinical laboratory, 60(5), 783–790.

[2316] Nuutinen, M., Uhari, M., Karvali, T., & Kouvalainen, K. (1994). Consequences of caustic ingestions in children. Acta paediatrica (Oslo, Norway : 1992), 83(11), 1200–1205.

[2317] Feldstein, S., Afshar, M., & Krakowski, A. C. (2015). Chemical Burn from Vinegar Following an Internet-based Protocol for Self-removal of Nevi. The Journal of clinical and aesthetic dermatology, 8(6), 50.

[2318] van Loon L. J. (2013). Role of dietary protein in post-exercise muscle reconditioning. Nestle Nutrition Institute workshop series, 75, 73–83.

[2319] Abdou et al (2021). Effect of high protein and fat diet on postprandial blood glucose levels in children and adolescents with type 1 diabetes in Cairo, Egypt. Diabetes & metabolic syndrome, 15(1), 7–12.

[2320] Bell et al (2015). Impact of Fat, Protein, and Glycemic Index on Postprandial Glucose Control in Type 1 Diabetes: Implications for Intensive Diabetes Management in the Continuous Glucose Monitoring Era. Diabetes Care, 38(6), 1008–1015.

[2321] Te Morenga et al (2017). The Effect of a Diet Moderately High in Protein and Fiber on Insulin Sensitivity Measured Using the Dynamic Insulin Sensitivity and Secretion Test (DISST). Nutrients, 9(12), 1291.

[2322] Park et al (2015). A high-protein breakfast induces greater insulin and glucose-dependent insulinotropic peptide responses to a subsequent lunch meal in individuals with type 2 diabetes. The Journal of nutrition, 145(3), 452–458.

[2323] Nilsson, M., Holst, J. J., & Björck, I. M. (2007). Metabolic effects of amino acid mixtures and whey protein in healthy subjects: studies using glucose-equivalent drinks. The American Journal of Clinical Nutrition, 85(4), 996–1004.

2324 Crovetti, R., Porrini, M., Santangelo, A., & Testolin, G. (1998). The influence of thermic effect of food on satiety. European journal of clinical nutrition, 52(7), 482–488. https://doi.org/10.1038/sj.ejcn.1600578

2325 Calcagno, M., Kahleova, H., Alwarith, J., Burgess, N. N., Flores, R. A., Busta, M. L., & Barnard, N. D. (2019). The Thermic Effect of Food: A Review. Journal of the American College of Nutrition, 38(6), 547–551. https://doi.org/10.1080/07315724.2018.1552544

[2326] Tsartsou et al (2019). Network Meta-Analysis of Metabolic Effects of Olive-Oil in Humans Shows the Importance of Olive Oil Consumption With Moderate Polyphenol Levels as Part of the Mediterranean Diet. Frontiers in nutrition, 6, 6.

[2327] Bozzetto et al (2016). Extra-Virgin Olive Oil Reduces Glycemic Response to a High-Glycemic Index Meal in Patients With Type 1 Diabetes: A Randomized Controlled Trial. Diabetes care, 39(4), 518–524.

[2328] Carnevale et al (2017). Extra virgin olive oil improves post-prandial glycemic and lipid profile in patients with impaired fasting glucose. Clinical nutrition (Edinburgh, Scotland), 36(3), 782–787.

[2329] Violi et al (2015). Extra virgin olive oil use is associated with improved post-prandial blood glucose and LDL cholesterol in healthy subjects. Nutrition & diabetes, 5(7), e172.

[2330] Bozzetto et al (2019). Gastrointestinal effects of extra-virgin olive oil associated with lower postprandial glycemia in type 1 diabetes. Clinical nutrition (Edinburgh, Scotland), 38(6), 2645–2651.

[2331] Madigan et al (2000) 'Dietary unsaturated fatty acids in type 2 diabetes: higher levels of postprandial lipoprotein on a linoleic acid-rich sunflower oil diet compared with an oleic acid-rich olive oil diet. ', Diabetes Care 2000;23(10):1472–1477.

[2332] Jenkins et al (2006). Almonds decrease postprandial glycemia, insulinemia, and oxidative damage in healthy individuals. The Journal of nutrition, 136(12), 2987–2992.

[2333] Josse et al (2007). Almonds and postprandial glycemia--a dose-response study. Metabolism: clinical and experimental, 56(3), 400–404.

[2334] Jenkins et al (2006). Almonds decrease postprandial glycemia, insulinemia, and oxidative damage in healthy individuals. The Journal of nutrition, 136(12), 2987–2992.

[2335] Viguiliouk et al (2018). Effect of dried fruit on postprandial glycemia: a randomized acute-feeding trial. Nutrition & Diabetes, 8(1).

[2336] Levine (2007) 'Exercise: A Walk in the Park?', Mayo Clinic Proceedings, Volume 82, Issue 7, July 2007, Pages 797-798.

[2337] Healy et al (2007). Objectively measured light-intensity physical activity is independently associated with 2-h plasma glucose. Diabetes care, 30(6), 1384–1389.

[2338] Stevenson et al (2006). Influence of high-carbohydrate mixed meals with different glycemic indexes on substrate utilization during subsequent exercise in women. The American journal of clinical nutrition, 84(2), 354–360.

[2339] Bryans et al (2007). The Effect of Consuming Instant Black Tea on Postprandial Plasma Glucose and Insulin Concentrations in Healthy Humans. Journal of the American College of Nutrition, 26(5), 471–477.

[2340] Anderson, R. A., & Polansky, M. M. (2002). Tea enhances insulin activity. Journal of agricultural and food chemistry, 50(24), 7182–7186.

[2341] Meng et al (2019). Effects and Mechanisms of Tea for the Prevention and Management of Diabetes Mellitus and Diabetic Complications: An Updated Review. Antioxidants (Basel, Switzerland), 8(6), 170.

[2342] Hirata et al (2017). Effect modification of green tea on the association between rice intake and the risk of diabetes mellitus: a prospective study in Japanese men and women. Asia Pacific journal of clinical nutrition, 26(3), 545–555.

[2343] Xu, R., Bai, Y., Yang, K., & Chen, G. (2020). Effects of green tea consumption on glycemic control: a systematic review and meta-analysis of randomized controlled trials. Nutrition & Metabolism, 17(1).

[2344] Iso et al (2006). The relationship between green tea and total caffeine intake and risk for self-reported type 2 diabetes among Japanese adults. Annals of internal medicine, 144(8), 554–562.

[2345] Park et al (2014). Green tea and type 2 diabetes. Integrative medicine research, 3(1), 4–10.

[2346] Ueda-Wakagi et al (2019). Green Tea Ameliorates Hyperglycemia by Promoting the Translocation of Glucose Transporter 4 in the Skeletal Muscle of Diabetic Rodents. International journal of molecular sciences, 20(10), 2436.

[2347] Liu et al (2013). Effect of green tea on glucose control and insulin sensitivity: a meta-analysis of 17 randomized controlled trials. The American journal of clinical nutrition, 98(2), 340–348.

[2348] Nagao (2009). A catechin-rich beverage improves obesity and blood glucose control in patients with type 2 diabetes. Obesity (Silver Spring, Md.), 17(2), 310–317.

[2349] Kim, H. M., & Kim, J. (2013). The effects of green tea on obesity and type 2 diabetes. Diabetes & metabolism journal, 37(3), 173–175.

[2350] Wang et al (2009). The effects of green tea (-)-epigallocatechin-3-gallate on reactive oxygen species in 3T3-L1 preadipocytes and adipocytes depend on the glutathione and 67 kDa laminin receptor pathways. Molecular nutrition & food research, 53(3), 349–360.

[2351] Raederstorff et al (2003). Effect of EGCG on lipid absorption and plasma lipid levels in rats. The Journal of nutritional biochemistry, 14(6), 326–332.

[2352] Mukai, K., Nagai, S., & Ohara, K. (2005). Kinetic study of the quenching reaction of singlet oxygen by tea catechins in ethanol solution. Free radical biology & medicine, 39(6), 752–761.

[2353] Hung et al (2005). Antimitogenic effect of green tea (-)-epigallocatechin gallate on 3T3-L1 preadipocytes depends on the ERK and Cdk2 pathways. American journal of physiology. Cell physiology, 288(5), C1094–C1108.

[2354] Wu et al (2003). Relationship among habitual tea consumption, percent body fat, and body fat distribution. Obesity research, 11(9), 1088–1095.

[2355] Butacnum et al (2017). Black tea consumption improves postprandial glycemic control in normal and pre-diabetic subjects: a randomized, double-blind, placebo-controlled crossover study. Asia Pacific journal of clinical nutrition, 26(1), 59–64.

[2356] Imran et al (2018). Exploring the potential of black tea based flavonoids against hyperlipidemia related disorders. Lipids in health and disease, 17(1), 57.

[2357] Hilker, D. M., & Somogyi, J. C. (1982). Antithiamins of plant origin: their chemical nature and mode of action. Annals of the New York Academy of Sciences, 378, 137–145.

[2358] Peng et al (2014). Hibiscus sabdariffa polyphenols alleviate insulin resistance and renal epithelial to mesenchymal transition: a novel action mechanism mediated by type 4 dipeptidyl peptidase. Journal of agricultural and food chemistry, 62(40), 9736–9743.

[2359] Ajiboye et al (2016). Hibiscus sabdariffa calyx palliates insulin resistance, hyperglycemia, dyslipidemia and oxidative rout in fructose-induced metabolic syndrome rats. Journal of the science of food and agriculture, 96(5), 1522–1531.

[2360] Peng et al (2011). Hibiscus sabdariffa polyphenolic extract inhibits hyperglycemia, hyperlipidemia, and glycation-oxidative stress while improving insulin resistance. Journal of agricultural and food chemistry, 59(18), 9901–9909.

[2361] Zemestani et al (2016). Chamomile tea improves glycemic indices and antioxidants status in patients with type 2 diabetes mellitus. Nutrition (Burbank, Los Angeles County, Calif.), 32(1), 66–72.

[2362] Chung et al (2010). Anti-diabetic effects of lemon balm (Melissa officinalis) essential oil on glucose- and lipid-regulating enzymes in type 2 diabetic mice. The British journal of nutrition, 104(2), 180–188.

[2363] Asadi et al (2019). Efficacy of Melissa officinalis L. (lemon balm) extract on glycemic control and cardiovascular risk factors in individuals with type 2 diabetes: A randomized, double-blind, clinical trial. Phytotherapy research : PTR, 33(3), 651–659.

[2364] Lee, H. J., Park, J. I., Kwon, S. O., & Hwang, D. D.-J. (2022). Coffee consumption and diabetic retinopathy in adults with diabetes mellitus. Scientific Reports, 12(1).

[2365] Mirmiran et al (2018). Long-term effects of coffee and caffeine intake on the risk of pre-diabetes and type 2 diabetes: Findings from a population with low coffee consumption. Nutrition, metabolism, and cardiovascular diseases : NMCD, 28(12), 1261–1266.

[2366] van Dam et al (2006). Coffee, caffeine, and risk of type 2 diabetes: a prospective cohort study in younger and middle-aged U.S. women. Diabetes care, 29(2), 398–403.

[2367] Lee et al (2016). Effect of Coffee Consumption on the Progression of Type 2 Diabetes Mellitus among Prediabetic Individuals. Korean journal of family medicine, 37(1), 7–13.

[2368] van Dam et al (2006) 'Coffee, Caffeine, and Risk of Type 2 Diabetes : A prospective cohort study in younger and middle-aged U.S. women', Diabetes Care 2006;29(2):398–403.

[2369] Fujii et al (2015). Ingestion of coffee polyphenols increases postprandial release of the active glucagon-like peptide-1 (GLP-1(7–36)) amide in C57BL/6J mice. Journal of Nutritional Science, 4.

[2370] Guasch-Ferré et al (2017). Dietary Polyphenols, Mediterranean Diet, Prediabetes, and Type 2 Diabetes: A Narrative Review of the Evidence. Oxidative medicine and cellular longevity, 2017, 6723931.

[2371] Dhir et al (2019). Neurological, Psychiatric, and Biochemical Aspects of Thiamine Deficiency in Children and Adults. Frontiers in Psychiatry, 10.

[2372] Bhupathiraju et al (2014). Changes in coffee intake and subsequent risk of type 2 diabetes: three large cohorts of US men and women. Diabetologia, 57(7), 1346–1354.

[2373] Chen et al (2022). Consumption of coffee and tea with all-cause and cause-specific mortality: a prospective cohort study. BMC Medicine, 20(1).

[2374] Robinson et al (2004). Caffeine Ingestion Before an Oral Glucose Tolerance Test Impairs Blood Glucose Management in Men with Type 2 Diabetes. The Journal of Nutrition, 134(10), 2528–2533.

[2375] Lane et al (2004). Caffeine impairs glucose metabolism in type 2 diabetes. Diabetes care, 27(8), 2047–2048.

[2376] Robertson et al (2018). Postprandial glycaemic and lipaemic responses to chronic coffee consumption may be modulated by CYP1A2 polymorphisms. The British journal of nutrition, 119(7), 792–800.

[2377] Cornelis et al (2006) 'Coffee, CYP1A2 genotype, and risk of myocardial infarction.' JAMA. 2006 Mar 8;295(10):1135-41.

[2378] Palatini et al (2009) 'CYP1A2 genotype modifies the association between coffee intake and the risk of hypertension.' J Hypertens. 2009 Aug;27(8):1594-601. doi: 10.1097/HJH.0b013e32832ba850.

[2379] Zhang et al (2013). Curcumin and diabetes: a systematic review. Evidence-based complementary and alternative medicine : eCAM, 2013, 636053.

[2380] Ghorbani et al (2014). Anti-hyperglycemic and insulin sensitizer effects of turmeric and its principle constituent curcumin. International journal of endocrinology and metabolism, 12(4), e18081.

[2381] Chuengsamarn et al (2012). Curcumin extract for prevention of type 2 diabetes. Diabetes care, 35(11), 2121–2127.

[2382] Chuengsamarn et al (2014). Reduction of atherogenic risk in patients with type 2 diabetes by curcuminoid extract: a randomized controlled trial. The Journal of nutritional biochemistry, 25(2), 144–150. /

[2383] Aggarwal B. B. (2010). Targeting inflammation-induced obesity and metabolic diseases by curcumin and other nutraceuticals. Annual review of nutrition, 30, 173–199.

[2384] Biswas et al (2005). Curcumin Induces Glutathione Biosynthesis and Inhibits NF-κB Activation and Interleukin-8 Release in Alveolar Epithelial Cells: Mechanism of Free Radical Scavenging Activity. Antioxidants & Redox Signaling, 7(1-2), 32–41. doi:10.1089/ars.2005.7.32

[2385] Tayyem et al (2006). Curcumin Content of Turmeric and Curry Powders. Nutrition and Cancer, 55(2), 126–131. doi:10.1207/s15327914nc5502_2

[2386] Sharma, R. A., Gescher, A. J., & Steward, W. P. (2005). Curcumin: The story so far. European Journal of Cancer, 41(13), 1955–1968. doi:10.1016/j.ejca.2005.05.009

[2387] Shoba et al (1998). Influence of Piperine on the Pharmacokinetics of Curcumin in Animals and Human Volunteers. Planta Medica, 64(04), 353–356. doi:10.1055/s-2006-957450

[2388] Padiya, R., Khatua, T. N., Bagul, P. K., Kuncha, M., & Banerjee, S. K. (2011). Garlic improves insulin sensitivity and associated metabolic syndromes in fructose fed rats. Nutrition & Metabolism, 8(1), 53. doi:10.1186/1743-7075-8-53

[2389] NIH (2020) 'Garlic', Accessed Online March 21st 2023: https://www.nccih.nih.gov/health/garlic

[2390] Reinhart, K. M., Talati, R., White, C. M., & Coleman, C. I. (2009). The impact of garlic on lipid parameters: a systematic review and meta-analysis. Nutrition Research Reviews, 22(1), 39–48. doi:10.1017/s0954422409350003

[2391] Gómez-Arbeláez et al "Aged Garlic Extract Improves Adiponectin Levels in Subjects with Metabolic Syndrome: A Double-Blind, Placebo-Controlled, Randomized, Crossover Study", Mediators of Inflammation, vol. 2013, Article ID 285795, 6 pages, 2013. https://doi.org/10.1155/2013/285795

[2392] Ansary et al (2020). Potential Health Benefit of Garlic Based on Human Intervention Studies: A Brief Overview. Antioxidants (Basel, Switzerland), 9(7), 619.

[2393] Wang et al (2017). Effect of garlic supplement in the management of type 2 diabetes mellitus (T2DM): a meta-analysis of randomized controlled trials. Food & nutrition research, 61(1), 1377571.

[2394] Shabani, E., Sayemiri, K., & Mohammadpour, M. (2019). The effect of garlic on lipid profile and glucose parameters in diabetic patients: A systematic review and meta-analysis. Primary care diabetes, 13(1), 28–42.

[2395] Bayan et al (2014). Garlic: a review of potential therapeutic effects. Avicenna journal of phytomedicine, 4(1), 1–14.

[2396] Thomson et al (2006). Including Garlic in the Diet May Help Lower Blood Glucose, Cholesterol, and Triglycerides. The Journal of Nutrition, 136(3), 800S-802S.

[2397] Borlinghaus et al (2014). Allicin: chemistry and biological properties. Molecules (Basel, Switzerland), 19(8), 12591–12618.

[2398] Jabbari et al (2005). Comparison between swallowing and chewing of garlic on levels of serum lipids, cyclosporine, creatinine and lipid peroxidation in Renal Transplant Recipients, Lipids in Health and Disease, 4(1), 11. doi:10.1186/1476-511x-4-11

[2399] Shin et al (2013). Short-term heating reduces the anti-inflammatory effects of fresh raw garlic extracts on the LPS-induced production of NO and pro-inflammatory cytokines by downregulating allicin activity in RAW 264.7 macrophages. Food and chemical toxicology: an international journal published for the British Industrial Biological Research Association, 58, 545–551.

[2400] Lawson et al (2018). Allicin Bioavailability and Bioequivalence from Garlic Supplements and Garlic Foods. Nutrients, 10(7), 812.

[2401] Hinnen, D. A. (2015). Therapeutic Options for the Management of Postprandial Glucose in Patients With Type 2 Diabetes on Basal Insulin. Clinical Diabetes, 33(4), 175–180.

[2402] He, L., Sabet, A., Djedjos, S., Miller, R., Sun, X., Hussain, M. A., Radovick, S., & Wondisford, F. E. (2009). Metformin and insulin suppress hepatic gluconeogenesis through phosphorylation of CREB binding protein. Cell, 137(4), 635–646. https://doi.org/10.1016/j.cell.2009.03.016

[2403] Liu, X. et al (2014) 'Discrete mechanisms of mTOR and cell cycle regulation by AMPK agonists independent of AMPK', PNAS, Vol 111(4), E435-E444.

[2404] Franciosi, M., Lucisano, G., Lapice, E., Strippoli, G. F., Pellegrini, F., & Nicolucci, A. (2013). Metformin therapy and risk of cancer in patients with type 2 diabetes: systematic review. PloS one, 8(8), e71583. https://doi.org/10.1371/journal.pone.0071583

[2405] Currie, C. J., Poole, C. D., & Gale, E. A. (2009). The influence of glucose-lowering therapies on cancer risk in type 2 diabetes. Diabetologia, 52(9), 1766–1777.

[2406] Kooy et al (2009) 'Long-term Effects of Metformin on Metabolism and Microvascular and Macrovascular Disease in Patients With Type 2 Diabetes Mellitus', Arch Intern Med. 2009;169(6):616-625.

[2407] Effect of intensive blood-glucose control with metformin on complications in overweight patients with type 2 diabetes (UKPDS 34). UK Prospective Diabetes Study (UKPDS) Group. (1998). Lancet (London, England), 352(9131), 854–865.

[2408] Konopka et al (2019) Metformin inhibits mitochondrial adaptations to aerobic exercise training in older adults. Aging cell, 18(1), e12880.

[2409] Campbell et al (2017). Metformin reduces all-cause mortality and diseases of ageing independent of its effect on diabetes control: A systematic review and meta-analysis. Ageing research reviews, 40, 31–44.

[2410] Claesen et al (2016). Mortality in Individuals Treated With Glucose-Lowering Agents: A Large, Controlled Cohort Study. The Journal of clinical endocrinology and metabolism, 101(2), 461–469.

[2411] Bannister et al (2014). Can people with type 2 diabetes live longer than those without? A comparison of mortality in people initiated with metformin or sulphonylurea monotherapy and matched, non-diabetic controls. Diabetes, obesity & metabolism, 16(11), 1165–1173.

[2412] Palmer et al (2016). Comparison of Clinical Outcomes and Adverse Events Associated With Glucose-Lowering Drugs in Patients With Type 2 Diabetes: A Meta-analysis. JAMA, 316(3), 313–324.

[2413] American Diabetes Association Professional Practice Committee (2022). 9. Pharmacologic Approaches to Glycemic Treatment: Standards of Medical Care in Diabetes-2022. Diabetes care, 45(Suppl 1), S125–S143.

[2414] Baggio and Drucker (2023) 'Glucagon-like Peptide-1 Analogs Other Than Exenatide', Medscape, Accessed Online March 29th 2023: https://www.medscape.org/viewarticle/578304

[2415] Ali et al (2016). The glucagon-like peptide-1 analogue exendin-4 reverses impaired intracellular Ca 2+ signalling in steatotic hepatocytes. Biochimica et Biophysica Acta (BBA) - Molecular Cell Research, 1863(9), 2135–2146.

[2416] Sattar et al (2021). Cardiovascular, mortality, and kidney outcomes with GLP-1 receptor agonists in patients with type 2 diabetes: a systematic review and meta-analysis of randomised trials. The lancet. Diabetes & endocrinology, 9(10), 653–662.

[2417] Zheng et al (2018). Association Between Use of Sodium-Glucose Cotransporter 2 Inhibitors, Glucagon-like Peptide 1 Agonists, and Dipeptidyl Peptidase 4 Inhibitors With All-Cause Mortality in Patients With Type 2 Diabetes: A Systematic Review and Meta-analysis. JAMA, 319(15), 1580–1591.

[2418] Singh, G., Krauthamer, M., & Bjalme-Evans, M. (2022). Wegovy (semaglutide): a new weight loss drug for chronic weight management. Journal of investigative medicine : the official publication of the American Federation for Clinical Research, 70(1), 5–13.

[2419] Amaro, A., Sugimoto, D., & Wharton, S. (2022). Efficacy and safety of semaglutide for weight management: evidence from the STEP program. Postgraduate medicine, 134(sup1), 5–17.

[2420] Phillips, A., & Clements, J. N. (2022). Clinical review of subcutaneous semaglutide for obesity. Journal of clinical pharmacy and therapeutics, 47(2), 184–193.

[2421] Müller, T. D., Blüher, M., Tschöp, M. H., & DiMarchi, R. D. (2022). Anti-obesity drug discovery: advances and challenges. Nature reviews. Drug discovery, 21(3), 201–223.

[2422] Marso et al (2016). Semaglutide and Cardiovascular Outcomes in Patients with Type 2 Diabetes. The New England journal of medicine, 375(19), 1834–1844.

[2423] Li et al (2003). Glucagon-like peptide-1 receptor signaling modulates beta cell apoptosis. The Journal of biological chemistry, 278(1), 471–478.

[2424] Goldenberg, R. M., & Steen, O. (2019). Semaglutide: Review and Place in Therapy for Adults With Type 2 Diabetes. Canadian journal of diabetes, 43(2), 136–145.

[2425] Dhillon S. (2018). Semaglutide: First Global Approval. Drugs, 78(2), 275–284.

340

[2426] Blundell et al (2017). Effects of once-weekly semaglutide on appetite, energy intake, control of eating, food preference and body weight in subjects with obesity. Diabetes, obesity & metabolism, 19(9), 1242–1251.

[2427] Doggrell S. A. (2018). Sgemaglutide in type 2 diabetes - is it the best glucagon-like peptide 1 receptor agonist (GLP-1R agonist)?. Expert opinion on drug metabolism & toxicology, 14(3), 371–377.

[2428] Sola et al (2015). Sulfonylureas and their use in clinical practice. Archives of medical science : AMS, 11(4), 840–848.

[2429] Olefsky, J. M., & Reaven, G. M. (1976). Effects of sulfonylurea therapy on insulin binding to mononuclear leukocytes of diabetic patients. The American journal of medicine, 60(1), 89–95.

[2430] Braun et al (2009). Somatostatin release, electrical activity, membrane currents and exocytosis in human pancreatic delta cells. Diabetologia, 52(8), 1566–1578.

[2431] Ramracheya et al (2010). Membrane potential-dependent inactivation of voltage-gated ion channels in alpha-cells inhibits glucagon secretion from human islets. Diabetes, 59(9), 2198–2208.

[2432] Gangji et al (2007). A systematic review and meta-analysis of hypoglycemia and cardiovascular events: a comparison of glyburide with other secretagogues and with insulin. Diabetes care, 30(2), 389–394.

[2433] Hirst et al (2013). Estimating the effect of sulfonylurea on HbA1c in diabetes: a systematic review and meta-analysis. Diabetologia, 56(5), 973–984.

[2434] Nestler J. E. (2008). Metformin in the treatment of infertility in polycystic ovarian syndrome: an alternative perspective. Fertility and sterility, 90(1), 14–16.

[2435] Kim et al (2012). Effect of berberine on p53expression by TPA in breast cancercells. Oncology Reports, 27, 210-215.

[2436] Lee, Y. S., Kim, W. S., Kim, K. H., Yoon, M. J., Cho, H. J., Shen, Y., … Kim, J. B. (2006). Berberine, a Natural Plant Product, Activates AMP-Activated Protein Kinase With Beneficial Metabolic Effects in Diabetic and Insulin-Resistant States. Diabetes, 55(8), 2256–2264. doi:10.2337/db06-0006

[2437] Yang, J., Yin, J., Gao, H., Xu, L., Wang, Y., Xu, L., & Li, M. (2012). Berberine Improves Insulin Sensitivity by Inhibiting Fat Store and Adjusting Adipokines Profile in Human Preadipocytes and Metabolic Syndrome Patients. Evidence-Based Complementary and Alternative Medicine, 2012, 1–9. doi:10.1155/2012/363845

[2438] Pérez-Rubio, K. G., González-Ortiz, M., Martínez-Abundis, E., Robles-Cervantes, J. A., & Espinel-Bermúdez, M. C. (2013). Effect of Berberine Administration on Metabolic Syndrome, Insulin Sensitivity, and Insulin Secretion. Metabolic Syndrome and Related Disorders, 11(5), 366–369. doi:10.1089/met.2012.0183

[2439] Melendez-Hevia, E., & Paz-Lugo, P. D. (2008). Branch-point stoichiometry can generate weak links in metabolism: the case of glycine biosynthesis. Journal of biosciences, 33(5), 771–780. https://doi.org/10.1007/s12038-008-0097-5

[2440] Kielty, C. M., Sherratt, M. J., & Shuttleworth, C. A. (2002). Elastic fibres. Journal of cell science, 115(Pt 14), 2817–2828. https://doi.org/10.1242/jcs.115.14.2817

[2441] Kaufman, M. J., Prescot, A. P., Ongur, D., Evins, A. E., Barros, T. L., Medeiros, C. L., Covell, J., Wang, L., Fava, M., & Renshaw, P. F. (2009). Oral glycine administration increases brain glycine/creatine ratios in men: a proton magnetic resonance spectroscopy study. Psychiatry research, 173(2), 143–149. https://doi.org/10.1016/j.pscychresns.2009.03.004

[2442] Sekhar, R. V., Patel, S. G., Guthikonda, A. P., Reid, M., Balasubramanyam, A., Taffet, G. E., & Jahoor, F. (2011). Deficient synthesis of glutathione underlies oxidative stress in aging and can be corrected by dietary cysteine and glycine supplementation. The American journal of clinical nutrition, 94(3), 847–853. https://doi.org/10.3945/ajcn.110.003483

[2443] Liao, Y. J., Lee, T. S., Twu, Y. C., Hsu, S. M., Yang, C. P., Wang, C. K., Liang, Y. C., & Chen, Y. A. (2016). Glycine N-methyltransferase deficiency in female mice impairs insulin signaling and promotes gluconeogenesis by modulating the PI3K/Akt pathway in the liver. Journal of biomedical science, 23(1), 69. https://doi.org/10.1186/s12929-016-0278-8

[2444] Yan-Do, R., Duong, E., Manning Fox, J. E., Dai, X., Suzuki, K., Khan, S., Bautista, A., Ferdaoussi, M., Lyon, J., Wu, X., Cheley, S., MacDonald, P. E., & Braun, M. (2016). A Glycine-Insulin Autocrine Feedback Loop Enhances Insulin Secretion From Human β-Cells and Is Impaired in Type 2 Diabetes. Diabetes, 65(8), 2311–2321. https://doi.org/10.2337/db15-1272

[2445] Yan-Do, R., & MacDonald, P. E. (2017). Impaired "Glycine"-mia in Type 2 Diabetes and Potential Mechanisms Contributing to Glucose Homeostasis. Endocrinology, 158(5), 1064–1073. https://doi.org/10.1210/en.2017-00148

[2446] El-Hafidi, M., Franco, M., Ramírez, A. R., Sosa, J. S., Flores, J. A. P., Acosta, O. L., Salgado, M. C., & Cardoso-Saldaña, G. (2018). Glycine Increases Insulin Sensitivity and Glutathione Biosynthesis and Protects against Oxidative Stress in a Model of Sucrose-Induced Insulin Resistance. Oxidative medicine and cellular longevity, 2018, 2101562. https://doi.org/10.1155/2018/2101562

[2447] Nguyen, D., Hsu, J. W., Jahoor, F., & Sekhar, R. V. (2014). Effect of increasing glutathione with cysteine and glycine supplementation on mitochondrial fuel oxidation, insulin sensitivity, and body composition in older HIV-infected patients. The Journal of clinical endocrinology and metabolism, 99(1), 169–177. https://doi.org/10.1210/jc.2013-2376

[2448] Cruz, M., Maldonado-Bernal, C., Mondragón-Gonzalez, R., Sanchez-Barrera, R., Wacher, N. H., Carvajal-Sandoval, G., & Kumate, J. (2008). Glycine treatment decreases proinflammatory cytokines and increases interferon-gamma in patients with type 2 diabetes. Journal of endocrinological investigation, 31(8), 694–699. https://doi.org/10.1007/BF03346417

[2449] Carvajal Sandoval, G., Medina Santillán, R., Juárez, E., RamosMartínez, G., & Carvajal Juárez, M. E. (1999). Effect of glycine on hemoglobin glycation in diabetic patients. Proceedings of the Western Pharmacology Society, 42, 31–32.

[2450] Gannon et al (2002). The metabolic response to ingested glycine. The American journal of clinical nutrition, 76(6), 1302–1307.

[2451] McCarty, M. F., DiNicolantonio, J. J., & O'Keefe, J. H. (2022). Nutraceutical Prevention of Diabetic Complications-Focus on Dicarbonyl and Oxidative Stress. Current issues in molecular biology, 44(9), 4314–4338. https://doi.org/10.3390/cimb44090297

[2452] Noe et al (2013) 'Effect of Glycine on Protein Oxidation and Advanced Glycation End Products Formation', Journal of Experimental & Clinical Medicine, Volume 5, Issue 3, June 2013, Pages 109-114.

[2453] Wang, Z., Zhang, J., Chen, L., Li, J., Zhang, H., & Guo, X. (2019). Glycine Suppresses AGE/RAGE Signaling Pathway and Subsequent Oxidative Stress by Restoring Glo1 Function in the Aorta of Diabetic Rats and in HUVECs. Oxidative medicine and cellular longevity, 2019, 4628962. https://doi.org/10.1155/2019/4628962

[2454] Lutchmansingh, F. K., Hsu, J. W., Bennett, F. I., Badaloo, A. V., McFarlane-Anderson, N., Gordon-Strachan, G. M., Wright-Pascoe, R. A., Jahoor, F., & Boyne, M. S. (2018). Glutathione metabolism in type 2 diabetes and its relationship with microvascular complications and glycemia. PloS one, 13(6), e0198626. https://doi.org/10.1371/journal.pone.0198626

[2455] Sekhar, R. V., McKay, S. V., Patel, S. G., Guthikonda, A. P., Reddy, V. T., Balasubramanyam, A., & Jahoor, F. (2011). Glutathione synthesis is diminished in patients with uncontrolled diabetes and restored by dietary supplementation with cysteine and glycine. Diabetes care, 34(1), 162–167. https://doi.org/10.2337/dc10-1006

[2456] NIH (2020) 'Chromium: Fact Sheet for Health Professionals', Dietary Supplement Fact Sheets, Accessed Online Jan 18 2021: https://ods.od.nih.gov/factsheets/Chromium-HealthProfessional/

[2457] Moradi, F., Kooshki, F., Nokhostin, F., Khoshbaten, M., Bazyar, H., & Pourghassem Gargari, B. (2021). A pilot study of the effects of chromium picolinate supplementation on serum fetuin-A, metabolic and inflammatory factors in patients with nonalcoholic fatty liver disease: A double-blind, placebo-controlled trial. Journal of Trace Elements in Medicine and Biology, 63, 126659. doi:10.1016/j.jtemb.2020.126659

[2458] Anderson, R. A., Cheng, N., Bryden, N. A., Polansky, M. M., Cheng, N., Chi, J., & Feng, J. (1997). Elevated intakes of supplemental chromium improve glucose and insulin variables in individuals with type 2 diabetes. Diabetes, 46(11), 1786–1791. https://doi.org/10.2337/diab.46.11.1786

[2459] Paiva, A. N., Lima, J. G. de, Medeiros, A. C. Q. de, Figueiredo, H. A. O., Andrade, R. L. de, Ururahy, M. A. G., ... Almeida, M. das G. (2015). Beneficial effects of oral chromium picolinate supplementation on glycemic control in patients with type 2 diabetes: A randomized clinical study. Journal of Trace Elements in Medicine and Biology, 32, 66–72. doi:10.1016/j.jtemb.2015.05.006

[2460] A. Santamaria, D. Giordano, F. Corrado, B. Pintaudi, M. L. Interdonato, G. Di Vieste, A. Di Benedetto & R. D'Anna (2012) One-year effects of myo-inositol supplementation in postmenopausal women with metabolic syndrome, Climacteric, 15:5, 490-495, DOI: 10.3109/13697137.2011.631063

[2461] D'Anna, R., Scilipoti, A., Giordano, D., Caruso, C., Cannata, M. L., Interdonato, M. L., Corrado, F., & Di Benedetto, A. (2013). myo-Inositol Supplementation and Onset of Gestational Diabetes Mellitus in Pregnant Women With a Family History of Type 2 Diabetes. Diabetes Care, 36(4), 854–857. https://doi.org/10.2337/dc12-1371

[2462] Matarrelli, B., Vitacolonna, E., D'angelo, M., Pavone, G., Mattei, P. A., Liberati, M., & Celentano, C. (2013). Effect of dietary myo-inositol supplementation in pregnancy on the incidence of maternal gestational diabetes mellitus and fetal outcomes: a randomized controlled trial. The Journal of Maternal-Fetal & Neonatal Medicine, 26(10), 967–972. https://doi.org/10.3109/14767058.2013.766691

[2463] Giordano, D., Corrado, F., Santamaria, A., Quattrone, S., Pintaudi, B., Di Benedetto, A., & D'Anna, R. (2011). Effects of myo-inositol supplementation in postmenopausal women with metabolic syndrome. Menopause, 18(1), 102–104. https://doi.org/10.1097/gme.0b013e3181e8e1b1

[2464] Costantino, D., Minozzi, G., Minozzi, E., & Guaraldi, C. (2009). Metabolic and hormonal effects of myo-inositol in women with polycystic ovary syndrome: a double-blind trial. European review for medical and pharmacological sciences, 13(2), 105–110.

[2465] Parthasarathy, L. K., Seelan, R. S., Tobias, C., Casanova, M. F., & Parthasarathy, R. N. (2006). Mammalian inositol 3-phosphate synthase: its role in the biosynthesis of brain inositol and its clinical use as a psychoactive agent. Sub-cellular biochemistry, 39, 293–314. https://doi.org/10.1007/0-387-27600-9_12

2466 Bizzarri, M., Fuso, A., Dinicola, S., Cucina, A., & Bevilacqua, A. (2016). Pharmacodynamics and pharmacokinetics of inositol(s) in health and disease. Expert opinion on drug metabolism & toxicology, 12(10), 1181–1196. https://doi.org/10.1080/17425255.2016.1206887

[2467] Asplin et al (1993) 'chiro-Inositol deficiency and insulin resistance: A comparison of the chiro-inositol- and the myo-inositol-containing insulin mediators isolated from urine, hemodialysate, and muscle of control and type II diabetic subjects, Proc. Natl. Acad. Sci. USA, Vol. 90, pp. 5924-5928, July 1993.

[2468] Sun, T., Heimark, D. B., Nguygen, T., Nadler, J. L., & Larner, J. (2002). Both myo-inositol to chiro-inositol epimerase activities and chiro-inositol to myo-inositol ratios are decreased in tissues of GK type 2 diabetic rats compared to Wistar controls. Biochemical and Biophysical Research Communications, 293(3), 1092–1098. https://doi.org/10.1016/s0006-291x(02)00313-3

[2469] Chang (2011) Mechanisms Underlying the Abnormal Inositol Metabolisms in Diabetes Mellitus. Thesis, ResearchSpace@Auckland.

[2470] Albert I Winegrad; Banting Lecture 1986: Does a Common Mechanism Induce the Diverse Complications of Diabetes?. Diabetes 1 March 1987; 36 (3): 396–406. https://doi.org/10.2337/diab.36.3.396

[2471] Olgemöller, B., Schwaabe, S., Schleicher, E. D., & Gerbitz, K. D. (1990). Competitive inhibition by glucose of myo-inositol incorporation into cultured porcine aortic endothelial cells. Biochimica et Biophysica Acta (BBA) - Molecular Cell Research, 1052(1), 47–52. https://doi.org/10.1016/0167-4889(90)90056-j

[2472] Haneda, M., Kikkawa, R., Arimura, T., Ebata, K., Togawa, M., Maeda, S., Sawada, T., Horide, N., & Shigeta, Y. (1990). Glucose inhibits myo-inositol uptake and reduces myo-inositol content in cultured rat glomerular mesangial cells. Metabolism, 39(1), 40–45. https://doi.org/10.1016/0026-0495(90)90145-3

[2473] Yorek, M. A., & Dunlap, J. A. (1989). The effect of elevated glucose levels on myo-inositol metabolism in cultured bovine aortic endothelial cells. Metabolism, 38(1), 16–22. https://doi.org/10.1016/0026-0495(89)90174-1

[2474] Greene, D. A., & Lattimer, S. A. (1982). Sodium- and energy-dependent uptake of myo-inositol by rabbit peripheral nerve. Competitive inhibition by glucose and lack of an insulin effect. Journal of Clinical Investigation, 70(5), 1009–1018. https://doi.org/10.1172/jci110688

[2475] Kanwar, Y. S., Wada, J., Sun, L., Xie, P., Wallner, E. I., Chen, S., Chugh, S., & Danesh, F. R. (2008). Diabetic nephropathy: mechanisms of renal disease progression. Experimental biology and medicine (Maywood, N.J.), 233(1), 4–11. https://doi.org/10.3181/0705-MR-134

[2476] Croze, M. L., & Soulage, C. O. (2013). Potential role and therapeutic interests of myo-inositol in metabolic diseases. Biochimie, 95(10), 1811–1827. https://doi.org/10.1016/j.biochi.2013.05.011

2477 Greenwood et al (2001) 'D-PINITOL AUGMENTS WHOLE BODY CREATINE RETENTION IN MAN', Journal of Exercise Physiologyonline, Volume 4 Number 4 November 2001, Accessed Online Sep 15 2021: https://www.asep.org/asep/asep/GreenwoodNOVEMBER2001.pdf

2478 Angeloff, L. G., Skoryna, S. C., & Henderson, I. W. (1977). Effects of the hexahydroxyhexane myoinositol on bone uptake of radiocalcium in rats: Effect of inositol and vitamin D2 on bone uptake of 45Ca in rats. Acta pharmacologica et toxicologica, 40(2), 209–215. https://doi.org/10.1111/j.1600-0773.1977.tb02070.x

2479 Bevilacqua, A., & Bizzarri, M. (2018). Inositols in Insulin Signaling and Glucose Metabolism. International Journal of Endocrinology, 2018, 1–8. doi:10.1155/2018/1968450

[2480] Larner J. (2002). D-chiro-inositol--its functional role in insulin action and its deficit in insulin resistance. International journal of experimental diabetes research, 3(1), 47–60. https://doi.org/10.1080/15604280212528

[2481] Gerasimenko, J. V., Flowerdew, S. E., Voronina, S. G., Sukhomlin, T. K., Tepikin, A. V., Petersen, O. H., & Gerasimenko, O. V. (2006). Bile acids induce Ca2+ release from both the endoplasmic reticulum and acidic intracellular calcium stores through activation of inositol trisphosphate receptors and ryanodine receptors. The Journal of biological chemistry, 281(52), 40154–40163. https://doi.org/10.1074/jbc.M606402200

[2482] Kukuljan, M., Vergara, L., & Stojilkovic, S. S. (1997). Modulation of the kinetics of inositol 1,4,5-trisphosphate-induced [Ca2+]i oscillations by calcium entry in pituitary gonadotrophs. Biophysical journal, 72(2 Pt 1), 698–707. https://doi.org/10.1016/s0006-3495(97)78706-x

[2483] Rapiejko, P. J., Northup, J. K., Evans, T., Brown, J. E., & Malbon, C. C. (1986). G-proteins of fat-cells. Role in hormonal regulation of intracellular inositol 1,4,5-trisphosphate. The Biochemical journal, 240(1), 35–40. https://doi.org/10.1042/bj2400035

[2484] Shen, X., Xiao, H., Ranallo, R., Wu, W. H., & Wu, C. (2003). Modulation of ATP-dependent chromatin-remodeling complexes by inositol polyphosphates. Science (New York, N.Y.), 299(5603), 112–114. https://doi.org/10.1126/science.1078068

2485 Eisenberg, F., & Parthasarathy, R. (1987). Measurement of biosynthesis of myo-inositol from glucose 6-phosphate. Cellular Regulators Part B: Calcium and Lipids, 127–143. doi:10.1016/0076-6879(87)41061-6

[2486] Holub (1986) 'Metabolism and Function of myo-Inositol and Inositol Phospholipids', Annual Review of Nutrition, Vol. 6:563-597.

[2487] Schlemmer, U., Frølich, W., Prieto, R. M., & Grases, F. (2009). Phytate in foods and significance for humans: Food sources, intake, processing, bioavailability, protective role and analysis. Molecular Nutrition & Food Research, 53(S2), S330–S375. Portico. https://doi.org/10.1002/mnfr.200900099

[2488] Clements, R. S., Jr, & Darnell, B. (1980). Myo-inositol content of common foods: development of a high-myo-inositol diet. The American journal of clinical nutrition, 33(9), 1954–1967. https://doi.org/10.1093/ajcn/33.9.1954

[2489] Ogura et al (2011). Effect of Grapefruit Intake on Postprandial Plasma Glucose. ANTI-AGING MEDICINE, 8(5), 60–68.

[2490] Pintaudi et al (2016). The Effectiveness of Myo-Inositol and D-Chiro Inositol Treatment in Type 2 Diabetes. International journal of endocrinology, 2016, 9132052.

[2491] Asimakopoulos et al (2020). Effect of dietary myo-inositol supplementation on the insulin resistance and the prevention of gestational diabetes mellitus: study protocol for a randomized controlled trial. Trials, 21(1).

[2492] Corrado, F., D'Anna, R., Di Vieste, G., Giordano, D., Pintaudi, B., Santamaria, A. and Di Benedetto, A. (2011), The effect of myoinositol supplementation on insulin resistance in patients with gestational diabetes. Diabetic Medicine, 28: 972-975. https://doi.org/10.1111/j.1464-5491.2011.03284.x

[2493] Schmidt et al (1981). The dawn phenomenon, an early morning glucose rise: implications for diabetic intraday blood glucose variation. Diabetes care, 4(6), 579–585.

[2494] Campbell et al (1985). Pathogenesis of the dawn phenomenon in patients with insulin-dependent diabetes mellitus. Accelerated glucose production and impaired glucose utilization due to nocturnal surges in growth hormone secretion. The New England journal of medicine, 312(23), 1473–1479.

[2495] Monnier et al (2012). Frequency and severity of the dawn phenomenon in type 2 diabetes: relationship to age. Diabetes care, 35(12), 2597–2599.

[2496] Monnier, L., Colette, C., Dejager, S., & Owens, D. (2015). The dawn phenomenon in type 2 diabetes: how to assess it in clinical practice?. Diabetes & metabolism, 41(2), 132–137.

[2497] Guo et al (2016). [Correlation study between obesity and dawn phenomenon in patients with type 2 diabetes] Zhonghua nei ke za zhi, 55(1), 16–20.

[2498] George M Bright, Terry W Melton, Alan D Rogol, William L Clarke; Failure of Cortisol Blockade to Inhibit Early Morning Increases in Basal Insulin Requirements in Fasting Insulin-dependent Diabetics. Diabetes 1 August 1980; 29 (8): 662–664.

[2499] Janež et al (2020). Insulin Therapy in Adults with Type 1 Diabetes Mellitus: a Narrative Review. Diabetes therapy : research, treatment and education of diabetes and related disorders, 11(2), 387–409.

[2500] Carr, R. D., & Alexander, C. M. (2014). Comment on Monnier et al. Magnitude of the dawn phenomenon and its impact on the overall glucose exposure in type 2 diabetes: is this of concern? Diabetes Care 2013;36:4057-4062. Diabetes care, 37(7), e161–e162.

[2501] Monnier et al (2007). The loss of postprandial glycemic control precedes stepwise deterioration of fasting with worsening diabetes. Diabetes care, 30(2), 263–269.

[2502] Zheng et al (2020). Effects of Exercise on Blood Glucose and Glycemic Variability in Type 2 Diabetic Patients with Dawn Phenomenon. BioMed research international, 2020, 6408724.

[2503] White, A. M., & Johnston, C. S. (2007). Vinegar Ingestion at Bedtime Moderates Waking Glucose Concentrations in Adults With Well-Controlled Type 2 Diabetes. Diabetes Care, 30(11), 2814–2815.

[2504] Atherton, P. J., & Smith, K. (2012). Muscle protein synthesis in response to nutrition and exercise. The Journal of physiology, 590(5), 1049–1057.

2505 Wycherley, T. P., Moran, L. J., Clifton, P. M., Noakes, M., & Brinkworth, G. D. (2012). Effects of energy-restricted high-protein, low-fat compared with standard-protein, low-fat diets: a meta-analysis of randomized controlled trials. The American journal of clinical nutrition, 96(6), 1281–1298. https://doi.org/10.3945/ajcn.112.044321

2506 Halton, T. L., & Hu, F. B. (2004). The effects of high protein diets on thermogenesis, satiety and weight loss: a critical review. Journal of the American College of Nutrition, 23(5), 373–385. https://doi.org/10.1080/07315724.2004.10719381

2507 Calcagno, M., Kahleova, H., Alwarith, J., Burgess, N. N., Flores, R. A., Busta, M. L., & Barnard, N. D. (2019). The Thermic Effect of Food: A Review. Journal of the American College of Nutrition, 38(6), 547–551. https://doi.org/10.1080/07315724.2018.1552544

2508 Westerterp K. R. (2004). Diet induced thermogenesis. Nutrition & metabolism, 1(1), 5. https://doi.org/10.1186/1743-7075-1-5

2509 Bray, G. A., Redman, L. M., de Jonge, L., Covington, J., Rood, J., Brock, C., Mancuso, S., Martin, C. K., & Smith, S. R. (2015). Effect of protein overfeeding on energy expenditure measured in a metabolic chamber. The American journal of clinical nutrition, 101(3), 496–505. https://doi.org/10.3945/ajcn.114.091769

2510 Crovetti, R., Porrini, M., Santangelo, A., & Testolin, G. (1998). The influence of thermic effect of food on satiety. European journal of clinical nutrition, 52(7), 482–488. https://doi.org/10.1038/sj.ejcn.1600579

[2511] Vander Wal, J. S., Marth, J. M., Khosla, P., Jen, K. L., & Dhurandhar, N. V. (2005). Short-term effect of eggs on satiety in overweight and obese subjects. Journal of the American College of Nutrition, 24(6), 510–515. https://doi.org/10.1080/07315724.2005.10719497

[2512] B Keogh, J., & M Clifton, P. (2020). Energy Intake and Satiety Responses of Eggs for Breakfast in Overweight and Obese Adults-A Crossover Study. International journal of environmental research and public health, 17(15), 5583. https://doi.org/10.3390/ijerph17155583

[2513] Pombo-Rodrigues, S., Calame, W., & Re, R. (2011). The effects of consuming eggs for lunch on satiety and subsequent food intake. International Journal of Food Sciences and Nutrition, 62(6), 593–599. https://doi.org/10.3109/09637486.2011.566212

2514 Weigle, D. S., Breen, P. A., Matthys, C. C., Callahan, H. S., Meeuws, K. E., Burden, V. R., & Purnell, J. Q. (2005). A high-protein diet induces sustained reductions in appetite, ad libitum caloric intake, and body weight despite compensatory changes in diurnal plasma leptin and ghrelin concentrations. The American journal of clinical nutrition, 82(1), 41–48. https://doi.org/10.1093/ajcn.82.1.41

2515 Hall K. D. (2008). What is the required energy deficit per unit weight loss?. International journal of obesity (2005), 32(3), 573–576. https://doi.org/10.1038/sj.ijo.0803722

2516 Bryner, R. W., Ullrich, I. H., Sauers, J., Donley, D., Hornsby, G., Kolar, M., & Yeater, R. (1999). Effects of resistance vs. aerobic training combined with an 800 calorie liquid diet on lean body mass and resting metabolic rate. Journal of the American College of Nutrition, 18(2), 115–121. https://doi.org/10.1080/07315724.1999.10718838

2517 Calbet, J. A. L., Ponce-González, J. G., Calle-Herrero, J. de L., Perez-Suarez, I., Martin-Rincon, M., Santana, A., … Holmberg, H.-C. (2017). Exercise Preserves Lean Mass and Performance during Severe Energy Deficit: The Role of Exercise Volume and Dietary Protein Content. Frontiers in Physiology, 8. doi:10.3389/fphys.2017.00483

2518 Vogels, N., & Westerterp-Plantenga, M. S. (2007). Successful Long-term Weight Maintenance: A 2-year Follow-up*. Obesity, 15(5), 1258–1266. doi:10.1038/oby.2007.147

2519 Muller, M. J., Bosy-Westphal, A., Kutzner, D., & Heller, M. (2002). Metabolically active components of fat-free mass and resting energy expenditure in humans: recent lessons from imaging technologies. Obesity Reviews, 3(2), 113–122. doi:10.1046/j.1467-789x.2002.00057.x

343

2520 Ravussin, E., Lillioja, S., Knowler, W. C., Christin, L., Freymond, D., Abbott, W. G., Boyce, V., Howard, B. V., & Bogardus, C. (1988). Reduced rate of energy expenditure as a risk factor for body-weight gain. The New England journal of medicine, 318(8), 467–472. https://doi.org/10.1056/NEJM198802253180802

2521 Rice, B., Janssen, I., Hudson, R., & Ross, R. (1999). Effects of aerobic or resistance exercise and/or diet on glucose tolerance and plasma insulin levels in obese men. Diabetes Care, 22(5), 684–691. doi:10.2337/diacare.22.5.684

2522 Janssen, I., Fortier, A., Hudson, R., & Ross, R. (2002). Effects of an Energy-Restrictive Diet With or Without Exercise on Abdominal Fat, Intermuscular Fat, and Metabolic Risk Factors in Obese Women. Diabetes Care, 25(3), 431–438. doi:10.2337/diacare.25.3.431

2523 Janssen, I., & Ross, R. (1999). Effects of sex on the change in visceral, subcutaneous adipose tissue and skeletal muscle in response to weight loss. International Journal of Obesity, 23(10), 1035–1046. doi:10.1038/sj.ijo.0801038

2524 Chomentowski, P., Dubé, J. J., Amati, F., Stefanovic-Racic, M., Zhu, S., Toledo, F. G., & Goodpaster, B. H. (2009). Moderate exercise attenuates the loss of skeletal muscle mass that occurs with intentional caloric restriction-induced weight loss in older, overweight to obese adults. The journals of gerontology. Series A, Biological sciences and medical sciences, 64(5), 575–580. https://doi.org/10.1093/gerona/glp007

2525 Miller, W. C., Koceja, D. M., & Hamilton, E. J. (1997). A meta-analysis of the past 25 years of weight loss research using diet, exercise or diet plus exercise intervention. International journal of obesity and related metabolic disorders : journal of the International Association for the Study of Obesity, 21(10), 941–947. https://doi.org/10.1038/sj.ijo.0800499

2526 METTLER, S., MITCHELL, N., & TIPTON, K. D. (2010). Increased Protein Intake Reduces Lean Body Mass Loss during Weight Loss in Athletes. Medicine & Science in Sports & Exercise, 42(2), 326–337. doi:10.1249/mss.0b013e3181b2ef8e

2527 Longland, T. M., Oikawa, S. Y., Mitchell, C. J., Devries, M. C., & Phillips, S. M. (2016). Higher compared with lower dietary protein during an energy deficit combined with intense exercise promotes greater lean mass gain and fat mass loss: a randomized trial. The American Journal of Clinical Nutrition, 103(3), 738–746. doi:10.3945/ajcn.115.119339

2528 Institute of Medicine (2005) 'Dietary Reference Intakes for Energy, Carbohydrate, Fiber, Fat, Fatty Acids, Cholesterol, Protein and Amino Acids', National Academy Press.

2529 Bilsborough, S., & Mann, N. (2006). A review of issues of dietary protein intake in humans. International journal of sport nutrition and exercise metabolism, 16(2), 129–152. https://doi.org/10.1123/ijsnem.16.2.129

2530 Layman, D. K., Anthony, T. G., Rasmussen, B. B., Adams, S. H., Lynch, C. J., Brinkworth, G. D., & Davis, T. A. (2015). Defining meal requirements for protein to optimize metabolic roles of amino acids. The American journal of clinical nutrition, 101(6), 1330S–1338S. https://doi.org/10.3945/ajcn.114.084053

2531 Campbell, W. W., Trappe, T. A., Wolfe, R. R., & Evans, W. J. (2001). The recommended dietary allowance for protein may not be adequate for older people to maintain skeletal muscle. The journals of gerontology. Series A, Biological sciences and medical sciences, 56(6), M373–M380. https://doi.org/10.1093/gerona/56.6.m373

2532 Morton, R. W., Murphy, K. T., McKellar, S. R., Schoenfeld, B. J., Henselmans, M., Helms, E., … Phillips, S. M. (2017). A systematic review, meta-analysis and meta-regression of the effect of protein supplementation on resistance training-induced gains in muscle mass and strength in healthy adults. British Journal of Sports Medicine, 52(6), 376–384. doi:10.1136/bjsports-2017-097608

2533 Hector, A. J., & Phillips, S. M. (2018). Protein Recommendations for Weight Loss in Elite Athletes: A Focus on Body Composition and Performance. International journal of sport nutrition and exercise metabolism, 28(2), 170–177. https://doi.org/10.1123/ijsnem.2017-0273

2534 Witard, O. C., Garthe, I., & Phillips, S. M. (2019). Dietary Protein for Training Adaptation and Body Composition Manipulation in Track and Field Athletes. International journal of sport nutrition and exercise metabolism, 29(2), 165–174. https://doi.org/10.1123/ijsnem.2018-0267

2535 Helms, E. R., Zinn, C., Rowlands, D. S., & Brown, S. R. (2014). A systematic review of dietary protein during caloric restriction in resistance trained lean athletes: a case for higher intakes. International journal of sport nutrition and exercise metabolism, 24(2), 127–138. https://doi.org/10.1123/ijsnem.2013-0054

2536 Aragon, A. A., Schoenfeld, B. J., Wildman, R., Kleiner, S., VanDusseldorp, T., Taylor, L., Earnest, C. P., Arciero, P. J., Wilborn, C., Kalman, D. S., Stout, J. R., Willoughby, D. S., Campbell, B., Arent, S. M., Bannock, L., Smith-Ryan, A. E., & Antonio, J. (2017). International society of sports nutrition position stand: diets and body composition. Journal of the International Society of Sports Nutrition, 14, 16. https://doi.org/10.1186/s12970-017-0174-y

2537 Helms, E. R., Aragon, A. A., & Fitschen, P. J. (2014). Evidence-based recommendations for natural bodybuilding contest preparation: nutrition and supplementation. Journal of the International Society of Sports Nutrition, 11, 20. https://doi.org/10.1186/1550-2783-11-20

2538 Beaudry, K.M., & Devries, M.C. (2019). Nutritional Strategies to Combat Type 2 Diabetes in Aging Adults: The Importance of Protein. Frontiers in Nutrition, 6.

2539 Stokes, T., Hector, A. J., Morton, R. W., McGlory, C., & Phillips, S. M. (2018). Recent Perspectives Regarding the Role of Dietary Protein for the Promotion of Muscle Hypertrophy with Resistance Exercise Training. Nutrients, 10(2), 180. https://doi.org/10.3390/nu10020180

2540 Campbell, A. P., & Rains, T. M. (2015). Dietary Protein Is Important in the Practical Management of Prediabetes and Type 2 Diabetes. The Journal of Nutrition, 145(1), 164S-169S.

2541 Janney, N. W. (1915). THE METABOLIC RELATIONSHIP OF THE PROTEINS TO GLUCOSE. Journal of Biological Chemistry, 20(3), 321–350.

2542 Conn JW, Newburgh LH. The glycemic response to isoglucogenic quantities of protein and carbohydrate. J Clin Invest. (1936)

2543 MacLean H. Modern Methods in the Diagnosis and Treatment of Glycosuria and Diabetes. London: Constable & Co. Ltd. (1924).

2544 Franz, M. J. (2002). Protein and diabetes: Much advice, little research. Current Diabetes Reports, 2(5), 457–464.

2545 Mary C Gannon, Frank Q Nuttall, Charles T Grant, Sean Ercan-Fang, Nacide Ercan-Fang; Stimulation of Insulin Secretion by Fructose Ingested With Protein in People With Untreated Type 2 Diabetes. Diabetes Care 1 January 1998; 21 (1): 16–22.

2546 Gannon et al (1992). Metabolic response to cottage cheese or egg white protein, with or without glucose, in type II diabetic subjects. Metabolism, 41(10), 1137–1145.

2547 Frank Q Nuttall, Arshag D Mooradian, Mary C Gannon, Charles Billington, Phillip Krezowski; Effect of Protein Ingestion on the Glucose and Insulin Response to a Standardized Oral Glucose Load. Diabetes Care 1 September 1984; 7 (5): 465–470.

2548 Te Morenga et al (2017). The Effect of a Diet Moderately High in Protein and Fiber on Insulin Sensitivity Measured Using the Dynamic Insulin Sensitivity and Secretion Test (DISST). Nutrients, 9(12), 1291.

2549 Park et al (2015). A high-protein breakfast induces greater insulin and glucose-dependent insulinotropic peptide responses to a subsequent lunch meal in individuals with type 2 diabetes. The Journal of nutrition, 145(3), 452–458.

[2550] Tian et al (2017). Dietary Protein Consumption and the Risk of Type 2 Diabetes: A Systematic Review and Meta-Analysis of Cohort Studies. Nutrients, 9(9), 982.

[2551] Ke, Q., Chen, C., He, F., Ye, Y., Bai, X., Cai, L., & Xia, M. (2018). Association between dietary protein intake and type 2 diabetes varies by dietary pattern. Diabetology & Metabolic Syndrome, 10(1).

[2552] Sluijs et al (2010). Dietary intake of total, animal, and vegetable protein and risk of type 2 diabetes in the European Prospective Investigation into Cancer and Nutrition (EPIC)-NL study. Diabetes care, 33(1), 43–48.

[2553] Song et al (2004). A prospective study of red meat consumption and type 2 diabetes in middle-aged and elderly women: the women's health study. Diabetes care, 27(9), 2108–2115.

[2554] DiNicolantonio, J. J., & O'Keefe, J. (2021). Low-grade metabolic acidosis as a driver of chronic disease: a 21st century public health crisis. Open heart, 8(2), e001730. https://doi.org/10.1136/openhrt-2021-001730

[2555] DiNicolantonio, J. J., & O'Keefe, J. H. (2021). Low-grade metabolic acidosis as a driver of insulin resistance. Open heart, 8(2), e001788. https://doi.org/10.1136/openhrt-2021-001788

[2556] Hamman et al (2006). Effect of Weight Loss With Lifestyle Intervention on Risk of Diabetes. Diabetes Care, 29(9), 2102–2107.

2557 Wanders, A. J., van den Borne, J. J., de Graaf, C., Hulshof, T., Jonathan, M. C., Kristensen, M., Mars, M., Schols, H. A., & Feskens, E. J. (2011). Effects of dietary fibre on subjective appetite, energy intake and body weight: a systematic review of randomized controlled trials. Obesity reviews : an official journal of the International Association for the Study of Obesity, 12(9), 724–739. https://doi.org/10.1111/j.1467-789X.2011.00895.x

2558 Clark, M. J., & Slavin, J. L. (2013). The effect of fiber on satiety and food intake: a systematic review. Journal of the American College of Nutrition, 32(3), 200–211. https://doi.org/10.1080/07315724.2013.791194

2559 Burton-Freeman B. (2000). Dietary fiber and energy regulation. The Journal of nutrition, 130(2S Suppl), 272S–275S. https://doi.org/10.1093/jn/130.2.272S

[2560] Hall et al (2021). Effect of a plant-based, low-fat diet versus an animal-based, ketogenic diet on ad libitum energy intake. Nature medicine, 27(2), 344–353.

[2561] Jakubowicz, D., & Froy, O. (2013). Biochemical and metabolic mechanisms by which dietary whey protein may combat obesity and Type 2 diabetes. The Journal of nutritional biochemistry, 24(1), 1–5.

[2562] Pereira et al (2002) 'Dairy Consumption, Obesity, and the Insulin Resistance Syndrome in Young Adults', JAMA. 2002;287(16):2081-2089.

[2563] Rideout, T.C., Marinangeli, C.P.F., Martin, H. et al. Consumption of low-fat dairy foods for 6 months improves insulin resistance without adversely affecting lipids or bodyweight in healthy adults: a randomized free-living cross-over study. Nutr J 12, 56 (2013).

[2564] Choi, H. K. (2005). Dairy Consumption and Risk of Type 2 Diabetes Mellitus in Men. Archives of Internal Medicine, 165(9), 997.

[2565] Liu et al (2006) 'A Prospective Study of Dairy Intake and the Risk of Type 2 Diabetes in Women', Diabetes Care 2006;29(7):1579–1584.

[2566] Rideout, T.C., Marinangeli, C.P.F., Martin, H. et al. Consumption of low-fat dairy foods for 6 months improves insulin resistance without adversely affecting lipids or bodyweight in healthy adults: a randomized free-living cross-over study. Nutr J 12, 56 (2013).

[2567] Ejtahed et al (2012). Probiotic yogurt improves antioxidant status in type 2 diabetic patients. Nutrition, 28(5), 539–543.

[2568] Madjd et al (2016). Comparison of the effect of daily consumption of probiotic compared with low-fat conventional yogurt on weight loss in healthy obese women following an energy-restricted diet: a randomized controlled trial. The American Journal of Clinical Nutrition, 103(2), 323–329.

[2569] Liljeberg Elmståhl, H., Björck, I. Milk as a supplement to mixed meals may elevate postprandial insulinaemia. Eur J Clin Nutr 55, 994–999 (2001).

[2570] Pal, S., Ellis, V., & Dhaliwal, S. (2010). Effects of whey protein isolate on body composition, lipids, insulin and glucose in overweight and obese individuals. British Journal of Nutrition, 104(5), 716–723.

[2571] Devries et al (2018). 'Changes in Kidney Function Do Not Differ between Healthy Adults Consuming Higher- Compared with Lower- or Normal-Protein Diets: A Systematic Review and Meta-Analysis. The Journal of Nutrition, 148(11), 1760–1775.

2572 Martin, W. F., Armstrong, L. E., & Rodriguez, N. R. (2005). Dietary protein intake and renal function. Nutrition & metabolism, 2, 25. https://doi.org/10.1186/1743-7075-2-25

2573 Friedman A. N. (2004). High-protein diets: potential effects on the kidney in renal health and disease. American journal of kidney diseases : the official journal of the National Kidney Foundation, 44(6), 950–962. https://doi.org/10.1053/j.ajkd.2004.08.020

[2574] Pedersen et al (2013). Health effects of protein intake in healthy adults: a systematic literature review. Food & Nutrition Research, 57(1), 21245.

[2575] Knight et al (2003). The impact of protein intake on renal function decline in women with normal renal function or mild renal insufficiency. Annals of internal medicine, 138(6), 460–467.

[2576] Krebs et al (2012). The Diabetes Excess Weight Loss (DEWL) Trial: a randomised controlled trial of high-protein versus high-carbohydrate diets over 2 years in type 2 diabetes. Diabetologia, 55(4), 905–914.

[2577] Beasley, J. M., & Wylie-Rosett, J. (2013). The role of dietary proteins among persons with diabetes. Current atherosclerosis reports, 15(9), 348.

[2578] Livesey et al (2013). Is there a dose-response relation of dietary glycemic load to risk of type 2 diabetes? Meta-analysis of prospective cohort studies. The American journal of clinical nutrition, 97(3), 584–596.

[2579] Willett, W., Manson, J., & Liu, S. (2002). Glycemic index, glycemic load, and risk of type 2 diabetes. The American journal of clinical nutrition, 76(1), 274S–80S.

[2580] Macdonald I. A. (2016). A review of recent evidence relating to sugars, insulin resistance and diabetes. European journal of nutrition, 55(Suppl 2), 17–23.

[2581] Greenwood et al (2013) 'Glycemic Index, Glycemic Load, Carbohydrates, and Type 2 Diabetes: Systematic review and dose–response meta-analysis of prospective studies', Diabetes Care 2013;36(12):4166–4171.

[2582] AlEssa H, Bupathiraju S, Malik V, Wedick N, Campos H, Rosner B, Willett W, Hu FB. Carbohydrate quality measured using multiple quality metrics is negatively associated with type 2 diabetes. Circulation. 2015; 1-31:A:20.

[2583] Tonstad et al (2009). Type of vegetarian diet, body weight, and prevalence of type 2 diabetes. Diabetes care, 32(5), 791–796.

[2584] Satija et al (2016). Plant-Based Dietary Patterns and Incidence of Type 2 Diabetes in US Men and Women: Results from Three Prospective Cohort Studies. PLoS medicine, 13(6), e1002039.

[2585] Du et al (2017). Fresh fruit consumption in relation to incident diabetes and diabetic vascular complications: A 7-y prospective study of 0.5 million Chinese adults. PLoS medicine, 14(4), e1002279.

[2586] Aune et al (2013). Whole grain and refined grain consumption and the risk of type 2 diabetes: a systematic review and dose-response meta-analysis of cohort studies. European journal of epidemiology, 28(11), 845–858.

345

[2587] Qian et al (2019). Association Between Plant-Based Dietary Patterns and Risk of Type 2 Diabetes. JAMA Internal Medicine, 179(10), 1335.

[2588] Schwingshackl et al (2017). Food groups and risk of type 2 diabetes mellitus: a systematic review and meta-analysis of prospective studies. European journal of epidemiology, 32(5), 363–375.

[2589] Iqbal et al (2021). Associations of unprocessed and processed meat intake with mortality and cardiovascular disease in 21 countries [Prospective Urban Rural Epidemiology (PURE) Study]: a prospective cohort study. The American Journal of Clinical Nutrition, 114(3), 1049–1058.

[2590] Skytte, M.J., Samkani, A., Petersen, A.D. et al. A carbohydrate-reduced high-protein diet improves HbA1c and liver fat content in weight stable participants with type 2 diabetes: a randomised controlled trial. Diabetologia 62, 2066–2078 (2019).

[2591] Accurso et al (2008). Dietary carbohydrate restriction in type 2 diabetes mellitus and metabolic syndrome: time for a critical appraisal. Nutrition & metabolism, 5, 9.

[2592] Boden et al (2005). Effect of a low-carbohydrate diet on appetite, blood glucose levels, and insulin resistance in obese patients with type 2 diabetes. Annals of internal medicine, 142(6), 403–411.

[2593] Volek et al (2004). Comparison of a very low-carbohydrate and low-fat diet on fasting lipids, LDL subclasses, insulin resistance, and postprandial lipemic responses in overweight women. Journal of the American College of Nutrition, 23(2), 177–184.

[2594] Bueno et al (2013). Very-low-carbohydrate ketogenic diet v. low-fat diet for long-term weight loss: a meta-analysis of randomised controlled trials. British Journal of Nutrition, 110(7), 1178–1187.

[2595] Brinkworth et al (2009). Long-term effects of a very-low-carbohydrate weight loss diet compared with an isocaloric low-fat diet after 12 mo. The American journal of clinical nutrition, 90(1), 23–32.

[2596] Dashti et al (2004). Long-term effects of a ketogenic diet in obese patients. Experimental and clinical cardiology, 9(3), 200–205.

[2597] Goldenberg et al (2021). Efficacy and safety of low and very low carbohydrate diets for type 2 diabetes remission: systematic review and meta-analysis of published and unpublished randomized trial data. BMJ (Clinical research ed.), 372, m4743.

[2598] Dyson, P. A., Beatty, S., & Matthews, D. R. (2007). A low-carbohydrate diet is more effective in reducing body weight than healthy eating in both diabetic and non-diabetic subjects. Diabetic medicine : a journal of the British Diabetic Association, 24(12), 1430–1435.

[2599] Guldbrand, H., Dizdar, B., Bunjaku, B. et al. In type 2 diabetes, randomisation to advice to follow a low-carbohydrate diet transiently improves glycaemic control compared with advice to follow a low-fat diet producing a similar weight loss. Diabetologia 55, 2118–2127 (2012).

[2600] Hernandez et al (2010). Lack of suppression of circulating free fatty acids and hypercholesterolemia during weight loss on a high-fat, low-carbohydrate diet. The American journal of clinical nutrition, 91(3), 578–585.

[2601] Yancy et al (2004). A low-carbohydrate, ketogenic diet versus a low-fat diet to treat obesity and hyperlipidemia: a randomized, controlled trial. Annals of internal medicine, 140(10), 769–777.

[2602] Daly et al (2006). Short-term effects of severe dietary carbohydrate-restriction advice in Type 2 diabetes-a randomized controlled trial. Diabetic Medicine, 23(1), 15–20.

[2603] Meckling et al (2004). Comparison of a low-fat diet to a low-carbohydrate diet on weight loss, body composition, and risk factors for diabetes and cardiovascular disease in free-living, overweight men and women. The Journal of clinical endocrinology and metabolism, 89(6), 2717–2723.

[2604] Sondike et al (2003). Effects of a low-carbohydrate diet on weight loss and cardiovascular risk factor in overweight adolescents. The Journal of pediatrics, 142(3), 253–258.

[2605] Foster et al (2003). A randomized trial of a low-carbohydrate diet for obesity. The New England journal of medicine, 348(21), 2082–2090.

2606 Hall, K. D., Guyenet, S. J., & Leibel, R. L. (2018). The Carbohydrate-Insulin Model of Obesity Is Difficult to Reconcile With Current Evidence. JAMA internal medicine, 178(8), 1103–1105. https://doi.org/10.1001/jamainternmed.2018.2920

2607 Gardner, C. D., Trepanowski, J. F., Del Gobbo, L. C., Hauser, M. E., Rigdon, J., Ioannidis, J. P. A., ... King, A. C. (2018). Effect of Low-Fat vs Low-Carbohydrate Diet on 12-Month Weight Loss in Overweight Adults and the Association With Genotype Pattern or Insulin Secretion. JAMA, 319(7), 667. doi:10.1001/jama.2018.0245

2608 Schoeller, D. A., & Buchholz, A. C. (2005). Energetics of obesity and weight control: does diet composition matter?. Journal of the American Dietetic Association, 105(5 Suppl 1), S24–S28. https://doi.org/10.1016/j.jada.2005.02.025

2609 Howell, S., & Kones, R. (2017). "Calories in, calories out" and macronutrient intake: the hope, hype, and science of calories. American journal of physiology. Endocrinology and metabolism, 313(5), E608–E612. https://doi.org/10.1152/ajpendo.00156.2017

[2610] Westman et al (2008). The effect of a low-carbohydrate, ketogenic diet versus a low-glycemic index diet on glycemic control in type 2 diabetes mellitus. Nutrition & metabolism, 5, 36.

[2611] Krebs et al (2010). Efficacy and safety of a high protein, low carbohydrate diet for weight loss in severely obese adolescents. The Journal of pediatrics, 157(2), 252–258.

[2612] Volek et al (2009). Carbohydrate restriction has a more favorable impact on the metabolic syndrome than a low fat diet. Lipids, 44(4), 297–309.

[2613] Tay et al (2008). Metabolic effects of weight loss on a very-low-carbohydrate diet compared with an isocaloric high-carbohydrate diet in abdominally obese subjects. Journal of the American College of Cardiology, 51(1), 59–67.

[2614] Brinkworth et al (2009). Long-term effects of a very-low-carbohydrate weight loss diet compared with an isocaloric low-fat diet after 12 mo. The American journal of clinical nutrition, 90(1), 23–32.

[2615] Jornayvaz et al (2010). A high-fat, ketogenic diet causes hepatic insulin resistance in mice, despite increasing energy expenditure and preventing weight gain. American journal of physiology. Endocrinology and metabolism, 299(5), E808–E815.

2616 Wanders, A. J., van den Borne, J. J., de Graaf, C., Hulshof, T., Jonathan, M. C., Kristensen, M., Mars, M., Schols, H. A., & Feskens, E. J. (2011). Effects of dietary fibre on subjective appetite, energy intake and body weight: a systematic review of randomized controlled trials. Obesity reviews : an official journal of the International Association for the Study of Obesity, 12(9), 724–739. https://doi.org/10.1111/j.1467-789X.2011.00895.x

2617 Clark, M. J., & Slavin, J. L. (2013). The effect of fiber on satiety and food intake: a systematic review. Journal of the American College of Nutrition, 32(3), 200–211. https://doi.org/10.1080/07315724.2013.791194

2618 Burton-Freeman B. (2000). Dietary fiber and energy regulation. The Journal of nutrition, 130(2S Suppl), 272S–275S. https://doi.org/10.1093/jn/130.2.272S

2619 Kristensen, M., Jensen, M. G., Aarestrup, J., Petersen, K. E., Søndergaard, L., Mikkelsen, M. S., & Astrup, A. (2012). Flaxseed dietary fibers lower cholesterol and increase fecal fat excretion, but magnitude of effect depend on food type. Nutrition & metabolism, 9, 8. https://doi.org/10.1186/1743-7075-9-8

2620 Uebelhack, R., Busch, R., Alt, F., Beah, Z. M., & Chong, P. W. (2014). Effects of cactus fiber on the excretion of dietary fat in healthy subjects: a double blind, randomized, placebo-controlled, crossover clinical investigation. Current therapeutic research, clinical and experimental, 76, 39–44. https://doi.org/10.1016/j.curtheres.2014.02.001

[2621] Yu et al (2014). The impact of soluble dietary fibre on gastric emptying, postprandial blood glucose and insulin in patients with type 2 diabetes. Asia Pacific journal of clinical nutrition, 23 2, 210-8 .

[2622] Weickert and Pfeiffer (2008) 'Metabolic Effects of Dietary Fiber Consumption and Prevention of Diabetes', The Journal of Nutrition, Volume 138, Issue 3, March 2008, Pages 439–442, https://doi.org/10.1093/jn/138.3.439

[2623] Kim et al (2020). Effect of the Intake of a Snack Containing Dietary Fiber on Postprandial Glucose Levels. Foods, 9(10), 1500.

[2624] Juntunen et al (2002) 'Postprandial glucose, insulin, and incretin responses to grain products in healthy subjects ', The American Journal of Clinical Nutrition, Volume 75, Issue 2, February 2002, Pages 254–262,

[2625] de Carvalho et al (2017). Plasma glucose and insulin responses after consumption of breakfasts with different sources of soluble fiber in type 2 diabetes patients: a randomized crossover clinical trial. The American Journal of Clinical Nutrition, 106(5), 1238–1245.

[2626] Juntunen et al (2003). Structural differences between rye and wheat breads but not total fiber content may explain the lower postprandial insulin response to rye bread. The American journal of clinical nutrition, 78 5, 957-64.

[2627] Anderson et al (2004). Carbohydrate and fiber recommendations for individuals with diabetes: a quantitative assessment and meta-analysis of the evidence. Journal of the American College of Nutrition, 23(1), 5–17.

[2628] USDA (2022) 'Broccoli, raw' FoodData Central, Accessed Online March 25th 2023: https://fdc.nal.usda.gov/fdc-app.html#/food-details/2345151/nutrients

[2629] USDA (2020) 'Apples, fuji, with skin, raw', FoodData Central, Accessed Online March 25th 2023: https://fdc.nal.usda.gov/fdc-app.html#/food-details/1750340/nutrients

[2630] Hatanaka (2020) '22 High Fiber Foods You Should Eat', Accessed Online March 25th 2023: https://www.healthline.com/nutrition/22-high-fiber-foods

[2631] Stewart, M. L., & Zimmer, J. P. (2018). Postprandial glucose and insulin response to a high-fiber muffin top containing resistant starch type 4 in healthy adults: a double-blind, randomized, controlled trial. Nutrition, 53, 59–63.

2632 Sanders, T. A. (2010), The role of fat in the diet – quantity, quality and sustainability. Nutrition Bulletin, 35: 138-146.

2633 Fats and oils in human nutrition. Report of a joint expert consultation. Food and Agriculture Organization of the United Nations and the World Health Organization. (1994). FAO food and nutrition paper, 57, i–147.

Made in the USA
Middletown, DE
02 May 2023